AF885666

THE SAVANT SYNDROME

INTELLECTUAL IMPAIRMENT, ASTONISHING CONDITION

Osvaldo Cairó Battistutti

Bibliographic data:
Osvaldo Cairó Battistutti
The Savant Syndrome: Intellectual Impairment, Astonishing Condition
Year of publication: 2021

All rights reserved:
This work is the intellectual property of its authors. This work in full or in part may not be reproduced in any form without the written permission of the copyright owners.

Cover design:
Graphic Designer: Lisandro Lazzaroni Battistutti (lisandrolazzaroni@gmail.com)

Cairó, Osvaldo Gabriel
The Savant Syndrome : Intellectual impairment, Astonishing condition / Osvaldo Gabriel Cairó. – 1a ed – Gobernador Crespo : Osvaldo Gabriel Cairó, 2021.
308 p. ; 24 x 17 cm.

ISBN 978-987-86-8316-4 (paperback)

1. Neurociencias. 2. Autismo. 3. Síndrome de Asperger. I. Título.
CDD 612.825

Dr. Osvaldo Cairó Battistutti
Instituto Tecnológico Autónomo de México (ITAM)

To all those with a different condition—your difference is what makes you remarkable.

ABOUT THE AUTHOR

Dr. Osvaldo Cairó Battistutti has been a Professor and Researcher at the Instituto Tecnológico Autónomo de México (ITAM) since 1988 and is a member of the National System of Researchers of Mexico. He is the author of several textbooks, including some which have become classics.

His research is focused on neuroscience and artificial intelligence, mainly in areas relating to knowledge, cognition, and intelligence. He has taken part in research projects financed by the National Council on Science and Technology (CONACYT) and the United Nations. He is a member of the Mexican Society of Artificial Intelligence (SMIA), an expert advisor to Argentina's National Scientific and Technical Research Council (CONICET), a consultant for the United Nations' Economic Commission for Latin America and the Caribbean (CEPAL), and a review editor for several international journals.

Some years ago, he was distinguished as one of the best teachers in engineering programs in Mexico, and in 2014 he earned the Academic Merit Prize, awarded in Mexico to the best academic in the area of engineering.

PREFACE

Savant syndrome is one of the most fascinating phenomena in the study of human differences and cognitive psychology. A savant, or individual with savant syndrome, is one who has been identified with a rare condition, mental disabilities, or certain disorders, including autism spectrum disorder (ASD), and who has one or more areas of extraordinary ability or brilliance, in stark contrast to serious individual general limitations. Their skills emerge spontaneously; they are literal, not symbolic; and they are not derived from practice. Savants have no idea of how they possess these skills. Their condition may be genetic, but may also be acquired in the pre-natal, perinatal, or postnatal stages. There are also cases in which savant syndrome is acquired later in life, following a blow to the head, a stroke, a central nervous system injury, or disease (Lythgoe et al., 2005).

The most dramatic examples of savant syndrome occur in individuals with exceptional skills in certain areas who simultaneously score very low on intelligence quotient (IQ) tests. It is paradoxical that individuals with a low intelligence quotient can perform extremely complex mathematical calculations that, in most cases, only individuals with a high IQ can perform. They may pose a challenge to many theories of intelligence, since their performance cannot be understood in terms of conventional intelligence (Pring, 2008).

Individuals with savant syndrome have a prodigious memory and spatial visualization abilities, are attracted to numbers and calendars, and are generally fascinated by music and art. Other skills, such as polyglottism, occur less frequently. The most common kind of savants are calendrical savants, also known as "human calendars," who can calculate the day of the week for any given date with remarkable speed and accuracy. It is disputed whether calculation, rather than memory alone, is involved (Cowan and Frith, 2009).

Although the concept of the syndrome is accepted, it is currently unrecognized by both the International Statistical Classification of Diseases and Related Health Problems (ICD-10), a medical classification list published by the World Health Organization, and the Diagnostic and Statistical Manual of Mental Disorders (DSM-5), published by the American Psychiatric Association.

Half of savants are autistic, while the other half has mental retardation, CNS injury or disease, or other types of disorders such as Williams' syndrome, Smith-Magenis syndrome, Prader-Willis syndrome, loss of corpus callosum, etc. On the other hand, approximately one in ten autistic people (10%) show savant abilities (Treffert, 2009). Savant syndrome is also approximately six times more frequent in men than in women (Geschwind and Galaburda, 1985). Hill (1978) calculated that of 105 individuals classified as savant in 63 publications, at least 85% were men.

One of the more plausible explanations for savant syndrome is associated with a dysfunction of the left hemisphere of the brain (Treffert, 2009; Sacks, 2007; Geschwind and Galaburda, 1985), whose skills are more abstract, logical, and symbolic, while the right hemisphere is used to compensate, leading to a cortical reorganization (Pulsifer et al., 2004).

There are many hypotheses associated with understanding more about the Savant syndrome, but none of them are completely sufficient. This is a very heterogeneous area of research historically dominated by anecdotal reports. Additionally, since each savant has their own peculiarities, most reviews take the shape of a collection of stand-alone descriptions. As Ammari (2011) has stated, "there is a lack of unifying definitions, diagnostic tools, age categories, and spectrum of prodigy all of which might be regarded as a disadvantage to savant syndrome."

This demonstrates once again the importance of using a uniform method to define savant status across domains. Considering all these factors, the purpose of the present essay is to analyze the different cases more rigorously, considering mainly persons with severe intellectual impairment who can perform in sharply circumscribed areas at a remarkable high level (Howlin et al., 2009).

ACKNOWLEDGMENTS

Many people helped, in one way or another, to make this project a reality, and some of them deserve special mention. Dr. Alejandro Hernández, ITAM's provost, Dr. Ante Salcedo, director of ITAM's Academic Division of Engineering, and Dr. Fernando Esponda, head of the Computer Science Department, were all enthusiastic from the beginning about the idea for this series of books and strongly supported me in bringing it to fruition.

Furthermore, the collaboration of savants, their families, and researchers was extraordinary and their enthusiasm and confidence was crucial to the successful completion of this project. I would especially like to thank Dr. Darold Treffert, the world's leading expert on savant syndrome, Dr. Alice Flaherty (Harvard Medical School), Dr. Laurence Becker, Dr. Makoto Yamaguchi (The University of Tokyo), Dr. Deirdre O'Connell (University of Sydney), Josephine Arader (Arader Galleries, New York), Franco Magnani, Gregory Blackstock, Dorothy Frisch (Gregory's cousin), Dr. Temple Grandin, Frances Passman (Tommy McHugh' partner of eight years), Gianni Bianchini (photographer and very good friend of Tommy McHugh), Mike Wawro (Richard Wawro's brother), Dr. Anthony Cicoria, Jon Sarkin, Paul Cary Goldberg (photographer and Sarkin's friend), Gloria Lenhoff, Sylvia Lenhoff (Gloria's mother), Alonzo Clemons, Nancy Mason (Alonzo Clemons), George Widener, Henry Boxer (Henry Boxer Gallery), Derek Amato, Geoff Harrison (Geoff Harrison Art), Patrick Fagerberg, Tony DeBlois, Janice DeBlois (Tony's mother), Stephen Wiltshire, Annette Wiltshire (Stephen's sister and Art Director at The Stephen Wiltshire Gallery), Ron Sandison, Derek Paravicini, Adam Ockelford (Director of the Applied Music Research Centre at the University of Roehampton in London), Daniel Tammet, Jérôme Tabet (photographer), Seth Chwast, Debra Chwast (Seth's mother), Herb Ascherman, Thristan Mendoza, Leland Lee, Karen

Chien (Leland's mother), Michele Chang (Leland Lee's language teacher), Matt Savage, Diane Savage (Matt's mother), Alex Abercrombie, Micah Gummel, Ping Lian Yeak, Sara Lee (Ping Lian's mother), Dr. Rosa Martinez (Strokes of Genius, Inc.), Buğra Cankir, Kamel Cankir (Buğra´s father), Dr. Sule Erden (Çukurova Üniversitesi Eğitim Fakültesi, Turkey), Rex Lewis-Clack, Cathleen Lewis (Rex's mother), Grant Maniér, Julie Coy (Grant's mother), Amanda LaMunyon, Sherry LaMunyon (Amanda's mother), Kodi Lee, Tina Lee (Kodi's mother), Jodi DiPiazza, Thomas DiPiazza (Jodi's father), Iris Grace Halmshaw, and Arabella Carter-Johnson (Iris's mother).

I would also like to extend my thanks to Elizabeth Collins and Noah Mazer, the curators of this book, who revised each line of the text so that it was almost perfect. Full credit for the book cover goes to graphic designer Lisandro Lazzaroni, who provided his brilliant solution based only on my simple description of the project. Finally, it is important to note that this work was partially founded by Asociación Mexicana de Cultura A.C.

TABLE OF CONTENTS

1

BRAIN, MIND, AND INTELLIGENCE

The human brain is undoubtedly the most impressive, complex, enigmatic, and intricate organ of the human body, having evolved over millennia. Despite the fact that it is likely the body's most studied organ, it is still the least understood, and is therefore the subject of unending fascination (Cairó, 2017).

Our brains are made up of more than 100 billion neurons or nerve cells that communicate through 1,000 trillion synaptic connections. The brain is housed in the skull and composed of the cerebrum (divided into two hemispheres), the brainstem (the posterior part of the brain), and the cerebellum (which plays an important role in motor control). All parts of the brain work together, but each part has its own special properties. The brain is responsible for controlling all of the body's functions as well as processing, integrating, and coordinating (often simultaneously) the information it receives from the outside world through the five senses: sight, smell, touch, taste, and hearing. It also gives rise to all the things that make us and define as human beings.

The mind, on the other hand, is the set of cognitive faculties which include consciousness, imagination, perception, thinking, judgment, language, and memory, housed (albeit virtually) in the brain. In this sense, the mind is not a physical object. It is like a magical, invisible state that can perceive and see what the eyes cannot. The mind can also be aware of the world. It is the essence of our being.

For years, there has been widespread discussion about what the mind means and what its properties are. A heated debate rages on the subject among theologians, philosophers, psychologists, and cognitive scientists. Researchers in different fields of science, including sociobiology, neuroscience, computer science, and artificial intelligence have also recently joined the debate. To this day, however, we have no consensus or neat definition that encompasses everything that the mind means.

A still-open question regarding the nature of the mind has been the mind-body problem, a legacy of Descartes' philosophy. Descartes argued that since both substances are of a completely different nature (physical and non-physical), it therefore is possible for one to exist without the other. What is clear from subsequent efforts to elucidate this problem is that misconceptions, false assumptions, varying arguments, and strong religious beliefs exist which can influence the analytical process and prevent us from reaching a commonly agreed-upon solution. It seems clear, however, that if the mind can exist independently of the brain, then there is a rational basis for hope in the soul's immortality, the existence of God, and life after death.

Since ancient times, a wide variety of theses have been submitted into discussion to tackle the brain-mind problem: among these are dualism (Cartesian duality—the mind exists independently of the brain); monism (unity of the origin of all things); idealism (reality is indistinguishable or inseparable from human understanding or perception); physicalism (everything is physical—mental phenomena are identical to neuronal phenomena); and functionalism (causal physicalism).

Like many other researchers with contemporary views, we focus mainly on functionalism and the computational theory of the mind (CTM) and will reduce the problem—whatever its nature—to a physical phenomenon known as neuronal activity. The brain (analogous to hardware) produces the mind (analogous to software: an information processing system similar to a Turing machine), which is ultimately what enables consciousness and intentionality toward everything that surrounds us. In this way, thinking, reasoning, and feelings are products of the mind, which later may result in attitudes and actions that define our behavior. When the brain dies, all brain functions permanently cease, and the mind ends as well.

This reduction does not preclude the adoption of various distinct approaches, which include connectionism, computationalism, and the Bayesian brain, among others. For the purposes of our study (which focuses on the world of savants), the reduction of the problem to neuronal activity does not interfere with other theses, and may even coexist with them. Kant, for instance, suggested that there is a set of *a priori* forms as a basis for understanding, such as space and time, "preloaded" or "pre-programmed" in the brain. Jerry Fodor, on the other hand, refers to computations operating on the syntax of the representations that make up the language of thought. The CTM thesis has not gone without scrutiny: philosophers, neuroscientists, and psychologists such as John Searle, Daniel Dennet, David Marr, Ulrich Neisser, and Fodor have all voiced criticisms of it. Criticism of the thesis, however, does not significantly affect the purpose of our reduction as regards the subjects we cover in this book. It should also be clear that this is by no means a unanimous opinion.

In this sense (reduction), each individual may have different hardware and software, and the differences that exist between them may be explained in these terms. The most intelligent would be those with heavily-wired hardware (brain) and very good software (mind). However, as Neisser et al. (1996) stated—and we concur—"a given person's intellectual performance will vary on different occasions, in different domains, as judged by different criteria."

With regards to mind and intellect, although the two are not independent of each other and generally work together, they are not quite synonymous, either. Intellect is a mental capacity, a decision-making faculty. It is the means by which the mind might be required to work (think) twice before making an intelligent decision. The concept of intelligence, on the other hand, covers many aspects of mental abilities, as well as the efficiency with which they are carried out. Intelligence is also marked by complex cognitive feats, comprehension of complex ideas, problem-solving, mathematical reasoning, learning from experience, adapting effectively to one's environment, and critical thinking. Again: although intellect and intelligence are highly-interrelated concepts, they are not exactly identical. While intelligence implies the ability to acquire skills and knowledge and use these appropriately, intellect implies abstract reasoning and the capacity to understand objectively: questioning and thinking. We should not accept ideas that lack logic or reason.

On December 13, 1994, in response to the controversial book *The Bell Curve* (Herrnstein and Murray, 1994), psychologist Linda Gottfredson published an article in *The Wall Street Journal* listing the 25 best definitions of intelligence. The first sentence, which gathered the consensus of 51 researchers, said:

> Intelligence is a very general mental capability that, among other things, involves the ability to reason, plan, solve problems, think abstractly, comprehend complex ideas, learn quickly and learn from experience. It is not merely book learning, a narrow academic skill, or test-taking smarts. Rather, it reflects a broader and deeper capability for comprehending our surroundings—'catching on,' 'making sense' of things, or 'figuring out' what to do (Gottfredson, 1997, p13).

One problem that frequently occurs when dealing with the concept of intelligence is that we tend to measure only what we actually know how to measure. Even when aware of this fact and its extreme limitations, we often establish our judgments based on these circumscribed measurements. For example, we do not know how to measure wisdom, creativity, or practical knowledge, which are intellectual abilities highly appreciated by humans (Cairó Battistutti, 2011). Sternberg (1985) stresses that there are three fundamental parts to intelligence: analytic, practical, and creative. At present, we can only measure analytics.

Regarding savants, the main subject of this book, it is worth noting that for many years it was thought that outstanding talent could only be found in intellectually exceptional individuals. Those with savant syndrome have now proven otherwise, and pose a serious challenge to theories that focus on general intelligence factors.

Individuals with a low intelligent quotient, who may even be considered mentally impaired or with serious developmental disabilities, may exhibit remarkable intelligence in some domains or islands of knowledge. This fact proves how far we are from a functional understanding of the brain. It seems that a hardware (brain) failure produces brilliant and hitherto inexplicable advances in software (mind) in certain domains of knowledge.

Savant syndrome is, of course, one of the most fascinating phenomena in the study of human differences and cognitive psychology. The savant skill is evidence of innate talent and a weakly coherent processing style. This essay carefully reviews and summarizes past and present world literature, current research findings, and new discoveries on the subject. It also reports known and recent cases and outlines future directions in the study of this impressive syndrome, in which a person demonstrates one or more areas of extraordinary ability or brilliance despite perceived disabilities in other mental areas.

2

SAVANTISM: A BRIEF HISTORY

One of the first cases of savant syndrome on record is that of Thomas Fuller (1710-1790), known as Negro Tom. Thomas, who was born in 1710 in the area of what is now known as Benin and Liberia, was stolen from his native Africa and sold to a Virginia planter as a slave at the age of 14.

Fuller was quickly nicknamed "the Virginia Calculator" because of his extraordinary ability for numbers and geometric progressions, although he was illiterate and unable to read or write in English. He was simply able to solve complex math problems in his head. Thomas was once asked how many seconds a man had lived who was 70 years, 17 days, and 12 hours old. He gave the correct answer—2,210,500,800 seconds—in just a minute and a half, even adjusting for the 17 leap years included (Rush, 1789). One of his examiners, who was using a pen and a piece of paper, advised Thomas that his result was not correct, to which the old man hastily replied, "stop, you forget the leap years." On adding the seconds of the leap years to the others, their sums agreed exactly (Benjamin Rush, Philadelphia, November 14, 1788).

Abolitionists also used Fuller as proof that Black people were not inferior to whites. When Fuller died in 1790, having never learned to read or write, the *Columbian Centinel*, a well-known daily of Boston, Massachusetts, published an article describing the life and mathematical feats of Thomas Fuller, an enslaved man who lived near Alexandria (Transcription source: *Columbian Centinel*, December 29, 1790, 123):

> DIED,—Negro Tom, the famous African calculator, aged 80 years. He was the property of Mrs. Elizabeth Cox, of Alexandria. Tom was a very black man. He was brought to this country at the age of fourteen and was sold as a slave with many of his unfortunate countrymen. This man was a prodigy. Though he could neither read nor write, he had perfectly acquired the use of enumeration. He could give the number of months, days, weeks, hours, minutes, and seconds, for any period of time that a person chose to mention, allowing in his calculations for all the leap years that happened in the time. He would give the number of poles, yards, feet, inches, and barley-corns in a given distance—say, the diameter of the earth's orbit—and in every calculation he would produce the true answer in less time than ninety-nine out of a hundred men would take with their pens. And what was, perhaps, more extraordinary, though interrupted in the progress of his calculations, and engaged in discourse upon any other subject, his operations were not thereby in the least deranged; he would go on where he left off, and could give any and all of the stages through which the calculation had passed.
>
> Thus died Negro Tom, this untaught arithmetician, this untutored scholar. Had his opportunities of improvement been equal to those of thousands of his fellow-men, neither the Royal Society of London, the Academy of Science at Paris, nor even a Newton himself need have been ashamed to acknowledge him a brother in science.

The first description of savant syndrome in a scientific paper appeared in the German scholarly journal *Gnothi Sauton* in 1783, describing the case of Jedediah Buxton (1707-1772). Jedediah could not write and had very limited knowledge, but was exceptionally talented with numbers and possessed a prodigious memory.

Buxton measured the whole lordship of Elmton, the town where he lived, an area of approximately 4km^2, simply by walking around it. He presented the exact area, not only in acres but also in square inches. Among the many examples of his arithmetical exploits is the calculation of the product of one farthing doubled 139 times. The result, expressed in pounds, is a 39-digit number. As if that calculation were not complex enough, Buxton afterwards multiplied this enormous number by itself.

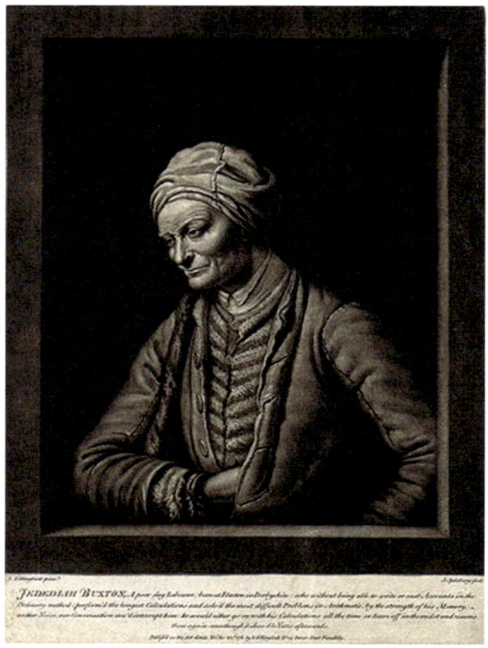

Figure 2.1 Jedediah Buxton (1707-1772).

Credit: Jedediah Buxton, a mental calculator. Mezzotint by J. Spilsbury, 1781, after B. Killingbeck. Credit: Wellcome Collection. Attribution 4.0 International (CC BY 4.0)

2.1 "Idiot Savant": Origins of the Term

While it is true that savant syndrome was first recognized by John Langdon Down (1828-1896), best known for his description of a relatively common genetic disorder (Down syndrome, which he classified in 1862), this type of disorder clearly did not originate at that time. The abovementioned cases of Thomas Fuller (cited by the American psychiatrist Benjamin

Rush) and Jedediah Buxton (cited by the German psychology journal) are proof of this.

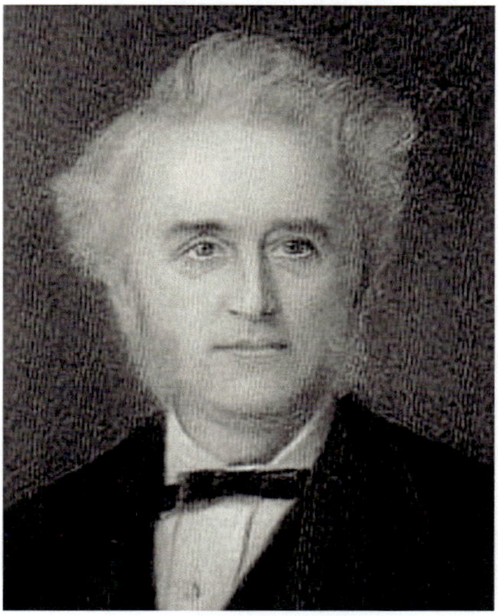

Figure 2.2 Portrait of John Langdom Down. First published ca. 1870.

Author: Sydney Hodges (1829-1900) Source: St. George's University of London (http://en.wikipedia.org/wiki/Image:JLHdown.jpg). Creative Commons CC0 License

Fuller and Buxton, however, with their sharp contrasts in intelligence, behavior, and motor function, and without the benefit of the advances in modern medicine and psychology we enjoy today, were considered in their own times to be strange beings possessed by a supernatural power.

The term "idiot savant" was first coined and used by John Down in the "Lettsomian Lecture on Some of the Mental Affections of Childhood and Youth," delivered at the invitation of the Medical Society of London in January 1887. Down stated that the term, derived from *savoir* (meaning "to know" in French), "has been applied to children who, while feeble-minded, exhibit special faculties which are capable of being cultivated to a very great extent" (Down, 1887).

In his lecture, Down presented several cases of children under his observation, characterized by impressive artistic, numerical, and musical skills (a group he identified as developmental in origin), differed markedly from cases of mental retardation which he was accustomed to seeing as a physician at the Earlswood Hospital. These individuals "exhibited outstanding abilities in specific areas, but their level of general ability was so poor that they were unable to live independently" (Howlin et al., 2009).

The term "idiot savant" was obviously unfortunate. While the word "idiot" is today considered pejorative, archaic, offensive, and imprecise, it was accepted scientifically in Down's day as referring to individuals with mental retardation and an IQ of less than 25. Those subjects with less serious manifestations were called "imbeciles," which mainly refers to the outcome of deteriorating organic causes, often senility. Down himself did not agree with the term, but thought that "idiot savant" should indeed be the disorder's scientific name, since "children who were afflicted by mental alienation or mental incapacity of any kind were placed in the category of idiots" (Down, 1887). Down himself stated:

> I have no great liking for the term idiot. It is so frequently a name of reproach. No one likes the name, and no mother will admit that her child deserves the title (Down, 1887).

All the cases reported by Down as idiot savants were men, and he never met with a female idiot savant. Idiot was formerly a technical term used in legal and psychiatric contexts to describe an individual with profound intellectual disability.

Barr suggested that with an idiot, any treatment would be useless, since no improvement could be expected. "The idiot is a form of human who sees nothing, feels nothing, hears nothing, does nothing and knows nothing, whereas imbeciles have the capacity to understand and reason" (Barr, 1910).

We may assume that among the cases detected by Down there were not only individuals with infantile mania, melancholia and delusions, moral insanity, epilepsy, and catalepsy, and idiots savants, but also autistic individuals, with Asperger syndrome and other rare conditions that had not yet been defined and would be considered later in redefining the term. In addition, in recent years, savants with IQs greater than 100 have been identified.

At about the same time, Forbes Winslow (1860), the most controversial psychiatrist of his time, published an extensive book entitled *On Obscure Diseases of the Brain and Disorders of the Mind.* Winslow wisely noted that as a general rule, "all diseases of the brain are very obscure in their origin, insidious in their progress, and most difficult to treat successfully." He described cases of individuals with a very low level of intelligence but with extraordinary memory.

> Idiots have exhibited the faculty of retention to a remarkable extent, and men of very limited and circumscribed powers of reasoning and of most defective judgment have had memories distinguished for their tenacity (Winslow, 1860).

Winslow supposed that there was a correlation, compensation, or other phenomenon that would need to be defined later, between a low intellectual coefficient and an extraordinary memory.

2.2 Other savants of the time

A few years later, Tredgold (1914) published a book titled *Mental Deficiency*, which included a chapter on these particular individuals who had remarkable intellectual disabilities but were simultaneously standing in other intellectual abilities. He described over 20 cases, reported by a variety of clinicians, of individuals with incredible ability or brilliance that contrasted starkly with their serious specific or general limitations. A Swiss gentleman named Gottfried Mind (1768-1814) was one of those cases.

> Gottfried could neither read nor write, he had no idea of the value of the money, and his general appearance was so obviously indicative of mental defect that his walks through the city were usually to the accompaniment of a crowd of jeering children (Tredgold, 1914).

However, he had an unparalleled talent for painting. He was known as "Raphael of Cats" because of his talent in depicting cats in art. His fascination for painting cats began when Mind met the painter Sigmund Freudenberger for the first time. It must be said that Mind learned the art of drawing and coloring with watercolors from Freudenberger. Once, as Sigmund was painting a cat, Mind, who was observing, told the painter that what he was producing was "not a cat." Freudenberger challenged Mind to do a better job, which Mind promptly did. After this incident, Mind devoted himself to painting not only cats, but also lions, rabbits, sheep, goats, deer, bears, etc., all with extraordinary mastery. One of his paintings was purchased by King George IV.

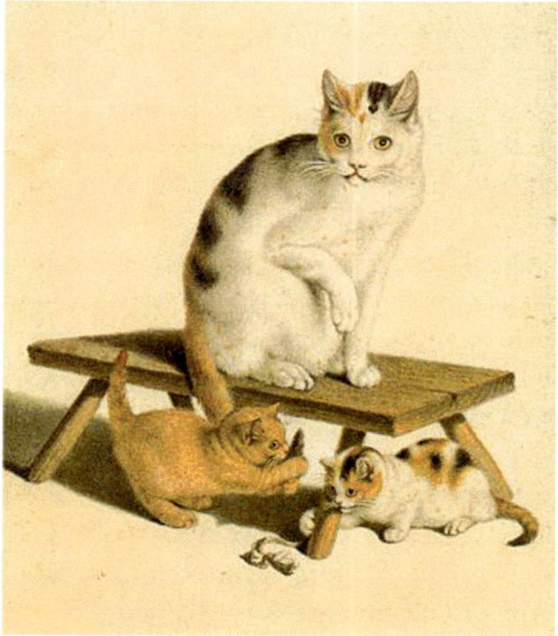

Figure 2.3 Cats, watercolour by Gottfried Mind Date: circa 1800

File source: http://www.hauspuma.de/History/LiteraturundKunst.html
Creative Commons CC0 License

In the same document, Tredgold also describes London-born James Henry Pullen (1835-1916), known as The Genius of Earlswood Asylum. Since

Pullen was practically lacking in language, was deaf, and was considered developmentally disabled, he was imprisoned in an asylum, in which he lived for 66 years, from age 15 until his death at 81, in 1916. He never learned to read or write.

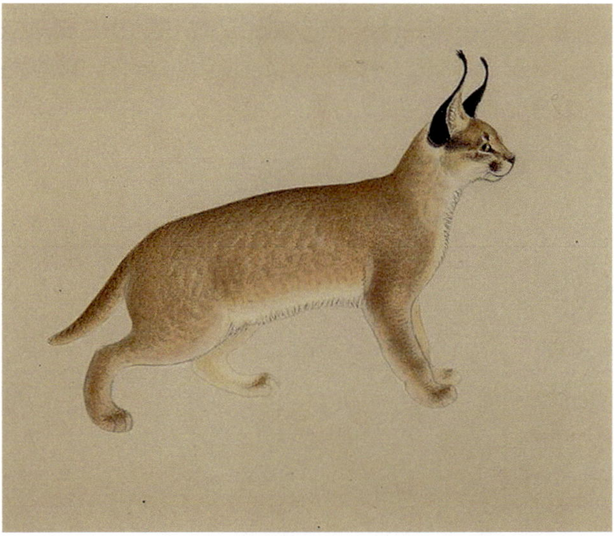

Figure 2.4 Lynx by Gottfried Mind, 1800-1814, 7 x 7 inches, watercolor over graphite drawing.
Photo courtesy of Josephine Arader and Arader Galleries, New York, USA.

Pullen had a very slow development, and since he spoke no words and was deaf, no school would admit him on the grounds that he would be unable to learn. For this reason, he remained with his parents, who were first cousins, until he was 12 years old. He was admitted to Essex Hall in Colchester in 1847 and then transferred to Earlswood Asylum for Idiots and Imbeciles in 1850. When Pullen was admitted there were 150 residents in the asylum, a population that swelled to 300 in 10 years, and to 500 in 20 years. He learned to spell his first word at age 14.

Pullen had an exceptional talent for carving in ivory and wood, and possessed marvelous mechanical and drawing abilities. Because of his expert craftsmanship, Pullen became all but a celebrity at Earlswood. He received two workshops where he could continue to develop his talent fully. In his daily life, he was well-behaved and, for the most part, seemed happy, although at times he could be intolerant, irascible, aggressive, once threatening to blow the place up. On another occasion, he even built a guillotine over the workshop door for uninvited visitors (Breathnach and Ward, 2015). The three doctors who treated him expressed different ideas about his disability, but they agreed on his unmatched talent.

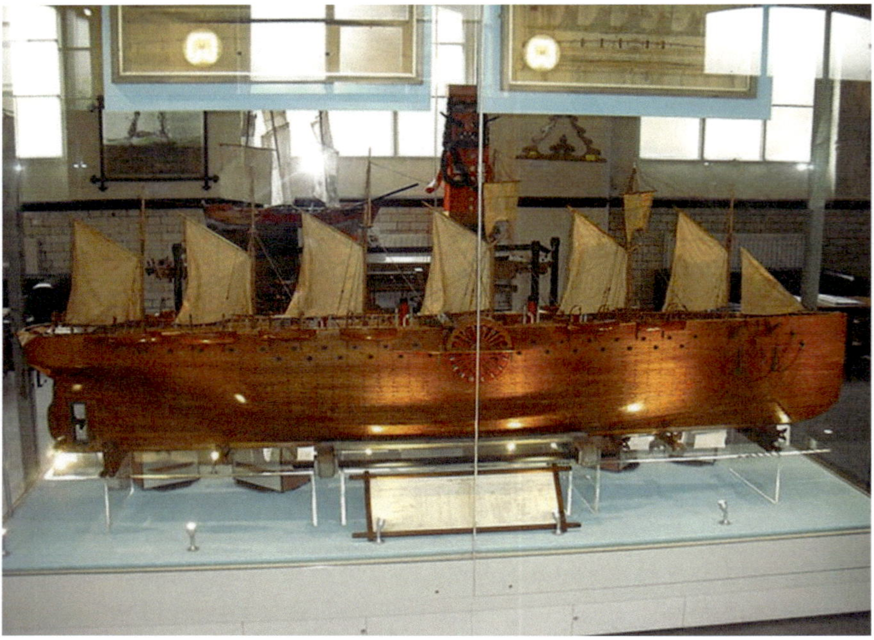

Figure 2.5 James Henry Pullen's model of SS Great Eastern on display at the Langdon Down Museum in Teddington, Middlesex, England. Author: P0mbal

Creative Commons Attribution-Share Alike 3.0 Unported license.

When Pullen died, his brain was preserved in ten percent (10%) formaldehyde for examination. Frederich Sano, one of his doctors, found that his brain weighted 1,190g (although to some extent, this reduced weight might be accounted for by a well-advanced senile deterioration) and that there was a notable difference in weight between the two hemispheres. Breathnach and Ward (2015) concluded that:

> ... his highly idiosyncratic artistic and technical skills combined with an explosive temper and difficulty in making social relationships indicate that he suffered from a pervasive developmental disorder and it is likely that he was an autistic savant.

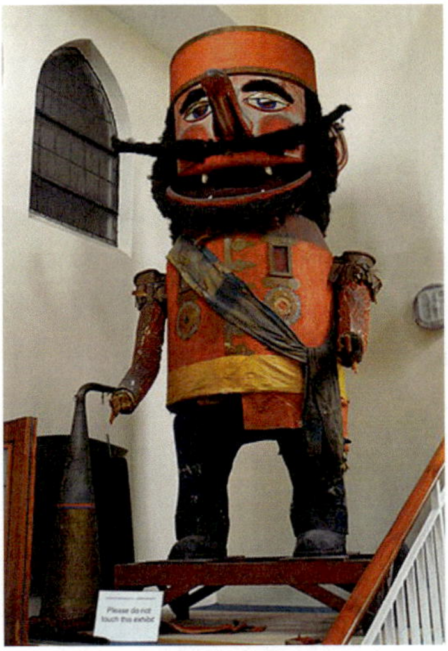

Figure 2.6 James Henry Pullen's giant Langdon Down Museum in Teddington, Middlesex, England. Made with wood (c. 1870s)

Author: Andy Scott. Source: Own work. https://commons.wikimedia.org/wiki/File:James_Henry_Pullen%27s_giant_Langdon_Down_Museum_in_Teddington.jpg

Source: Creative Commons Attribution Share Alike 4.0 International license.

Another important figure of the time who is now recognized as an autistic savant was Thomas Greene Wiggins (1849-1908). Better known as Blind Tom, Thomas was an African-American musical prodigy who is regarded one of the best-known American performing pianists in history. Although he never learned or spoke more than 100 words, he could play more than 7,000 pieces on the piano, including 100 of his own composition. Such was Thomas's skill on the piano, that he was referred to as "the eighth wonder of the world."

Thomas was born blind to enslaved parents on the Wiley Edward Jones plantation in Harris County, Georgia. When he was nine months old, he was sold in an auction at no extra cost alongside his parents, Charity and Domingo Wiggins, and his two sisters, to Colonel James Bethune (sometimes called General) of Columbus, Georgia. The family was initially meant to be separated for sale, but Colonel Bethune took pity on them and purchased them together. Bethune was a veteran of the American Indian Wars, a practicing lawyer, and a newspaper editor for the *Columbus Times*. Bethune was responsible for changing Tom's name to Thomas Wiggins Bethune, as it was customary at that time for enslaved women and their children to be given their slaveholder's last name. Since Thomas was born blind and was presumed mentally handicapped, it seemed clear that he would be able to carry out the tasks the enslaved were charged with and would not have any economic value to his owners. This prompted an initial proposal to simply kill him. Fortunately, this did not happen, and Thomas spent much of his early years wandering freely and playing in Colonel Bethune's plantation.

Thomas was known on the Bethune plantation for his ability to almost perfectly imitate, either vocally or musically, any sound he heard, from the crowing of a rooster to a ten-minute conversation between individuals, although he did not understand what it meant. For this reason, many contemporaries described him as nothing more than a human parrot. Thomas was likeable and moved in a funny and strange way, and had other amusing peculiarities. All these characteristics contributed to him being treated as a pet.

Charity, his mother, was allowed to bring him with her to the main house where she worked. Colonel Bethune's family and wife had seven children who enjoyed singing and playing the piano. Having once heard the general's daughters play the piano, Thomas trembled with ecstasy and immediately displayed a rapt fascination with music. Once given access to the keyboard by himself, Thomas astounded the Bethune family by performing the music he had heard. The general was delighted with little Tom and told his mother (presumably with what he thought of as good intentions) that her son was even smarter than the family dog. To demonstrate that what he said was true, Colonel Bethune told Thomas "Tom, sit down," and "Tom, get up."

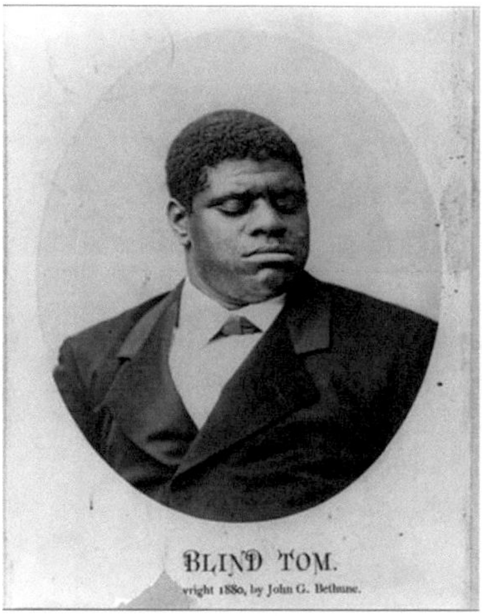

Figure 2.7 Blind Thomas Wiggins (c. 1880)

Photoprint by Golder & Robinson, N.Y. Copyrighted by John G. Bethune.

This image is available from the United States Library of Congress's Prints and Photographs division under the digital ID cph.3b30858. Creative Commons CC0 License

By the age of five, Thomas had written his first composition, "The Rain Storm." By the time Thomas was six, Colonel Bethune recognized his prodigious musical talent and made a piano available to him in a room next to his home. This was partly because the family was unable to keep little Thomas out of the room where the general's children's piano was kept. Thomas was already an expert on the piano and even wrote his own compositions. He claimed that the wind, the rain, or the birds had taught him the melodies of his compositions (a beautiful statement). Perhaps already thinking of his business possibilities, the general hired a music teacher for Thomas. This turned out not to be very useful, since little Thomas was more skillful than the teacher. The teacher suggested to the general that the best course of action was simply to let Thomas listen to the music of Beethoven, Bach, Mendelssohn, Verdi, Chopin, Bach, and other masters, since the boy was able to reproduce it perfectly after hearing it just once. Bethune agreed, and that was what they did.

When Thomas turned eight, Colonel Bethune, aware of the diamond in the rough he had in his hands and recognizing Thomas's talent as a potential source of income, hired Thomas to tour the length and breadth of the United States to promote his skill on the piano. "His managers promoted him as an untutored, natural musician who could repeat any composition, no matter how difficult, after a single hearing" (O'Connell, 2009).

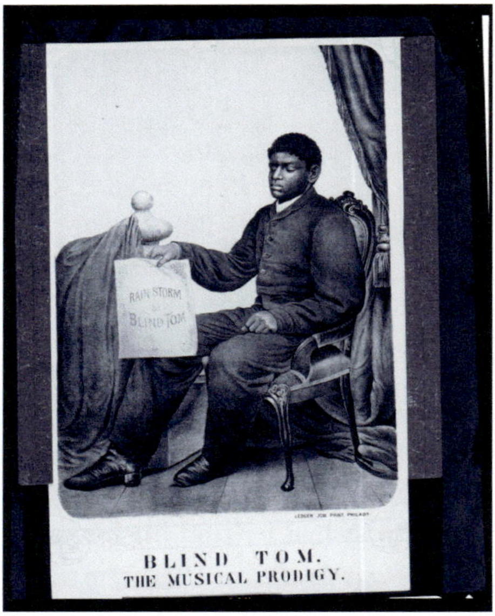

Figure 2.8 Blind Tom, the musical prodigy. The New York Public Library Digital Collections. 1879. http://digitalcollections.nypl.org/items/510d47db-c6d9-a3d9-e040-e00a18064a99

The boy performed as often as four times a day, which allowed him to earn fabulous sums of money. It should be noted, however, that most of the money went to the coffers of Bethune and his business partner, the concert promoter

Perry Oliver. Thomas was exploited, deceived, robbed, and manipulated (O'Connell, 2009). It is estimated that the income Bethune and Oliver obtained at that time reached $50,000 a year, a fortune at the time (the equivalent of $5 million dollars today).

Thomas was not only a genius on the piano: he composed masterfully, wrote music, and sold his scores. In 1860, he visited Congress and performed at the White House before President James Buchanan. The press referred to him as the greatest pianist of the age, whose skills surpassed Mozart. The celebrated writer Mark Twain (1835-1910) was enthralled with Thomas's remarkable abilities, and attended many of Blind Tom's performances. In 1866, General Bethune took Thomas on a tour of Europe, to great acclaim.

Blind Tom excelled as both a formidable composer ("The Battle of Manassas," "Oliver Galop," and "Virginia Polka" are some of his masterpieces) and a virtuoso pianist, playing pieces of music by the great geniuses of his time. Thomas did many surprising things in his musical career, but one of his most remarkable feats was the performance of three pieces of music at once. He played "Fisher's Hornpipe" with one hand, "Yankee Doodle" with the other, and sang "Dixie," all at once.

Thomas was under the legal guardianship of Bethune family members for his entire life, until suffering a powerful stroke in April 1908 and dying in June of the same year, at 59 years old. He was buried in the Cemetery of the Evergreens in Brooklyn, New York. After his death, he was awarded several posthumous recognitions.

2.3 Autism

The first relevant descriptions of what we currently know as autism were provided by Leo Kanner (1943) and Hans Asperger (1944), although it was not until 1980 that autism was first recognized as a new type of mental disorder. The term autism, however, was first used by the Swiss psychiatrist and eugenicist Paul Eugen Bleuler (1857-1939), who also coined other psychiatric terms, including schizophrenia, schizoid, and depth psychology.

In 1938, Kanner began to study children "whose condition differ[ed] so markedly and uniquely from anything reported so far" (Kanner, 1943) and with captivating and intriguing peculiarities. While many of these children had been diagnosed with some of the basic schizophrenia phenomena, Kanner noted dramatic differences from all other known instances of childhood schizophrenia in these cases.

These children exhibited extreme isolation from practically the beginning of their lives and did not respond to anything that came from the outside world. Additionally, these children showed no affective contact with people, though they had excellent relationships with objects which did not threaten to interfere with their loneliness. They also displayed a tendency to echo language (echolalia).

As the children grew and approached the age of six, their language became more communicative, they began to play in groups—though still never with the other members of the play group, and at least on the periphery alongside the group (Kanner, 1943). They tolerated noise and movement better, even though their desire for solitude remained unchanged.

Today autism is considered a neurobiological and developmental condition that begins in childhood (usually appearing by age two or three). It is considered a life-long disability which in many cases prevents individuals from living independently. It encompasses a broad range of conditions and varies widely in the way it affects people: how they behave, interact with others, communicate, and learn. An autistic person tends to engage in restrictive and repetitive patterns of behavior and usually lives in their own world. As Temple Grandin points out:

> In 2013, the American Psychiatric Association revised the diagnostic criteria for autism and greatly broadened the spectrum. It now ranges from brilliant scientists, artists, and musicians to an individual who cannot dress himself or herself (Grandin's website).

Clearly, there is a considerable difference between a brilliant scientist and a mentally retarded individual. "The problem with autism is you've got a spectrum that ranges from Einstein to someone with no language and intellectual disability," said Grandin (Grandin's website).

> In spite of its name—from the Greek noun 'autos' meaning 'self'—autistic men and women are neither selfish nor self-absorbed: many fall in love, raise children, form lasting friendships. Many, too, alongside parents and carers, have silently or publicly fought decades of prejudice and discrimination on the basis of behaviours judged abnormal (Tammet, 2016b).

Diagnosing an individual with autism is not the same as determining if someone has AIDS or coronavirus, in which a test result is either positive or negative. Here, the breadth of the spectrum is still vast, and at some point, we will need to define either a new taxonomic categorization or classification based on similar conditions to in order to determine better treatments for each group, which will allow a better quality of life for individuals. It is obvious that placing a very large set of individuals under the same umbrella is not working for everyone.

One of the problems caused by having such a broad spectrum is associated with the school that an autistic child will attend. If an autistic child goes to a mainstream school, the school is likely not to recognize their special needs, and they will be teased incessantly by his classmates, causing different kinds of frustration. On the other hand, if the child attends a school for children with special needs, they will have to be in the same classes, for instance, as children suffering from mental retardation or Down syndrome. These children will not be representative of the child's condition, and this will also end up frustrating the child.

Many autistic children obviously think differently than other children do, and this factor poses unique challenges to both teachers and schools. In fact, they think differently from each other. Grandin (2006) wrote:

> There were three types of specialized thinking: a) Visual Thinkers like she is, who think in photographically-specific images; b) Music

and Math Thinkers – who think in patterns and may be good at mathematics, chess, and programming computers, and c) Verbal Logic Thinkers – who think in word details, and she noted that their favorite subject may be history.

A crucial element in the school learning process is that teachers be flexible enough with autistic students. Strict rules and habits create barriers, when what is in fact needed is the tearing down of all kinds of barriers. Educational approaches must be tailored to meet students' needs. If they want their children to advance, parents will have to accept that their children must leave their comfort zones and face daily challenges that will push them to interact, socialize, and communicate with others. This must, however, take place in a controlled environment that takes into account each child's abilities and special needs. Temple Grandin has noted the potential detriment of educational approaches that do not challenge autistic children:

> It hurts because they don't have enough expectations for the kids. I see too many kids who are smart and did well in school, but they're not getting a job because when they were young, they didn't learn any work skills, Grandin said (Grandin's website).

In order to make room for inclusion, it is extremely important to break down barriers; barriers which in many cases purport to separate the supposedly normal from the abnormal, though it remains unclear how or by whom these barriers were created. Only in this way can these children acquire a quality education and reach their full potential.

No single cause of autism has yet been determined, and its etiology is multifaceted. Research shows that the disorder is supported both by the environment and, primarily, by genetics, but the problem is that its causes may be different in different individuals. Presumably there are some "circuits," so to speak, that work badly in the brain, but so far, those faulty circuits have not been detected and cause an impressive number of behavioral signs. The most common medical condition associated with autism is epilepsy; a substantial percentage of autistic people have this condition. This in some way suggests that both conditions share an underlying biology and an excited brain. Viscidi et al. (2013) reported that "the average prevalence of epilepsy in children with ASD 2-17 years was 12.5%; among children aged 13 years and older, 26% had epilepsy." In a study of 6,975 children with ASD, Ewen et al. (2019) found that 10% had epilepsy.

Regarding the etiology of autism, current research and accumulated evidence indicate that abnormalities of the cerebellum might be associated with autism. The cerebellum supports not only cognitive functions, including language and executive functions, but also affective regulation (Becker and Stoodley, 2013) and sensory processing (Grandin, 1992). What has been shown so far is that "the cerebellum is structurally and functionally abnormal in patients diagnosed with autism or within the ASD spectrum" (Rogers et al., 2013; Fatemi et al., 2008). "MRI studies also report that autistic children have smaller cerebellar vermal volume as compared to typically developing children" (Webb et al., 2009). Besides this, "cerebellar neuroanatomical alterations are among the most replicated findings in postmortem brain samples of patients with autism" (Fernández et al., 2019). Townsend and Westerfield (2010) reported neuroanatomic abnormalities in a recent review of 58 postmortem cases. The most consistent findings are in the cerebellum and brain stem. In particular, a reduced number of Purkinje neurons were found in the cerebellar vermis and hemispheres (Bauman and Kemper, 2005; Bailey et al., 1998b). Cerebellar anatomic abnormalities were found in 21-25 of all 29 examined cases. Abnormality in limbic structures was present in a majority of autism cases examined (Townsend and Westerfield, 2010; Bauman and Kemper, 2005; Guerin et al., 1996). They were found to be reduced both in neuron size and neuron number (Schumann and Amaral, 2006).

According to CDC (US Centers for Disease Control and Prevention), the prevalence rate of autism spectrum disorder was 16.9 per 1,000 births (1 in 59 children) in 2018. Four times as many boys are autistic than girls, although studies also show that when autism occurs in girls, cognitive impairment is more severe. In general, autism spectrum disorder is present in 1 in 40 boys and in 1 in 185 girls. Furthermore, approximately 56% have an intellectual disability (an IQ < 85) and just 44% have an IQ score above 85 (IQ > 85).

Referring to prognosis, Howlin and Magiati (2017) point out that approximately 48% of the autistic population cannot live independently (poor or very poor outcomes), and just 20% (but with 95% confidence intervals varying from 14 to 27% across studies) were deemed to have good or very good outcomes which allow them to hold a good job and live independently. Finally, as Grandin (2008) said:

> In an ideal world the scientist should find a method to prevent the most severe forms of autism but allow the milder forms to survive. After all, the really social people did not invent the first stone spear. It was probably invented by an Aspie who chipped away at rocks while the other people socialized around the campfire. Without autism traits we might still be living in caves.

Grandin also wrote of Albert Einstein, Ludwig Wittgenstein, Vincent van Gogh, and Charles Darwin "as figures with autistic characteristics, individuals without whose abilities the modern world would be unthinkable" (Murray, 2008).

2.4 Asperger Syndrome (AS)

Hans Asperger, an Austrian pediatrician, eugenicist, and medical theorist, at about the same time as Kanner, observed a group of children who exhibited a pattern of behavior and abilities that included "a lack of empathy, little ability to form friendships, one-sided conversations, intense absorption in a special interest, and clumsy movements" (Atwood, 1997). Unaware of Kanner's work, Asperger chose to name this pattern "autistic psychopathy, using the latter word in the technical sense of abnormality of personality" (Wing, 1981). Unknowingly, both Asperger and Kanner independently delineated two developmental disorders that primarily afflicted young boys (Baskin et al., 2006).

Asperger also noticed that some of these children had no problems with language and that their cognitive development was normal. They also developed highly grammatical speech (which sometimes gave the impression of having been learned from memory or copied from others or from a book), curiosity about their environment, self-help skills, and great talent in their youth, and bordered on the pedantic when explaining their lines of reasoning. They had successful careers, like Elfriede Jelinek, winner of the 2004 Nobel Prize in Literature. The pattern of behavior observed by Asperger is now called Asperger syndrome. Asperger's work was virtually ignored in the English-speaking world until Lorna Wing's (1981) seminal article on the subject was published.

Wing highlights that many of these children may be bullied at school, consequently becoming anxious and fearful, while those who are more fortunate may be accepted as eccentrics because of their unusual abilities and because they follow their own interests, in spite of instructions and activities provided by their teachers. In recent years, it has been noted that lack of empathy is possibly the most dysfunctional aspect of this syndrome (Baron-Cohen and Wheelwright, 2004). It is also known that people with Asperger syndrome may have serious difficulties in understanding irony, humor, sarcasm, or certain facial gestures in which surface meaning is completely contrary to underlying meaning. Regardless of the behavior of each of these individuals, the problem in most cases is serious enough to be treated in a psychiatric clinic.

Wing (1981) also stated that in the last part of adolescence or in early adult life, anxiety, attention deficit hyperactivity disorder (ADHD), and varying degrees of depression have also been observed in several individuals with Asperger syndrome. Wolff and Chick (1980) found that in a study of 22 people with Asperger syndrome, five had attempted suicide by early adulthood. Cassidy et al. (2014) also reported a surprisingly high prevalence of suicidal ideation and suicide plans or attempts among adults with Asperger syndrome. Among 374 adults (256 men and 118 women) diagnosed with Asperger syndrome, 243 (66%) of 367 respondents self-reported suicidal ideation and 127 (35%) of 365 respondents self-reported plans or attempts at suicide (Cassidy et al., 2014).

Gillberg et al. (2016) examined comorbid psychiatric and neurodevelopmental disorders in fifty adult males with Asperger syndrome and found that 47 of these men met criteria for comorbid psychiatric and neurodevelopmental disorders, most commonly either ADHD, depression, or both.

As with autism, the exact causes of Asperger syndrome are not fully understood. Both the environment and genes can play an important interplay role and favor this disorder, but not much more is known. Brain imaging has also failed to identify a common underlying condition.

Regarding the prevalence of this syndrome, Vos et al. (2016) estimated that AS affects 37.2 million people globally. Fombonne and Tidmarsch (2003) reported a prevalence of 28.5 per 10,000 (1519 children aged 7-16 years) in a study conducted in Gothenburg, Sweden. Frombonne and Tidmarsch (2003) also showed the results of six studies conducted in Europe. In this case, the prevalence rate ranges from 0.3 to 48.4 per 10,000, reflecting the differences between the methodologies used across the studies. Mattila et al. (2007) presented the results of an epidemiological study of 5,484 eight-year-old children in Finland. The prevalence rates per 10,000 were 25, according to Gillberg and Gillberg's (1989) criteria.

Asperger syndrome is very difficult to diagnose. In general, one might venture to say children with the syndrome are either: a) of normal intelligence, but possess some problems with social interaction and nonverbal communication and display clumsy and uncoordinated gross motor movements, obsessiveness (a trademark of this disorder), and an extreme interest in organized subjects like maps; or b) autistic children with very strong language and cognitive development, great talent, and extreme curiosity about certain topics. Asperger's is therefore very similar to a high-functioning autism. What is true is that "Asperger's syndrome can be found in varying degrees in the normal population" (Wing, 1981) or hidden within the group of individuals with a schizoid personality.

The point is that while the diagnosis of autism is unquestionable today (albeit within a wide range), Asperger syndrome raises certain doubts, as some researchers suggest that they are varieties of the same underlying abnormality, as we ourselves commented above. Klin (2006) reported that "there are indications that AS is currently functioning as a residual diagnosis given to normal-intelligence children with a degree of social disabilities." Tantam (1988) put this more bluntly, saying that "Asperger seems to have been describing children who were less severely impaired and more intelligent than those described by Kanner." This helps illustrate the ambiguous boundaries that persist between AD and Asperger's.

Finally, it is fair to state that "controversy remains as to what constitutes AS and whether it should be declared a separate disease or higher-functioning autism" (Baskin et al., 2006). The syndrome was removed from the Diagnostic and Statistical Manual of Mental Disorders (DSM-5) of the American Psychiatric Association in 2013, and is considered to be within autism spectrum disorder (ASD), together with autism and pervasive developmental disorder not otherwise specified (PDD-NOS). One might say that it differs from other ASDs in that subjects possess relatively normal language and intelligence. It should be noted that Asperger's formally remains within the international statistical classification of diseases and related health problems of the World Health Organization (ICD-10) which is used in other countries as a subtype of ASD.

> ICD-10 F84.5 Asperger syndrome (version 2019: https://icd.who.int/browse10/2019/en#/F84.0): "A disorder of uncertain nosological validity, characterized by the same type of qualitative abnormalities of reciprocal social interaction that typify autism, together with a restricted, stereotyped, repetitive repertoire of interests and activities. It differs from autism primarily in the fact that there is no general delay or retardation in language or in cognitive development. This disorder is often associated with marked clumsiness. There is a strong tendency for the abnormalities to persist into adolescence and adult life. Psychotic episodes occasionally occur in early adult life."

2.5 Autism Spectrum Disorder (ASD)

ASD is a developmental and neurological disability affecting people who range from gifted to severely challenged. It refers to a family of conditions characterized by broad variability in clinical presentations, symptomatology, and degree of affectedness (Klin, 2006)—the spectrum—although it revolves around aspects of the socialization process; that is, how a person acts and socializes with others, causing problems in social interaction and communication. ASD also involves restricted interests and repetitive patterns of behavior. The level of disability and the combination of symptoms varies tremendously from person to person. ASD is included under the broad heading Pervasive Developmental Disorder (PDD).

ASD is considered a developmental disorder because the first symptoms are observed in the first years of life and persist throughout a person's life. In some cases, a reliable diagnosis can be even obtained between 18 and 24 months of age. Autism spectrum disorder has no single known cause. It is assumed that genes and environmental factors play a fundamental role in their development, but the weight of each factor is unknown. Tick et al. (2016) estimated that between 64% and 91% of risk lies in family history.

There is currently no cure, nor any one standard treatment, for ASD. Some treatments do exist which work very well in some individuals and greatly improve their quality of life by increasing a child's ability to grow and learn new skills. The main features of ASD are:

- Impairment of socialization processes (social interaction and communication).
- Repetitive and limited patterns of behaviour.
- Focused interest.
- Symptoms that affect individuals' behavior and inhibit their ability to function well in school, at home and their own lives.

ASD encompasses disorders that were previously considered separate, including severe autism, functioning autism, Asperger syndrome, and pervasive developmental disorder not otherwise specified (PDD-NOS). Recently, the DSM-5 redefined ASD to encompass autism, Asperger syndrome, PDD-NOS, and childhood disintegrative disorder (CDD). Although the diagnosis of ASD has changed, it is still correct to continue using the terms autism and Asperger syndrome.

PDD-NOS (Walker et al., 2004; de Bruine et al., 2007), on the other hand, is a diagnosis used for severe and pervasive socialization process without any intellectual deficit or repetitive and limited patterns of behaviour. In some cases, behavioural patterns may occur, but they are not severe. For instance, a child with PDD-NOS may want to have friends but not know how to form friendships. They also fail to respond or react to facial gestures, jokes, sarcastic comments, or emotional cues such as laughter, crying, or facial gestures. They want to do something, but their problem is that they do not quite know how. Some call this syndrome an atypical autism or milder autism because "looks like" autism or Asperger syndrome, but does not fit all the symptoms. PDD-NOS may also vary widely or occur in conjunction with a broad spectrum of intellectual ability. What is certain is that not all children with PDD-NOS have the same symptoms. A diagnosis of PDD-NOS is more accurate once a child has reached the age of three or four.

In a comparative study, Walker et al. (2004) found that "on measures of level of functioning (communication, daily living and social skills, IQ, and age of acquisition of language) and on various symptoms of autism (impaired communication and reciprocal social interaction and a preference for repetitive and stereotyped activities)," out of 270 children (21 with PDD-NOS, 33 with Asperger Syndrome, and 216 with Autism diagnosis):

> PDD-NOS children had scores that were between those of the children with autism and those of the children with AS. In contrast, the PDD-NOS group had fewer autistic symptoms, especially repetitive stereotyped behaviours, than both the autism and AS groups (Walker et al., 2004).

Frombonne (2009) stated that the prevalence for PDD not otherwise specified is around 30/10,000 in recent surveys.

Regarding childhood disintegrative disorder (Charan, 2012; Fombonne, 2002; Volkmar and Rutter, 1995), also known as Heller's syndrome and disintegrative psychosis, Charan stated:

> This is a rare and devastating pervasive developmental disorder characterized by late onset (>3 years of age) of developmental delays or regression of developmental ability in language, social function, and motor skills (Charan, 2012).

This is clearly the strangest and most unsettling developmental condition of unknown etiology that we may encounter. In such cases, children develop well until they are three or four years old (even up to the age of ten, in some cases) and then, practically in a matter of days, gradually or abruptly begin to lose language, motor, social, and other skills that they have already learned. CDD affects many different areas of the child's development and bears some similarity to autism (it is sometimes considered a low-functioning form of autism). However, autism does not involve severe regression after several years of normal development. Heller, an Austrian educator, described this disorder in 1908, 35 years before Kanner's and Asperger's reports.

So far, the causes of this disorder are unknown, but there are grounds to believe that it develops in the neurobiology of the brain. Charan (2012) stated that "about half the children diagnosed with CDD have an abnormal electroencephalogram (EEG)." Mehra et al. (2019) pointed out a possible link with genetic and autoimmune neurobiological mechanisms. There is still no cure for CDD and its treatment is very similar to that of autism. One experimental treatment uses steroids to slow the progression of the condition.

Fombonne (2009) has reported that:

> ... the pooled estimate based on eight identified cases and a total surveyed population of 406,660 children, was 2.0/100,000. The upper-bound limit of the associated confidence interval (4.0/100,000) indicates that CDD is a very rare condition, with about one case to occur for every 103 cases of autistic disorder.

More recently, Mehra et al. (2019) showed a prevalence of 1.1 to 9.2 per 100,000. These results are drawn from a cross-sectional study with 96 participants (80 men and 16 women). Their conclusion is that CDD is very rare and that its prevalence is 60 times lower than that of autistic disorder.

2.6 Autistic Savant and Savant Syndrome

Once autistic disorder was formally recognized, the term "idiot savant" was discontinued and replaced by "autistic savant." This term, however, was also short-lived. Although savant syndrome is strongly associated with autism, only 50% of savants form part of the autistic population (it is known that one in ten people with autistic disorder is a savant, however). In other words, not all savants are autistic, and not all autistic persons are savants. The term autistic savant was therefore a misnomer and was renamed "savant syndrome," which is now widely used.

Regarding the prevalence of autism in the savant population, Miller (1998) noted that of the 45 individuals described in his review, 22 had autism. Treffert (2000) also concluded that approximately "50 per cent of individuals with savant skills described in the literature appeared to meet criteria for autism."

On the other hand, Rimland (1978) reported that "from 5,400 autistic children from the US and 39 other countries, 531 (9.83%) were classified as idiot savants."

> Of those with reported skills, the most common were music (53%), memory (40%), mathematical/calculating skills (25%) and art (19%); 53 per cent had multiple special abilities (Rimland & Fein 1988).

Bölte and Poustka (2004) noted that in a study of 254 individuals with autism, 33 (13%) were identified with at least one special skill and 29 individuals had multiple savant skills. Howlin et al. (2009) also stated that of 137 autistic individuals (mean age 24 years, 100 males and 37 females), "thirty-nine participants (28.5%) met criteria for either a savant skill or an exceptional cognitive skill: 15 for an outstanding cognitive skill; 16 for a savant skill based on parental report; 8 met criteria for both a cognitive and parental rated savant skill." Meilleur et al. (2015) have recently found unusual data in a large sample size of autistic individuals, five or six times greater than what appears in the literature. Of 254 autistic individuals, 62.5% showed outstanding skills, including special isolated skills (SIS). Meilleur et al. concluded the prevalence of SIS increased with intelligence and age due to experience. Although the data show some coherence, they also differ from each other, and this is especially because autistic talents vary depending on the criteria used to define them.

There is substantial knowledge currently available about savants and numerous papers, describing dozens of cases, have been published in the scientific literature. Still, savant syndrome is not recognized as a mental disorder within the DSM-5, and the condition affects only about one in a million people (Hyltenstam, 2016).

3

SAVANT SKILLS

The repertoire of mastery among savants falls within a circumscribed range, although as Snyder (2001) has said, "art, music and mathematics are often presumed to be the supreme expressions of the creative mind." Other skills, such as polyglotism, mechanical virtuosity, touch, or vision, including synesthesia and sensory sensitivity, occur less frequently. Savants generally possess a single special skill, but in some instances several skills exist simultaneously. Rimland and Fein (1988) point out that the incidence of multiple skills appeared to be higher in savants with autism than in savants with other developmental disabilities.

Darold Treffert (2009) has also drawn distinctions on the spectrum of savant skills. The definitions of each of these categories are presented exactly as Treffert describes them.

a. Splinter skills: "The most common. Include obsessive preoccupation with, and memorization of, music and sports trivia, license plate numbers, maps, historical facts or obscure items such as vacuum cleaner motor sounds, for example" (Treffert, 2009).
b. Talented savants: "Those cognitively impaired persons in whom the musical, artistic or other special abilities are more prominent and highly honed, usually within an area of single expertise, and are very conspicuous when viewed in contrast to overall disability" (Treffert, 2009).
c. Prodigious savants: "This is a term reserved for those extraordinary rare individuals for whom the special skill is so outstanding that it would

> be spectacular even if it were to occur in a non-impaired person" (Treffert, 2009).

The skills at which savants most commonly excel are generally those described below. However, as we will point out further on, some doubts exist about certain skills, especially those found in mathematical and linguistic savants. These doubts exist because these abilities related to functions of the brain are found in the left hemisphere, which is the more academic, analytical, and logical side of the brain.

3.1 Calendrical Savants

Calendrical savants are one of the most common kinds of savants. They can calculate the day of the week for any given date (past, present, or future) with remarkable speed and accuracy, even considering that the calendar is characterized by many internal regularities such as different monthly structures, cyclical repetitions and leap years. In the Gregorian calendar a year is a leap year if:

a. the year is evenly divisible by 400; or
b. the year is evenly divisible by 4, but not by 100.

Most calendar calculating skills seem to appear between the ages of eight and 15 (Dubischar-Krivec et al., 2009). Whether calculation rather than only memory is involved is a matter of dispute (Cowan and Frith, 2009). Calendrical savants are often associated with autism spectrum disorder, non-specific learning disabilities, and even individuals who have undergone brain surgery (Heavey et al., 2012).

One of the main arguments against mere calculation is their apparent lack of arithmetical skills on an IQ test and that "several savants are known to spend a lot of time studying calendars" (Cowan et al., 2003). Most calendrical savants fail in the calculation of simple arithmetic expressions but have very short response times, so the use of an algorithm or internalized formulae is unlikely (Dubischar-Krivec et al., 2009; Horwitz et al., 1969). "Some savants have provided evidence of memorizing calendars by naming the colors of the dates on calendar" (Howe and Smith, 1988).

As Cowan et al. (2003) has said:

> [...] researchers have generally believed calendrical savants do not use internalized formulae. They have rejected internalized formulae as a basis for savants' skills because to learn and use these formulae requires competence in reading and arithmetic beyond the savants' abilities.

Another argument against calculation is that savants are typically unable to give an account of how they solve date questions (O'Connor and Hermelin, 1989; Howe and Smith, 1988). The inability of savants to articulate their methods has been taken as evidence that they do not use conscious calculation and have no method other than reliance on memory. From this point of view, rote memorization of the calendar coupled with extensive practice might explain the skills of calendrical savants (Dubischar-Krivec et al., 2009).

This is hardly conclusive, however. We hypothesize that savants have some skills that go far beyond rote memory. A good tennis player can perform an excellent two-handed backhand or smash and be barely able to explain exactly how they did so. That the tennis player does not know how to explain their skill in detail does not mean they do not have that skill. An animal might also mimic nature in order to go unnoticed and to protect their species from predators; like the tennis player, the animal cannot explain how it does this. Moreover, people may unconsciously imitate the language and gestures of people with whom they interact to provoke empathy in order to favor personal relationships. Again, the fact that we are not currently able to explain a skill does not mean that it cannot be done. This may be an innate ability that is enhanced by practice. Cowan et al. (2003) postulated that the abilities of calendrical savants suggest the existence of a modular mathematical intelligence or unconscious integer arithmetic. Snyder (2009) has argued that savants have privileged access to lower level, less-processed information before it is packaged into holistic concepts and meaningful labels.

Furthermore, when testing the assumption that individuals with savant syndrome can memorize a complete calendar, one must bear in mind that books and perpetual calendars do not cover more than 400 years in the Gregorian period (Cowan and Frith, 2009). Therefore, an individual with savant syndrome should not be able to answer questions about dates more than 400 years in the future. Horwitz et al. (1969), however, presented results in which a twin savant correctly answered questions about any date between the years 4,100 and 40,400 AD. O'Connor et al. (2000) also showed similar results. One savant could correctly answer questions about years further in the future than the year 8000 AD.

One piece of evidence in favor of the argument that savants use calculation is the systematic error made with leap years in centennial years. Most savants calculate as if all century years were leap years and make mistakes which increase linearly and significantly the further away the year in question is (Hermelin and O'Connor, 1986). If savants were in fact to memorize the complete calendar, they would not make these kinds of errors. Another phenomenon that allows us to hypothesize that savants use calculation is that they need more time to calculate dates that are more remote from the present (Cowan et al., 2003).

Dorman (1991) cites similar results. R.D. (Verbal IQ: 81, Perf. IQ: 81, Full scale IQ: 84), an 18-year-old male at the time of investigation, with porencephalic cavitation of a large portion of the left hemisphere (his entire hemisphere was excised at the age of eight in order to relieve intractable seizures) who remained hemiparetic on his right side and had a right hemianopsia, was able to calculate any day of the week in the past, present, or the near future, but it took him longer to solve the problem as the date increased or decreased in distance from the current year, presumably because the number of serial additions or subtractions would increase. "The suggestion that date calculation does involve at least some calculation process is consistent with recent functional magnetic resonance imaging data," according to Cowan and Frith (2009).

Ho et al. (1991) also described a calendrical savant who performed poorly on the Wechsler Adult Intelligence Scale-IV (WAIS arithmetic) but was very successful on tests that required only calculations. They conclude that his difficulty on the WAIS arithmetic test was in understanding the story context of each problem.

After analyzing several cases and reading virtually all the literature available on the subject, we argue that calendrical savants use memorized dates and calculation skills as well as rule-based strategies (which govern the structure of the Gregorian calendar) when previous strategies are inefficient for calculating dates. The more remote the date, especially in the future, the more difficulties savants have, and the longer it takes them to perform the corresponding calculation. Snyder and Mitchell (1999) "proposed that mathematical savants, including calendrical savants, depend on privileged access to some previously unsuspected lower level of integer processing" (Cowan et al., 2003). Questions about the roots of a calendrical savant's abilities remain unanswered at present.

3.2 Mnemonist Savants

One of the outstanding features of other savants is their prodigious memory. While all savant skills are usually combined with a colossal memory, mnemonic skills also represent a savant domain *per se* (Neumann et al., 2010). Mnemonist savants have been known to memorize entire books, population statistics, public transport schedules, maps, area and zip codes, sports statistics, license plate numbers, and even telephone directories.

Although their interests may focus on different domains of knowledge, they do not necessarily exhibit good memory outside of their specific area of special knowledge (Neumann et al., 2010; Wallace et al., 2009). O'Connor and Hermelin (1989) reported that mnemonist savants exhibit a semantic organization of their long-term memory different from that of other individuals. Neumann et al. (2010) also found "an early activation in right occipital areas during the processing of pseudowords that did not occur in the control group," although this may be due to a visual processing style of verbal material.

Savant syndrome should not be confused with hyperthymestic syndrome or with mnemonists (those with learned skills), although the specific differences between them have yet to be resolved.

Hyperthymestic syndrome is a rare neurological condition in which a person shows a surprisingly detailed memory for specific and general events and remembering dominates their life. These individuals live in the past and are barely able to attend to the present or the future. Parker et al. (2006) described the case of a woman whose remembering dominated her life: "Her memory is nonstop, uncontrollable, and automatic." Individuals with hyperthymestic syndrome are often exhausted. Although experts do not yet have a clear explanation for this new syndrome, they believe that it is a subconscious process in which individuals encode information involuntarily and retrieve it automatically (Wang, 2018). This is unquestionably an indeliberate act. Recent findings have led experts to speculate that the amygdala likely supports the encoding and retrieval of autobiographical memory and is therefore linked to hyperthymesia (Ally et al., 2013). Other results reveal that individuals with hyperthymesia have an enlarged temporal lobe and caudate nucleus. Based on case studies, there are only around 60 identified cases of individuals with hyperthymesia in the entire world.

Figure 3.1 A synesthetic person might associate a color with letters and numbers.

Author: Mysid. Source: Self-made in Inkscape based on en:Image:Synesteticwiki3.png
https://en.wikipedia.org/wiki/Synesthesia#/media/File:Synesthesia.svg
Licensing: Creative Commons CC0 License.

Mnemonists, on the other hand, are individuals with extraordinary talent and learned skills. Their years of deliberate practice allow them to remember and recall unusually long lists of data and numbers, unfamiliar names, entries in books, etc. They use mnemonic strategies, such as the method of loci, to perform their memory feats. Bower (1970) explained that the method of loci is "the use of an orderly arrangement of locations into which one could place the images of things or people that are to be remembered." Maguire et al. (2003) have stated that the method of loci leads to changes in brain activation during memorization, mainly in the medial parietal cortex, retro splenial cortex, and right posterior hippocampus. The neuropsychologist Luria reported that Solomon Shereshevsky, a mnemonist who participated in many behavioral studies, used synesthesia to associate numbers and words as visual images or colors to encode information presented to him.

The most visible difference between individuals with savant syndrome, hyperthymestic syndrome, and mnemonists is that the former have serious intellectual, neurological, and/or sensory disabilities, while the latter two have no neurological disorders beyond an extreme obsession with remembering, either as a deliberate or non-deliberate act. Kim Peek and Howard Potter are two extraordinary cases of mnemonist savants.

3.3 Mathematic Savants

Mathematical savants can perform mind-boggling mathematical calculations at breakneck speeds. They arrive at answers virtually instantly and excel mainly in hypercalculia and numerosity.

> Hypercalculia is a specific developmental condition in which the ability to perform mathematical calculations is significantly superior to general learning ability and to school attainment in maths (Boucher, 2017).

Hypercalculia is an extremely heightened mathematical talent. Joseph Sullivan, one of two autistic savants who served as the principal prototypes for Dustin Hoffman's portrayal of Raymond Babbitt in *Rain Man*, was asked "What number times what number gives 1,234,567,890?" In four seconds, Sullivan responded with 137,174,210 x 9 (Snyder and Mitchell, 1999). It is obvious that such people do not memorize or perform calculations in the same way or at the same pace as neurotypical individuals.

Numerosity, on the other hand, is a multisensory concept, a numerical intuition which allows humans (including infants) and different species of animals to estimate many objects without counting them. The main difference between savants and the rest of individuals is that they push the level of numerosity to a complexity bordering on perfection.

Among animals, an approximate number system has been found in several species, including fish, rats, birds, dogs, monkeys, ants, and wild rodents (Kilian et al., 2003; Emmerton et al., 1997; Woodruff and Premack, 1981). The capacity for some numerical operations, e.g. addition, has been demonstrated in many species, including rats, ants, and great apes. The ability to manage and add fractions has been demonstrated in chimpanzees (Hersch, 1998). Ants have been shown to be able to count up to 20 and add and subtract numbers by up to 5 (Reznikova and Ryabko, 2011).

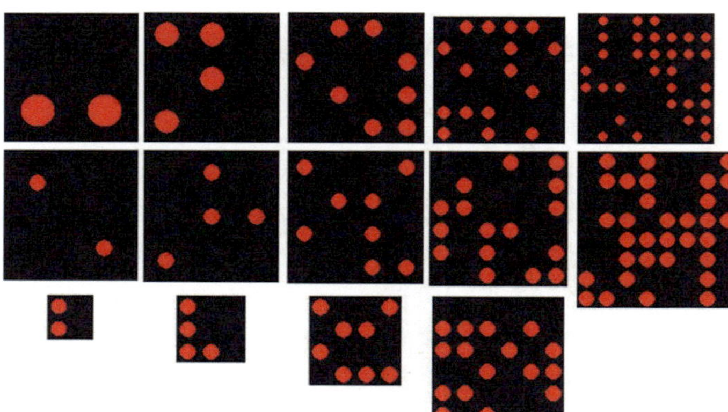

Figure 3.2 "Examples of dot arrays for the numerosities tested in Macaque: 2, 4, 8, 16, and 32. Stimuli with the same average total number of pixels are in the first row; same radius and overall extent in the second row; and same radius and density in the third row" (Roitman et al., 2007).

Source: https://doi.org/10.1371/journal.pbio.0050208.g002.
Author: Jamie D Roitman, Elizabeth M Brannon, Michael L Platt. Creative Commons Attribution-Share Alike 4.0 International license

Concerning savants, Sacks (2009) reported autistic twins who instantly guessed the exact number of matchsticks that had just fallen on the floor, saying in unison "one hundred and eleven." Piazza et al. (2004) have stated that whenever we engage in calculations, the left and right intraparietal regions of the brain are systematically activated. After studies in human neuroimaging and development psychology, Dehaene et al. (2004) and Butterworth (2005) have also convincingly shown that the parietal cortex, particularly the bilateral intraparietal sulcus, is related with numerosity estimation.

Most mathematical savants can also see numbers as shapes with colors, textures, and emotions, and answers to calculations emerge in their minds. This condition in which a perceptual experience in one sensory or cognitive stream leads to automatic, involuntary experiences in a second sensory or cognitive pathway is known as synesthesia (Brogaard et al., 2013; Ward et al, 2006; Baron-Cohen and Harrison, 1997). Today, the link between mathematical savants, autism, and synesthesia is seen as being closer than had been originally imagined.

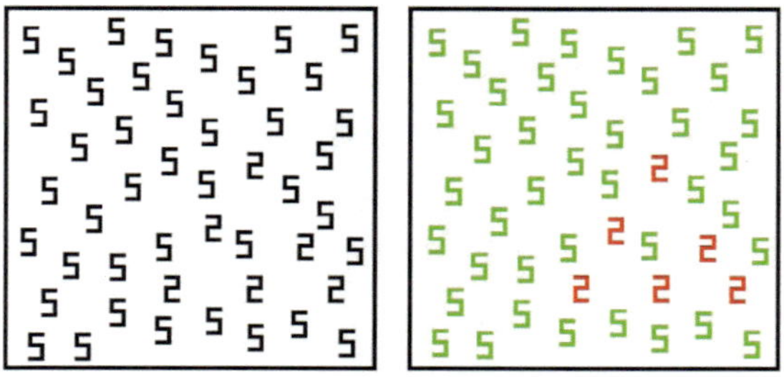

Figure 3.3 "This image demonstrates the logic of one test used to demonstrate the reality of synesthesia. On the left is the image presented to participants, in which a triangle composed of 2s is embedded among a field of 5s. For non-synesthetes this triangle would be hard to identify (displays were presented for one second). However, for someone who experiences 2s as red and 5s as green, the triangle should be more easily identified" (Ramachandran et al., 2001). Image Credit: Edward M. Hubbard (Ramachandran et al., 2001).

https://commons.wikimedia.org/wiki/File:Synaesthesiatest.jpg
Creative Commons Attribution 2.5 Generic license.

Azoulai et al. (2005) have suggested that synesthesia assists memory and that the shapes and colors housed in a mathematical savant's memory allow them to perform superfast computations without consciously doing math. Although the results of these investigations are encouraging, more evidence is needed to confirm the acquisition of savant abilities in autistic and synesthetic individuals. Talent can present itself in different ways. Excellent attention to detail caused by sensory hypersensitivity might lead to rules that govern common areas of savant abilities, but these areas are also characterized by irregularities and unpredictability (Bouvet et al., 2014).

Daniel Tammet is one of the best-known math savants in the entire world. He can "see" and "feel" numbers. Tammet says: "When I multiply numbers I do not calculate; I see two forms and a third emerges – the result. It's like doing math without thinking" (Tammet, 2017; Johnson, 2005).

In Tammet's mind, numbers have unique shapes, colors, textures, and emotions. Each digit from zero to 10,000 is pictured in his mind as a 3-dimensional shape with a specific color and texture. He describes the number 289 as ugly, 333 as attractive, and pi as beautiful. Tammet is capable of astronomical calculations. He holds the European record for calculating decimals of pi, with 22,514 digits. "To him, pi isn't an abstract set of digits; it's a visual story, a film projected in front of his eyes" (Johnson, 2005).

Tammet is a particular savant. Most savants cannot explain the things they do, while Daniel can describe everything he sees in his head. Tammet argues that savant abilities are not supernatural but rather an outgrowth of natural, instinctive ways of thinking about numbers and words.

> Tammet suggests that part of the mystery is what he terms hyper connectivity, an unusual communication between different parts of the brain and unusual convergence of ideas and feelings and concepts, such as imagining a number as having a color (Wilson, 2009).

The classification of mathematical savants is not without controversy. Numerical and scientific skills are found mainly in the left hemisphere of the brain. Since research indicates that savants generally have damage in the left hemisphere and use the right to compensate, damage to the left hemisphere can be expected to cause a deficit in all functions related to this hemisphere, including mathematical functions.

There is also another way to analyze and see the problem. It is a fact that most calculations involve networks that link multiple brain areas. We can even find overlaps in some cases, so determining clear answers is difficult. Most studies suggest that arithmetic depends on the left parietal lobe and the intraparietal sulcus. Logic depends largely on the prefrontal cortex. Geometry, on the other hand, requires spatial functions and depends on the right parietal lobe. What is evident is that humans often use logic in conjunction with arithmetic and geometry in order to solve mathematical problems. For this reason, we say that mathematical problem-solving involves networks that link multiple brain areas, and therefore involves collaboration between different skills in the two hemispheres.

3.4 Artistic Savants

Artistic savants are those savants who have an extraordinary ability to draw, paint, or sculpt. For them, their intrinsic abilities come as naturally as sleeping or breathing. Artistic savants handle their media correctly and easily. Selfe (1977) has highlighted the capacity of artistic savants to produce visually correct, complex artistic outputs, in some cases several months after seeing an initial image. One theory about this unusual and outstanding skill focuses on the exceptional eidetic and photographic memory of these individuals. This ability allows them to recall extraordinarily detailed images from memory with remarkable precision after only a few instances of exposure.

In truth, eidetic memory is the ability to see and retain an object soon after one looks away from it. In most people, memory of a viewed object lasts no more than a few seconds. Eidetic memory "is reported to occur in a small number of children and generally not found in adults" (Hudmon, 2009). Although the terms *eidetic* and *photographic memory* are popularly used interchangeably, they do not signify precisely the same thing. Hudmon (2009) reported that:

> Examples of people with a photographic-like memory are rare. Eidetic imagery is the ability to remember an image in so much detail, clarity, and accuracy that it is as though the image were still being perceived. It is not perfect, as it is subject to distortions and additions (like episodic memory), and vocalization interferes with the memory.

Some researchers argue that we all possess eidetic memory, but that some individuals are masterfully and unconsciously able to transfer this memory to a longer-term storage bank. Simola (2015), on the other hand, has stated that photographic memory "is the ability to recall pages of text, numbers, or similar, in great detail, without the visualization that comes with eidetic memory." Although the idea seems reasonable, this conjecture (photographic memory) has so far never been proven, and some point out that it is impossible, or nothing but a myth.

Myth or not, it's obvious that there are things we know exist without yet knowing how they work. What we cannot understand or clearly explain can cause considerable confusion. While most researchers do not believe photographic memory exists and that eidetic memory does not go beyond a few seconds, Stephen Wiltshire is able to draw a landscape or a city from memory after seeing it just once from a plane. Nobody can explain it.

Mendez (2004) has stated that patients with frontotemporal dementia (FTD) with predominant left temporal involvement have experienced increased artistic activity. In marked contrast, FTD patients with predominant right temporal involvement have been unable to manifest the core elements of art. These results, besides suggesting a neuroanatomical schema for artistic creativity, are congruent with the most plausible explanation for savant syndrome, which is associated with a dysfunction of the left hemisphere of the brain and its compensation by the right hemisphere. Since artistic sense—visuospatial abilities, geometric patterns, visual rhythms, balance, shape and proportion—is located the right hemisphere, a dysfunction or decrease in semantic abilities in the left hemisphere would result in increased abilities in the right hemisphere. Miller et al. (1996) noted that most FTD patients with enhanced creativity have had asymmetrical left anterior temporal dysfunction and poor verbal skills.

3.5 Musical Savants

Musical savants are those individuals who possess absolute or perfect pitch and excellent instrumental skills which contrast starkly with serious individual and general limitations. There are also some cases of individuals who acquired these extraordinary musical abilities after a serious brain or central nervous system injury or disease. This does not mean that anyone who suffers a heavy blow to the head acquires superpowers. In most cases, these accidents do not have such happy endings. The case of Tony Cicoria, for example, is extraordinary: after his accident, he became an acquired savant. Most musical savants are focused on the piano, but there are reports of savants playing various instruments. Thristan Mendoza is a Filipino autistic savant and marimba prodigy.

Absolute pitch (AP) is a rare condition and is generally inherited or "pre-loaded," manifesting before the age of five and not acquired through musical training. Saffran and Griepentrog (2001) have found reason to believe that infants possess absolute pitch early in life but change to relative pitch later on (Andrade and Bhattacharya, 2003). Absolute pitch allows a person to name and recognize isolated auditory stimuli based on a note itself without any external reference. This skill cannot be turned off. While the ability is more common in autistic people (the incidence may be 1 in 20) and individuals with Williams Syndrome, most savants have a high degree of absolute pitch (possibly 1 in 3) (Heaton, 2009; Sacks et al., 1995; Rimland and Fein, 1988). In contrast, researchers estimate the occurrence of AP to be 1 in 10,000 in the general population (Sacks et al., 1995).

On the other hand, it is known that many musicians have quite good relative pitch, a skill that can be learned through ear training, and that this level of relative pitch may be enough to make one an excellent musician and composer. As Slonismky (2002) stated:

> The lack of perfect pitch does not exclude musical talent, or even genius. Neither Wagner nor Tchaikovsky had absolute pitch while a legion of mediocre composers possessed it to the highest degree.

Sacks (2007) has noted that the corpus callosum, which connects the brain's two hemispheres, is bigger in professional musicians, "and people with absolute pitch (that is, those who can immediately name a heard note) have an asymmetric enlargement in a part of the auditory cortex." The question is whether or not this marked characteristic is innate or acquired through training. Wieser (2003) also points out that most composers who can continue to work in spite of degenerative disease or with localized damage are cases that involve the left hemisphere.

> The composers Shebalin and Langlais suffered strokes in the left temporal-parietal regions which, despite inducing aphasia, did not negatively influence note reading or musical composing abilities (Miller et al., 2000; Sergent, 1993).

Cavallera et al. (2012) stated that the composer Maurice Ravel's symptoms of Pick's disease and pre-senile dementia which affected his left hemisphere may have been the origin of the obsessive structure of his orchestral piece *Boléro.* In marked contrast, McFarland and Fortin (1982) described a prominent organist who lost all his musical faculties after suffering infarction of the right superior temporal and supramarginal gyri.

3.6 Linguistic Savants

Linguistic or polyglot savants are extremely rare. Polyglot savants are able to speak up to six languages fluently and with utter ease. People who speak eleven or more languages are considered hyperpolyglots. They have the ability to learn and master multiple languages as an avocation. Although this may seem extraordinary, according to Tucker (1999), "it is believed that multilingual speakers outnumber monolingual speakers in the world's population."

Multilingualism is common in some regions of the world. In Eritrea, for instance, it is common for an educated individual to speak at least five languages perfectly. 70% of Eritrea's residents speak three of its nine native languages: Tigrinya, Tigre, and Dahlik. Educated people also speak Arabic and English, and many understand Italian. In New Guinea, where 871 languages and 200 dialects are spoken (making it the most linguistically diverse place on Earth) multilingualism is highly common: educated individuals there have developed the linguistic proficiency to speak at least four languages (Tucker, 1999).

What most draws the attention is that the mastery of multiple foreign languages is demonstrated in most cases with a low IQ, without formal instruction, and in stark contrast to other overall handicaps (Ammari, 2011; Morgan et al., 2007; Heaton and Wallace, 2004; Smith and Tsimpli, 1995).

Christopher [last name omitted] is one of the most studied cases of linguistic savantism (Smith and Tsimpli, 1995). He can speak, write, and translate at least 16 different foreign languages with varying degrees of knowledge, including Danish, Dutch, German, French, Italian, Portuguese, Spanish, Polish, Finnish, Hindi, Greek, Turkish, Welsh, Russian, Norwegian, and even Epun, an artificial language with peculiar properties that does not exist in the real world and could not be acquired by any normal child (Bates, 1997). He is also able to identify various other languages by their alphabets, including Bengali, Chinese, Czech, Arabic, Hebrew, Japanese, Icelandic, and Gujarati. Despite his brilliance in the linguistic domain, Christopher cannot properly communicate with others and has severe difficulties in non-verbal cognitive domains (Morgan et al., 2007).

Christopher's case is unique in that it contradicts some of what we know about savant syndrome. Savants generally have damage or dysfunction in the left hemisphere, while the right hemisphere attempts to compensate. The problem in this case is that Cristopher has damage to his left hemisphere and has developed an extraordinary skill which belongs to the same hemisphere. As Ammari (2011) has stated, "the acquisition of languages would be out of question in the case of savants since it is purely a left-brain function." Bates

(1997) suggested that this characterization raises an important question: is Christopher a linguistic savant, or simply a man with exceptional language skills who is at the same time severely impaired in visual and spatial terms? To date, although we can never underestimate the brain's plasticity or its ability to reorganize and adapt as a result of experience, we have no perfect answer for this question.

Whatever the answer, and perhaps because we still do not have enough knowledge about the domain of savantism, we are approaching an all-encompassing definition and putting all individuals with intellectual difficulties who also possess extraordinary abilities under the same umbrella. "Consequently, conflicting views, conceptual diversity and overlapping boundaries have led to a lack of a delineated clear-cut distinction pertinent to savant syndrome" (Ammari, 2011).

4

INSIDE THE BRAIN OF A SAVANT

Recent studies have offered some clues as to the obscure origin of savantism, but how exactly their findings clarify the larger picture remains unclear.

Intriguingly, the existence of "Acquired savant syndrome" suggests that the potential for incredible mental abilities resides in all of us, but that a serious injury to the brain is required in order for it to manifest itself (Treffert, 2009). The arrival of new techniques like neural imaging (fMRI) and Transcranial Magnetic Stimulation (TMS) has opened new paths for studying savant syndrome.

Although there are many hypotheses associated with savant syndrome, no single theory is adequate to explain the facts surrounding the syndrome. This is a very heterogeneous area of research and has historically been dominated by anecdotal reports. One of the more plausible explanations for savant syndrome associates the syndrome with a dysfunction of the left hemisphere of the brain which the right hemisphere attempts to compensate for. While well-established as a theory, lateralization (looking to the left hemisphere) does not account for certain cases (linguistic savants).

Three current theories—weak central coherence, enhanced perceptual functioning, and hyper-systemizing theory—attempt to deal with both autism and savants. The fact that savant skills are inextricably linked to ASD suggests that, as Wallace (2008) noted, "neuropsychological models of autism spectrum disorders may help to explain the raised incidence of savant skills in this population." Transcranial magnetic stimulation provides a way to temporarily simulate the condition of a savant in normal individuals by creating a reversible injury. The procedure effectively inhibits, temporarily, the normal functioning of the left frontotemporal lobe. The left hemisphere is disconnected, while the right one is used to compensate. These and other new developments may help us to understand the neural origins underlying the phenomenon of savantism.

4.1 Lateralization: Looking to the Left Hemisphere

Individuals with autism and those with savant syndrome both have damage or dysfunction in the left hemisphere. This leads to compensatory activity by the right hemisphere, which is specialized for literal, non-symbolic skills (Treffert, 2009; Sacks, 2007; Geschwind and Galaburda, 1985). In many of these cases, the right hemisphere is larger than the left, since increased function is correlated with increased volume (Bókkon et al., 2013; Corrigan et al., 2012; Erikson et al., 2011).

The left hemisphere is the more logical and verbal side of the brain and is responsible for control of the right side of the body. Logic, reasoning, analytic thought, number skills, science, mathematics, and language are functions of the left hemisphere. In contrast, the right hemisphere which controls the left side of the body and is more visual, emotional, and intuitive. Creativity, intuition, arts, rhythm, insight, music awareness, and imagination are functions of the right hemisphere. Both hemispheres work together and complement each other to perform all vital bodily processes. They are connected by the corpus callosum, a wide, thick nerve tract beneath the cerebral cortex, creating an information highway. The skills most often seen in savants are those associated with the right hemisphere, while those most lacking are skills associated with the left hemisphere.

Treffert and Wallace (2002) reported that "a 1975 pneumoencephalogram study found left hemispheric damage in 15 of 17 autistic patients; four of them had savant skills." Rimland and Fein (1988), who have compiled the largest database of autistic individuals (more than 34,000), also observed that most autistic savants have damage in the left hemisphere, while the right hemisphere is used to compensate and shows savant-associated skills. Miller et al. (2000) reported on 12 individuals with FTD and left anterior temporal dysfunction who developed extraordinary savant art and musical abilities as their dementia progressed. Dorman (1991) also reported exceptional calendar calculation ability in an eight-year-old boy after early left hemispherectomy.

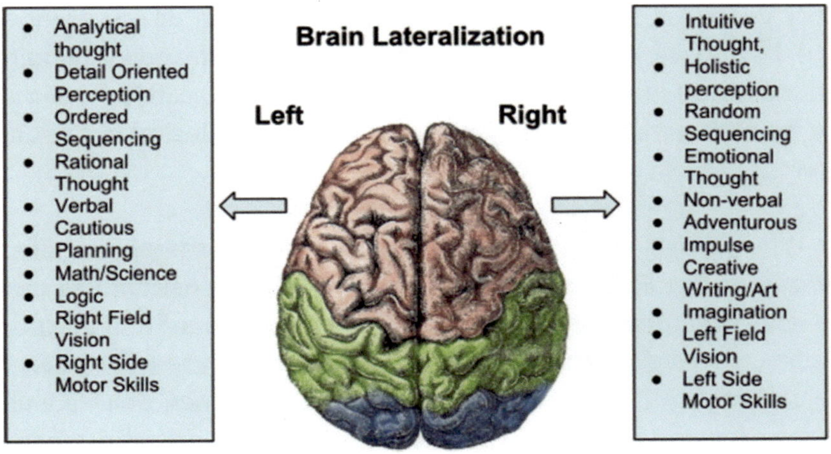

Figure 4.1 Brain Lateralization. This picture demonstrates the lateralization of the human brain, which is divided into two hemispheres. The left brain controls functions that have to do with logic and reason, while the right brain controls functions involving creativity and emotion. Author: Own work.

source: http://en.wikipedia.org/wiki/File:Cerebral_lobes.png Creative Commons Attribution-Share Alike 3.0 Unported license.

> R.D. was born of normal pregnancy but developed a porencephalic cavitation of a large part of the left hemisphere. At age eight his entire left hemisphere was excised in order to relieve intractable seizures. Following the surgery, R.D. developed extraordinary calendar calculation skills (Dorman, 1991).

Brink (1980) reported the case of Mr. Z, who was born in rural Mexico and possessed an intelligence that was at least normal. As a boy, he had suffered a wound from a pistol in his left temple. "For two years Mr. Z was mute, deaf, and paralyzed on the right side. Gradually he regained his hearing and the use of his limbs" (Brink, 1980).

Following that injury, unusual skills—gardening, carpentry, and mechanical work—emerged, presumably from the undamaged right hemisphere (an injury to the left hemisphere stimulated the increased development of the right hemisphere). "Without instruction [Mr. Z] dismantled, reassembled and modified several multi-gear bicycles" (Brink, 1980). Similarly, in the case of a prodigious musical savant, scans and neuropsychological test results also showed left brain damage (Treffert, 2009).

When a part of the hemisphere or the entire hemisphere suffers any damage, its functions can sometimes be assumed by a neighboring region in the same hemisphere or by the corresponding region in the other hemisphere (leading to a cortical reorganization), depending upon the area damaged and the patient's age (Pulsifer, et al., 2004). Most brain injuries, which are unique, obviously involve multiple cognitive deficits (usually social deficits for autistic and individuals with savant syndrome). The left hemisphere (which we are dealing with) is responsible for expression in all its senses. This is to say that the left hemisphere controls activities such as speaking, reading, writing, and logic, as well as the faculties necessary to transform a set of information (analysis and interpretation) into words, gestures, and thoughts.

Geschwind and Galaburda (1985), of Harvard University, have offered a set of hypotheses about the biological mechanism of lateralization that leads to asymmetries and might explain this kind of brain. They suggested that some cognitive processes tend to be more dominant in one hemisphere than the other. The left and right hemispheres are distinct from each other but entities which interact with each other through signals crossing the corpus callosum and other hemispheric bridges (Garavan et al., 1999).

Geschwind and Galaburda (1985) paid particular attention to the role of the intrauterine environment as a determinant of the pattern of asymmetries and in particular sex hormones, e.g. testosterone, or related factors. This may explain why disorders involving the disruption of the left hemisphere of the brain (savant syndrome, dyslexia, autism) occur so much more often in male individuals than in female.

> The left hemisphere typically completes its development later than the right hemisphere, so it is susceptible to prenatal influences for a longer period. Therefore, in the developing male fetus, circulating testosterone can slow the growth of the left hemisphere (Geschwind and Galaburda, 1985).

Mell et al. (2003) and Miller et al. (2000) have observed that the emergence of new skills in the context of dementia suggests that loss of function in one area of the brain can give rise to new functions elsewhere. They stated that loss of function in the left anterior temporal lobe may lead to facilitation of artistic or musical skills as the dementia progresses.

4.2 Linguistic Savants and the Left Hemisphere

The left hemisphere hypothesis works well to account for most savant cases, but there are other cases which it cannot explain and which may even contradict this hypothesis. Linguistic skills, for instance, are found in the left hemisphere of the brain. This is one of the best-established facts about the brain: frontal and temporo-parietal regions of the left hemisphere play a crucial role in language processing. Since theories on the origins of savantism point out that savants generally have damage in the left hemisphere and use the right to compensate, damage to the left hemisphere can be expected to cause a deficit in all functions related to this hemisphere, including language. If we were to take the left hemisphere hypothesis literally, we should not expect to encounter linguistic or polyglot savants—we know, however, that they do exist.

Although we should never underestimate the brain's plasticity, its ability to reorganize and adapt, or its bilateral activations as a result of experience, to date we have no perfect answer to this conundrum.

> Historically, the right hemisphere has been associated with spatial processing and the left hemisphere with verbal processing; however the picture is more complex than this (Arsalidou and Taylor, 2011).

Recent evidence from the field of cognitive neuroscience may help to shed some light on the neural basis of language comprehension and change what for years was considered fact. On the one hand, some misconceptions exist on this subject that must be clarified. On the other, there are some conjectures currently being tested which may yield coherent results in the coming years.

Regarding misconceptions, it must be said that it is not only the left hemisphere that is involved in language processing; the right hemisphere also plays an important role (Lindell, 2006; Jung-Beeman, 2005).

> The evidence reviewed challenges the notion that language is solely a function of the 'verbal' left hemisphere, indicating that the right cerebral hemisphere makes significant and meaningful contributions to normal language processing as well (Lindell, 2006).

Firstly, some patients with RH brain damage have subtle deficits in comprehending natural language (Jung-Beeman, 2005; Bookheimer, 2002; Beeman, 1998). Some well-founded results also indicate that as language processing becomes complex, both the anterior temporal region and the right hemisphere become involved (Xu et al., 2005; Démonet et al., 2005; Jung-Beeman, 2005; Humphries et al., 2001). Finally, Jung-Beeman (2005) has also pointed out that the right hemisphere is highly active when metaphors are understood (Mashal et al., 2007; Bottini et al., 1994), jokes are told (Goel and Dolan, 2001), grammatical errors are repaired mentally (Meyer et al., 2000), and even when inconsistencies are detected in stories (Ferstl et al., 2005). Mitchell and Crow (2005) also reported that some language functions are mediated by the right hemisphere rather than the left.

> These functions include discourse planning/comprehension, understanding humour, sarcasm, metaphors and indirect requests,

and the generation/comprehension of emotional prosody (Mitchell and Crow, 2005).

With regard to conjecture, although most savants have damage to the left hemisphere, there are no data which contradict the fact that an individual may suffer an injury or damage to the right hemisphere and use the left in an attempt to compensate. Unquestionably, however, "most of these studies concur that patients with lesions to the left hemisphere have greater overall impairment than the right hemisphere lesion group" (Semenza and Benavides-Varela, 2018). This finding should not surprise us greatly, since we know that in normal individuals, the left hemisphere dominates the right.

Cohen et al. (2004) reported the case of an eleven-year-old girl who learned to read and write without her left occipital lobe, due to a left occipitotemporal resection for a Sturge-Weber angioma at the age of four. The girl already knew how to speak, but had to learn to read and write again. Vargha-Khadem et al. (1997) published astonishing results regarding Alex, an eight-and-a-half-year-old boy who recovered speech and language skills after a left hemispherectomy to treat Sturge-Weber Syndrome which was affecting his left hemisphere. Alex's advances were measured periodically for any of their selective aspects, including phonology, from age of nine until he was 15 years old (Vargha-Khadem et al. (1997). Gazzaniga (1983) also reported results on patients with different right-hemisphere linguistic competence ranges after early left-hemisphere brain damage and a brain bisection.

There is further conjecture which is quite reasonable, based on evidence from birds, especially the impressive Clark's nutcracker (Nucifraga columbiana), which may apply to other animals and humans. The Clark's nutcracker is a bird with extraordinary memory skills, to the point of being considered a mnemonist savant. The Clark's nutcracker survives mainly by burying seeds in the ground during summer, retrieving them in the winter by memory. This means that it is able to remember where it has stored thousands of separate caches of food in order to get them back when needed some months later.

O'Dwyer (2016) remarked that "the prodigious memory of the Clark's nutcracker seems to be accompanied by an enlarged hippocampus compared with related species of birds that have not developed caching abilities, but in all other respects the bird seems to function normally. The hippocampus is a brain structure that is crucial for memory formation." This implies that "its hyper-performance in one domain does not appear to come at a cost in another" (O'Dwyer, 2016). There do not appear to be compensatory social deficits.

Today we know that there are very gifted people with extremely high IQs all over the world. These individuals are said to possess "hyperbrains." They are not considered savants because they do not meet the established criteria, i.e., either visible mental impairments or serious developmental disabilities. However, without appropriate test data, we cannot assume that they do not have certain abnormalities in different components of the brain which explain their extraordinary abilities without the accompanying burden of a noticeable deficit in social skills.

A hyperbrain is known to be a predictive indicator of educational success and a high level of income. Eminent geniuses have changed the world, developing groundbreaking ideas which live on long after their deaths.

> Many of them, however, possess overexcitabilities in various domains that may predispose them to certain psychological disorders as well as physiological conditions involving elevated sensory and altered immune and inflammatory responses (hyperbody) (Karpinski et al., 2018).

In recent years, numerous studies have reported a correlation between high intelligence and mental impairments (Karpinski et al., 2018; Wraw et al., 2016; Rommelse et al., 2016; Clarke et al., 2016; Smith et al., 2015). This conjecture linking individuals with a high IQ (hyperbrain), to subsequent psychological disorders and savantism is new and requires further study.

Finally, there is a third hypothesis that, with further exploration, may yield interesting results for the study of savantism: bilateral activation. Some functions of the brain are known to take place predominantly in one of the two hemispheres. This is commonly referred to as lateralization. However, when one of the hemispheres is affected for some reason (by an accident, a blow, degradation, stroke, etc.), one or both of them can react, rewire, and assume tasks that normally do not engage them. The underlying assumption here is that all areas (components) of the brain work together to both solve problems and master cognitive challenges.

Bilateral activation is often found in older adults. It has suggested that this is because the brain compensates for degradation or rearranges itself due to problems with other parts of the brain (Park and Reuter-Lorenz, 2009). Bilateral activation also occurs when there is a stroke or damage to one of the hemispheres (Arsalidou and Taylor, 2011; Calautti et al., 2007; Jung-Beeman, 2005; Small et al., 2002).

For years, it was thought that the brain was "prewired," so to speak, according to our genetic endowments. It is now understood that the brain may come slightly "wired," but is quite plastic and its "rewiring" is based on experience. Understanding left and right hemisphere processes as well as bilateral activation with electroencephalography (EEG) and functional magnetic resonance imaging (fMRI) will be essential for unraveling many of the mysteries of savants. We must also be fair in our assessment: although much remains to be done, progress in recent years has been enormous.

4.3 Weak Central Coherence Theory (WCC)

It is known that savant populations contain a high proportion of individuals with autism. Treffert and Rebedew (2015) reported that 75% of individuals in whom savant syndrome was present in childhood had an autism-related condition as the underlying disorder. Therefore, as Heaton and Wallace (2004) stated:

> It is not unreasonable to consider that theoretical models of the savant syndrome might be evaluated and outlined within the context of our current understanding of cognitive characteristics well documented in autistic spectrum disorder.

Mottron et al. (2013) have also noted that knowledge about the anatomical and functional brain characteristics observed in autism can enhance our understanding of savant syndrome.

The weak central coherence (WCC) theory attempts to explain how it is that some people with autism can show outstanding ability in subjects like numbers, music and art, while simultaneously suffering from major problems in social interaction and communication which lead them to live in completely isolated worlds (Happé, 1996). Even though this theory is related to autism spectrum disorders, it explains what happens to most people with savant syndrome (50% of savants are autistic).

Neuropsychological theory suggests that weak central coherence, a common cognitive feature (a cognitive style) in autistic people, can produce information-processing advantages (Happé et al., 2001). Frith (1989) pointed out that autistic people think and see the smallest parts of the world in detail (excellent attention to detail), yet have great difficulties in grasping the bigger picture. This is to say that they perform exceptionally well on tasks that may benefit from failure to perceive gestalt (such as the embedded figures test and the block design task), but have an impaired ability to perceive an integrated coherent whole (such as the visual-motor integration task, which places demands on global processing). "[Frith's] hypothesis is that autistic children actually perceive details better than neurotypical people, but 'cannot see the wood for the trees'" (Frith, 2008; Happé and Frith, 2006).

The WCC theory is one of the most prominent theories that try to explain the abnormalities of autistic individuals on tasks involving local and global cognitive processes. However, other researchers disagree based on their conflicting data. Ozonoff et al. (1994), for instance, pointed out that "autistic subjects performed as well as controls on tasks requiring global-local processing and inhibition of neutral responses." Lopez and Leekan (2003) presented results in which children with autism do not fail to process information in context. Plaisted (2015) and Rinehart et al. (2000) noted that people with autism are able to process holistically, but that they tend to process information locally when not instructed to do it globally. Mottron et al. (1999) concluded that "contrary to expectations based on the central coherence and hierarchisation deficit theories, [our] findings indicate intact holistic processing among persons with autism."

Considering these contradictory findings, it is clear that while an eye for detail is part of the cognitive phenotype of autism, it is not the be-all and end-all of the disorder (Happé, 2018). Recent findings have emphasized superior local perception, as well as suggesting intact global integration (Booth and Happé, 2018; Koldewyn et al., 2013). As D'Souza et al. (2016) stated, individuals with these neurodevelopmental disorders (i.e. ASD and WS) cannot simply be characterized as having a local or global processing style. "The use of 'local' or 'global' processors for explaining neurodevelopmental studies needs to be reconceptualized" (D'Souza et al. (2016).

4.4 Enhanced Perceptual Functioning (EPF)

The enhanced perceptual functioning (EPF) model (Mottron et al., 2006) is one of the leading theories for interpreting cognitive and fMRI data in autism. EPF is also the most predominant theory in accounting for the observation that autistic individuals have relative peaks of ability in both the visual and auditory modalities.

EPF theory focuses on the fact that perception (auditory and visual perceptual processes) plays a different and superior role in autistic cognition, rather than social or higher order cognitive processes (Mukerji et al., 2013). Mottron et al. (2009) stated that individuals with ASD manifest highly developed, low-level perceptual skills, mainly due to a hyper-functioning of regions of the brain typically associated with primary perceptual functions. The theory retains the idea of local bias, as with WCC, but attributes this local bias to a superiority *per se* of low-level perceptual operations (Mottron et al., 2009; Mottron et al., 2006). From this point of view, one emerging cognitive deficit tends to strengthen others "that are practiced and over-learned to the point of becoming one or more restricted interests" (Wallace, 2008). This gives rise to savant abilities.

Mottron et al. (2009) have suggested that:

> [...] perception as a whole should be viewed as an integral part of the mechanism of savant abilities, in as much as these unexpectedly strong skills are intrinsic manifestation of autistic behavior, learning and intelligence.

However, it is not yet clear to what extent the mechanisms of primary perception are associated with the skill peaks of the autistic and the emergence and character of savant abilities. Moreover, despite its strengths, the model predicts a single, isolated area of skill in savants, despite the fact that, in some individuals, several skills exist simultaneously (incidence is higher in autistic savants).

4.5 Hyper-systemizing Theory

The hyper-systemizing theory is another theory which links autism, savants, and talent. Given the high incidence of autism in the savant population, any theory or model which explains autism could help explain the amazing abilities possessed by savants.

Darius (2007) stated that there are six features that crop up continually in studies of savantism: testosterone, systemizing skill, heredity, extraordinary memory, interest, and practice. Systemizing—the drive to analyze or construct a system—is the core part of this theory, but is also strongly related to other theories.

Exceptional attention to detail is, not surprisingly, an essential feature of the hyper-systemizing theory, since systemization implies attention to tiny details. Baron-Cohen (2006) observed that "what defines a system is that it follows rules, and when we systemize we are trying to identify the rules that govern the system, in order to predict how the system will behave."

Systems may be mechanical, abstract, natural, collectible, motoric, or even social. The main difference between the weak central coherence theory and the hyper-systemizing theory is that in the former, the central objective is attention to detail, whereas in the latter, details are the main reason for understanding the system. This allows individuals to see the big picture and to understand the laws and control the variables that govern the system.

The cognitive style of the hyper-systematization theory is strongly associated with Asperger syndrome. The fact that hyper-systemizing predisposes individuals to show talent might explain why individuals with Asperger syndrome can have successful professional lives, despite living them in isolation.

According to Baron-Cohen et al. (2003):

> ... the existence of talented mathematicians with AS, such as Richard Borcherds, is proof that such individuals can integrate the details into a true understanding of the system.

Individuals with Asperger syndrome are as intelligent or more intelligent than other people, but have much more trouble with social skills. Today, Asperger syndrome is technically part of the autism spectrum disorder and is often considered a high-functioning type of ASD.

On the other hand, the empathizing–systemizing (E-S) theory (Baron-Cohen, 2009a) explains the deficits in empathy and the intact, even superior, skill in systemizing present in autistic individuals or those with Asperger syndrome. In fact, it is the discrepancy between E and S that determines whether one develops an autism-spectrum condition.

The theory suggests that people may be classified on the basis of their scores, using the Empathy Quotient (EQ) and Systemizing Quotient (SQ), in two dimensions: empathizing (E) and systemizing (S) (Baron-Cohen et al., 2009). Systemizing has been described above. Empathizing has both a cognitive and an affective component, which involve an emotional response that arises from the understanding the emotional life of other individuals (Eisenberg,

2002). The test scores sort brains into five different types. The profile E>S is more common in females, while the profile S>E is more common in males.

The latter is the reason Baron-Cohen and his team claim that men tend to choose areas of knowledge related to science, technology, engineering, and mathematics. Billington et al. (2007) noted that E-S theory is a better predictor than gender of who chooses STEM subjects. They evaluated the performance of 415 students (203 men, 59% of whom were from the field of science and 212 women, 73% of whom from the were field of humanities) on activities related to empathy and systemizing. The results confirmed the earlier findings: the women achieved superior results in the EQ test, while the men performed better in the SQ test. Billington et al. (2007) stated that "individuals with strong systemizing drive are more likely to enter the physical sciences, irrespective of their sex."

Baron-Cohen's critics, however, are not hard to find. Nash and Grossi (2007) have criticized the theory of sex differences, arguing that boys and girls develop in similar ways. They show that findings of differences in math and science performance are not reliable, vary depending on the measures used, and come from poorly designed studies with equivocal findings. Fine (2010) used Baron-Cohen's views as an example of "neurosexism." Autism researchers say that his work is biased towards higher-functioning individuals with autism spectrum disorders who have good language capabilities and at least average intelligence. These researches suggest that this diminishes the utility of the sample as a test of the hypothesis (Buchen, 2011). At first glance it is not obvious that this applies to low-functioning individuals. Baron-Cohen, on the contrary, accepts that the data are not sufficient. He remains open to new hypotheses and does not see a problem in introducing the empathizing-systemizing theory before all the evidence is in.

4.6 Transcranial Magnetic Stimulation (TMS)

TMS (Horvath et al., 2011, Barker et al., 1985) is a noninvasive technique of brain stimulation, applied in 40-minute sessions, which uses magnetic fields to stimulate cortical sites. TMS requires no anesthesia or sedation and has no systemic side effects. Magnetic fields pass readily across the scalp and the skull and produce currents in the induced electrical field lying parallel to the plane of the coil. These currents are able to excite neural processes lying in the plane of the induced field in a manner roughly analogous to direct cortical stimulation with electrodes (Wassermann, 2002). TMS is a mainly used in the treatment of autism, depression, schizophrenia, and Alzheimer's disease.

Snyder et al. (2006) reported that TMS treatments significantly and rapidly improve intellectual capacity, enabling patients to understand scientific theories and solve complex mathematical problems. A meta-analysis by Luber and Lisanby (2014) of over 60 studies concluded that TMS in healthy people produces significant improvements in speed, accuracy, and superior performance in tasks involving attention, memory, and language. Using this information, Snyder (2009) concluded that savant skills are latent in all of us.

> This suggests why savant skills might arise spontaneously in otherwise normal people, and why such skills might be artificially induced by low-frequency repetitive transcranial magnet stimulation (Snyder, 2009).

The utility of TMS theory is presumed to reflect the fact that when one side of the brain is damaged, the other completely unleashes its abilities to such a degree that it can regain the individual's previous intellectual capacity. Savants are clear examples of this theory. Snyder suggested that if his theory about the origin of exceptional numerical savant skills were to be verified, any person in the future would be likely able to perform extremely complex calculations (Fox, 2002).

One of the experiments to demonstrate the above was conducted by Snyder at the Center for the Mind in Sydney, Australia. Snyder temporarily simulated the condition of a savant in normal individuals by creating a "virtual" (reversible) injury (Steven and Pascual-Leone, 2006; Hoffman and Cavus, 2002). This meant using TMS to briefly inhibit the left fronto-temporal lobe, responsible for linguistic and oral production, movements of the phono articulatory organs, and memory. The left hemisphere section is disconnected because savant syndrome is basically associated with a left-brain dysfunction, while the right hemisphere is used to compensate.

Twelve volunteer students (five men, seven women) from the University of Sydney, ranging from 19 to 33 years of age, participated in the experiment and were tested before, during, and after TMS treatment. Each of the participants in the study was shown 50 to 150 oval-shaped discrete elements distributed evenly on a monitor for 1.5 seconds.

> They have to accurately guess the absolute number of discrete elements displayed on a monitor. Both the spatial position of the elements and their number were randomly generated by computer for every presentation (Snyder et al., 2006).

The results were impressive. Ten students immediately acquired a skill like that of a savant after the application of TMS. The skills of eight of the ten students decreased an hour later, as the effect of TMS wore off. In another experiment, 40% of the volunteers developed extraordinary intellectual abilities in 15 minutes that allowed them to solve complex mathematical problems. The results of these experiments are consistent with others previously reported in drawing (Snyder et al., 2003), proofreading skills, and induced numerosity (Snyder et al., 2006). In these cases, individuals who did not show any talent for these areas acquired these abilities after TMS treatment. Luber and Lisanby (2014) have also stated that multiple sessions of high frequency (rTMS: greater than 1 Hz) combined with TMS/task performance can induce Hebbian-like learning, which can prolong the enhancement's effects.

Adverse Effects

Although TMS is generally regarded as safe, caution is advised. Wassermann (2002) points out that while behavioral effects may be greater, potential risks may be as well. The more prominent the nonspecific behavioral and attentional effects are, the more difficult the results may be to interpret. Fitzgerald and Daskalakis (2013) warn of the possibility that adverse short-term effects may occur, such as transient hearing loss, transient impairment of working memory, transient induction of hypomania, and even the rare occurrence of syncope and seizures.

In addition, selecting the frequency (Grosbras and Paus, 2002; Boroojerdi et al., 2001; Maeda et al., 2000), intensity (Lewald et al., 2002; McConnell et al., 2001; Stewart et al., 2001) and duration of stimulation, (Maeda et al., 2000; Wasermann, 1998; Pascual-Leone et al., 1994) which often determines the success or failure of a study (Robertson et al., 2003), is a difficult process and frequently can be an arbitrary decision. Knowing what precisely you are stimulating (Bohning et al., 1999) and the exact anatomical localization of the stimulation site are other substantial problems (Herwig et al., 2001). This follows from the fact that stimulating a specific area of the brain may have functional consequences not only at the site but also throughout the neuronal circuit (Robertson et al., 2003).

Although the results of TMS are preliminary and require that independent researchers replicate the findings, the use of the technique has gained popularity in different fields of health around the world. The use of TMS was approved for treatment of migraines (Drues, 2014), depressive disorders (Voineskos et al., 2016; Hu et al., 2016), epilepsy (Gersner et al., 2016), Parkinson's disease (Dileone et al., 2017; Torres et al., 2015), autism (Oberman et al., 2016), panic disorder (Li et al., 2014), traumatic brain injury and stroke (Shin et al., 2014), post-stroke recovery (Bashir et al., 2010), and the enhancement of human cognitive performance in healthy people (Luber and Lisanby, 2014).

4.7 Findings in a Chromosomal Region

Chromosomal region 15q11-q13 is of particular interest to autism genetics, since several published results, obtained using genetic exploration and methods, show chromosomal abnormalities in individuals with an autism phenotype (Wang et al., 2018; Hollis et al., 2017; Hogart et al., 2010; Dykens et al., 2004; Nurmi et al., 2003). There is also a suggestive link between a savant's skill and chromosome 15q11-q13. This chromosome is particularly important because it may give rise to a cognitive style or pattern of cognitive impairment, even when the skill itself may be due to other genetic or environment factors (Darius, 2007).

Similar types of skills have been noted in individuals with Prader-Willi syndrome, which results from deletions of this chromosomal region. Hogart et al. (2010) and Dyckens et al. (2004) also pointed out that paternally or maternally derived deficiencies of 15q11-q13 result in Prader-Willi or Angelman syndromes. Dyckens et al.(2004) are currently using a global approach to review potential autism susceptibility genes in the 15q11-q13 region. Ma et al. (2005) also found increased evidence for linkage in this region in a subgroup of 21 autism families (total families = 94) stratified, based on a savant skill factor from the Autism Diagnostic Interview. However, their findings do not support savant skills as an informative phenotypic subset for linkage in these data.

Accurately described phenotypes are crucial for fine mapping of the 15q11-q13 region and understanding genetic variation in autism. Nurmi et al. (2003) also stated that the higher occurrence rate of savant skills in autism suggests that a savant skill may be an autism-specific phenotype feature. More recently, Ruthsatz et al. (2015) also identified a suggestive and potential genetic link, a shared locus, between autism, savants, and chromosome 1, in a region known as 1p31-q21.

Although these new findings are promising, they must be replicated in further studies. It is also important to define whether this region is related only to autistic individuals or also to individuals with savant syndrome.

4.8 Other Findings

Some other findings show a strong genetic component in people with autism disorder, which has given rise to interest in the broader autism phenotype (Happe et al., 2001). Landa et al. (1991) reported that the parents of children with autism told rather more fragmented and less coherent spontaneous narratives than did control parents (Happé et al., 2001). Yirmiya et al. (2001) and Bailey et al. (1998a) conclude that there is strong evidence that both parents and male relatives of autistic children show an increased incidence of social peculiarities and communication difficulties.

Baron-Cohen's research on relatives of people with Asperger syndrome and autism found that their fathers and grandfathers are twice as likely to be engineers as the general population (Baron-Cohen and Hammer, 1997). These findings are interesting because they suggest a link between a male feature and the broader phenotype of autism, as well as suggesting a sex difference in certain aspects of information processing.

> These data also suggest that genetics and the environment play a role in autism prevalence, and children with technically minded parents are therefore more likely to be diagnosed with autism (Baron-Cohen, 2012).

Finally, Pellicano et al. (2006) supported the emerging consensus: the need to invoke several coexisting cognitive capabilities/deficits to account for the extant heterogeneity in autism, evident at the genetic, neurobiological, and behavioral levels. Happé et al. (2006) also argue that there is no single (genetic, neural, or cognitive) cause for the diverse symptoms which define autism. Replication with larger samples will be necessary to confirm all these hypotheses and contribute to our understanding the pathogenesis of autism.

5

CASE STUDIES, SKILLS, AND IMPAIRMENTS

In this chapter, we will profile thirty six notable savants who are more remarkable for their extreme skills and strengths than for their limitations. In most cases, their abilities are superior to those exhibited by highly intelligent normal individuals.

This is the first time that so many profiles have been brought together in a single paper or book. Twenty-nine of these savants are men and seven are women. Twenty-four of them are from the United States, six are from England, and one each is from Scotland, Italy, Turkey, the Philippines, Taiwan, and Malaysia. Seven of the people profiled here are acquired savants whose abilities emerged after a CNS injury or disease.

These profiles were drafted in a sincere effort to remain neutral and objective, neither defaming nor sensationalizing our subjects. We have also avoided invading individuals' privacy and based much of their respective content on publicly-available information from high-quality sources; mainly research articles, books, and newspaper notes. Wherever possible, we have quoted the savants themselves, without any kind of filter or intervention. In the interests of balanced investigation, however, when most of the public information available on a savant came solely from the savant themselves, we were unable to include their profile here.

We acknowledge the very real possibility of unintentional mistakes, given that the information we found may not have been accurate (as we all know, even information from reliable sources is not always 100% certain). In this case, we extend a sincere apology to the savants and their families and hope they will assist us in correcting them in future editions of the book.

5.1 Franco Magnani (born 1934)

I greatly appreciate the contributions of Franco Magnani in the detailed review of this profile.

Magnani was born in Pontito, near Florence, Italy in 1934. He is a painter and an acquired savant. His memory is, simply stated, extraordinary: although he has not lived in Italy for 30 years, Magnani is able to remember and capture every detail of his home town in his paintings. Although his childhood was happy, his father passed away in an accident when Magnani was eight years old. World War II came soon afterwards. Magnani's world crumbled when the Nazis occupied his home town. His mother was forced to work in the fields, while he and his brothers took care of the housework.

Magnani came to the U.S. in the 1960s. Having settled in San Francisco, he experienced a strange and sudden illness, which is still something of a mystery. The disease caused fever and delusions. Confined to his bed, Magnani was swept up in dreams so vivid that he could smell and hear the sounds of his childhood in his hometown and was unable to think of anything else. He was seized with an irresistible desire to paint, and he suddenly found that was able to capture these dreams in precise detail, despite never having practiced painting in his life.

Magnani married his beloved wife Ruth, also a painter, in 1975 and together they opened the Pontito Gallery. The gallery closed in 1988, when Ruth passed away.

Oliver Sacks, the famous neurologist, met Magnani in 1988. He was struck by the fact that Magnani's paintings were practically identical to photographs of his town Pontito, taken by Susan Schwartzenberg in 1987. Sacks discovered that Magnani lived in the past and did not have the luxury most of us take for granted—to stop remembering.

In 1990, Magnani returned to Pontito and soon had a premonition that it would be overcome in the future by a nuclear attack. One way of preserving the identity of the town was to make dozens of paintings that captured all the details of his native town, which was what he began to do.

Impairments: Acquired savant. Hyperthymestic syndrome. He suffered a mysterious illness with characterized by fever and delusions that confined him to his bed. It also brought dreams so vivid that he could smell and hear the sounds of his childhood in his hometown and was unable to think of anything else.

Skills: Artist, painter. He is able to capture his vivid dreams, which returned him to in his childhood in Pontito, Italy, in an extraordinarily accurate manner.

Below are references, links to some videos, and additional reading about Franco Magnani.

- Franco Magnani's official website: https://francomagnani.net/
- Piechowski-Jozwiak, B., & Bogousslavsky, J. (2020). Painting in Neurology. In *Brain and Art* (pp. 41-52). Springer, Cham.
- Chatterjee, A. (2015). The neuropsychology of visual art. *Art, Aesthetics, and the Brain, 341.*
- Sacks, O. (2012). *An anthropologist on Mars: Seven paradoxical tales.* Vintage.
- Michaud, J. (2010). Back Issues: Franco Magnani. The New Yorker. August 24, 2010. https://www.newyorker.com/books/double-take/back-issues-franco-magnani
- Warner, J. (2009). Franco Magnani and JG Ballard. Identity Theory. May 10, 2009. http://www.identitytheory.com/franco-magnani-and-jg-ballard/
- Chatterjee, A. (2006). The neuropsychology of visual art: Conferring capacity. *International Review of Neurobiology, 74,* 39-49.
- Franco Magnani. https://www.youtube.com/watch?v=5RzBKp-Pbhc
- 10 People Who Became GENIUSES from BRAIN DAMAGE. https://www.youtube.com/watch?v=DrYNJkwVwC4&t=5s

5.2 George and Charles Finn (born 1939)

George and Charles Finn, known as the "Bronx Calendar Twins," are autistic twin brothers born in 1939 in the United States. Horwitz et al. (1965) described the brothers as "self-taught with an IQ in the range of 60-70's." They concentrate exclusively on numbers and calendars—anything beyond this is impossible for them. These identical twins became famous in the 1960s for their skills in calendar computing, in interviews with famed journalist Morley Safer on radio and television, and for their encounters with Oliver Sacks, described in his book *The Man Who Mistook His Wife for a Hat* (1985).

George and Charles can calculate the day of a specific calendar date thousands of years backwards or forwards and are also able to precisely recall the weather on each day of their life. George is regularly correct, and Charles usually so.

> Although Charles is completely accurate only for this century (twentieth century), George can project his calendar identifications to centuries before and centuries beyond our present perpetual calendars (Horwitz et al., 1965).

For example, when asked: "in which years does April 21st fall on a Sunday?", each will answer correctly: 1968, 1957, 1963, 1946, and so on. George can continue as far back as 1700 (Horwitz et al., 1965). The brothers say that the answers suddenly appear in front of them. Their explanation seems logical, since neither of them can perform the simplest of arithmetic operations. They do not use paper, pencil, or any other tools to perform their calculations; only their minds.

For the Finn brothers, answering these questions is as simple as remembering what you had for breakfast today. Of course, they can also answer this question for each day of their life. Morley Safer (1931-2016), a Canadian-American broadcast journalist, reporter, and correspondent for CBS News, introduced viewers to George Finn.

Much has been speculated about the twins' numerical prowess and the mechanisms that operate in their brains to deliver such results. The most astonishing and interesting essay on them, although not without criticism in recent years (Tammet, 2016; Yamaguchi, 2009; Dehaene, 2001), was published by Oliver Sacks in his book *The Man Who Mistook His Wife For a Hat* (Sacks, 1985). Sacks first met the twins at a state mental hospital when they were 26 years old. He was impressed by seeing them: they seemed indistinguishably grotesque, identical in their faces, body movements, personalities, intelligence, and brain stigmata (Sacks, 1985). He considered them obsessive and schizoid.

Sacks says that his first sight of the twins' natural ability came spontaneously.

> A box of matches on their table fell, and discharged its contents on the floor: '111,' they both cried simultaneously... I counted the matches – it took me some time – and there were 111. ... 'How did you work that out?' I said. ... They indicated, as best they could, in poor, insufficient terms—but perhaps there are no words to correspond to such things—that they did no 'work it out', but just 'saw' it, in a flash (Sacks, 1985).

Sacks also points out the twins' ability to generate 6-digit prime numbers. Sacks challenged them to generate more complex primes, giving them a ten-digit prime number that he found in a book he possessed. The twins then came to generate numbers of up to 12 digits (Sacks, 2009). As Sacks tells it, in one of his visits, he came upon them:

> [...] seated in a corner together, with a mysterious, secret smile on their faces, a smile I had never seen before, enjoying the strange pleasure and peace they now seemed to have... John would say a number—a six-figure number. Michael would catch the number, nod, smile and seem to savour it. Then he, in turn, would say another six-figure number, and now it was John who received, and appreciated it richly... (Sacks, 1985).

Sacks returned to his home. Checking the figures against his book, Sacks found that they were all prime numbers. Intrigued, he went to visit again the next day, carrying his book.

> After a few minutes I decided to join in, and ventured a number, an eight-figure prime. They both turned towards me, then suddenly became still, with a look of intense concentration and perhaps wonder on their faces... suddenly, simultaneously, they both broke into smiles... Then John, who always took the lead, thought for a very long time...and brought out a nine-figure number; and after a similar time his twin Michael responded with a similar one. And then I, in my turn, after a surreptitious look in my book, added my own rather dishonest contribution, a ten-figure prime I found in my book. There was again, and for even longer, a wondering, still silence; and then John, after a prodigious internal contemplation brought out a twelve-figure number. I had no way of checking this (Sacks, 1985).

According to Sacks (2009), the twins do not seem to operate with numbers, at least not as a calculator does. They are not interested in calculations, nor can they understand calculations—they see numbers directly, as a huge natural landscape. It is impossible to think that the twins arrive at the numbers using trial divisions, when they cannot perform the simplest of arithmetic operations.

In recent years, Sacks' claims about the twins' abilities have been the subject of much criticism, and some have questioned whether his report is true at all. Yamaguchi (2009) pointed out that it takes 65 divisions to find the smallest of the 6-digit primes (100003) and more than 150 divisions to find 7-digit primes. Trial divisions are therefore ruled out in the case of twins. Sacks also reported that the 6, 8, and 10-digit numbers were taken from a table in a book he had on prime numbers. In recent years it was mentioned that such a book never existed (nobody knows of one, in any case) and that it would furthermore be impossible for a book to contain all the prime numbers of up to 10 digits, since these would reach 50 million numbers in the best of cases (Yamaguchi, 2009). Yamaguchi stressed that:

> We are regrettably forced to conclude that the details of that report cannot be trusted. Considering the sincerity of Oliver Sacks in his other reports, I am inclined to believe that at least the twins really generated 6-digit primes (Yamaguchi, 2009).

Daniel Tammet (2016) also referred to Sacks' statements on the Finn brothers when analyzing Silberman's (2015) book, *Neurotribes: The Legacy of Autism and the Future of Neurodiversity.*

> The problem is, the story, so seductive to a generation of journalists including Silberman, has no basis in reality. As other commentators have noted (Yamaguchi, 2007), there is no known mechanism by which such mental arithmetic might be possible, and even the existence of a tome of mathematical tables large enough to contain every prime number as long as eight digits has been placed in doubt (Tammet, 2016).

Although Sacks' text on the Finn twins was ultimately questioned, no one doubts the abilities of George and Charles Finn. The abilities of savants arise spontaneously on many occasions, and no one has yet been able to say what mechanisms the brain employs to achieve this.

Impairment: Autism. George and Charles cannot add, subtract, multiply, or divide even simple single digit numbers. For instance, they cannot solve the abstract equation 2 + 2.

Skills: Calendar calculation, memory, sense of smell. They can accurately state the day of any date to centuries before and centuries beyond our present perpetual calendars, but this ability is not reflected in other parts of their learning. They do not know the difference between the Gregorian and Julian calendars. When asked how they perform calculations, they simply reply that they see the numbers (the result) in their heads. Extraordinary memory for weather. Both can remember exactly what the weather was like on any day of their lives. They can also pick out their own clothes among 1,000 other garments at a laundromat by smell alone.

Below are references, links to some videos, and additional reading about George and Charles Finn.

- Silberman, S. (2017). *Neurotribes: The legacy of autism and how to think smarter about people who think differently*. Atlantic Books.
- Tammet, D. (2016). Autism: a spectrum of speculation. *Brain, 139*(3), 999-1000.
- Silberman, S. (2015). How Oliver Sacks helped introduce the world to autism. BuzzFeed. August 30, 2015. https://www.buzzfeed.com/ssilberman/how-oliver-sacks-introduced-the-world-to-autism
- Silberman, S. (2015b). *Neurotribes: The legacy of autism and the future of neurodiversity*. Penguin.
- Dehaene, S. (2011). *The number sense: How the mind creates mathematics*. OUP USA.
- Sacks, O. (2009). *The man who mistook his wife for a hat*. London: Picador.
- Yamaguchi, M. (2009). Savant syndrome and prime numbers. *Polish Psychological Bulletin, 40*(2), 69.
- Yamaguchi, M. (2007). Response to Snyder's "Comments on Priming Skills of Autistic Twins and Yamaguchi (2006) Letter to the Editor:'Questionable Aspects of Oliver Sacks'(1985) Report,'" Journal of Autism and Developmental Disorders. *Journal of Autism and Developmental Disorders, 37*(7), 1401-1401.
- Snyder, A. (2007). Comment on Priming Skills of Autistic Twins and Yamaguchi (2006) Letter to the Editor:" Questionable Aspects of Oliver Sacks'(1985) Report", Journal of Autism and Developmental Disorders. *Journal of Autism and Developmental Disorders, 37*(7), 1398-1399.
- Sacks, O. (2002). El hombre que confundió a su mujer con un sombrero. Editorial Anagrama: Barcelona.
- Spitz, H. (1995). Calendar calculating idiots savants and the smart unconscious. *New Ideas in Psychology, 13*(2), 167-182.
- Horwitz, W., Deming, W. and Winter, R. (1969). A further account of the idiots savants, experts with the calendar. *American Journal of Psychiatry*, 126(3), 412-415.
- Hamblin, D. (1966). They are idiot savants: wizards of the calendar. *Life, 60*, 106-8.

- Horwitz, W., Kestenbaum, C., Person, E. and Jarvik, L. (1965). Identical Twin—" idiot savants"—calendar calculators. *American Journal of Psychiatry*, 121(11), 1075-1079.
- Brain Man. 60 Minutes. January 28, 2007. https://www.cbsnews.com/news/brain-man/
- 60 Minutes, CBS. Morley Saffer interviews the Finn brothers. https://www.youtube.com/watch?v=q9eVqoRctkk
https://www.youtube.com/watch?v=zew9UXSV51g

5.3 Gregory Blackstock (born 1946)

I greatly appreciate the contributions of Dorothy Frisch, Gregory's cousin, in writing and reviewing this profile.

Gregory Blackstock was born in 1946 in Seattle, Washington. He is an autistic savant and artist. Blackstock was born at a time when autism had not yet been identified as a mental disorder, and therefore suffered its full consequences. Autism only began being treated as such in the 1980s, so Blackstock lived most of his life without knowing or understanding exactly what was happening to him. It should be said that his parents, educated and of sufficient means, did not understand the problem either (they were given a diagnosis of paranoid schizophrenia) and for this reason enrolled their son in a school for children with special needs, where Blackstock spent five years institutionalized in California far from his family. After completing school, he spent most of his life working in menial jobs, including 25 years spent working as dishwasher at the Washington Athletic Club in Seattle. He retired in 2001.

Blackstock had two passions: music and drawing. His story with music really began when he had his first accordion lesson at the age of ten. From that moment on, he was always fascinated by accordions—he began regular lessons in 1961 after his return to Seattle, and he received his first instrument of his own in 1963. He also displayed an early fascination with art and had the habit of drawing everything that was around him, mainly with graphite, permanent marker, and colored pencil on paper. He did not gain widespread attention,

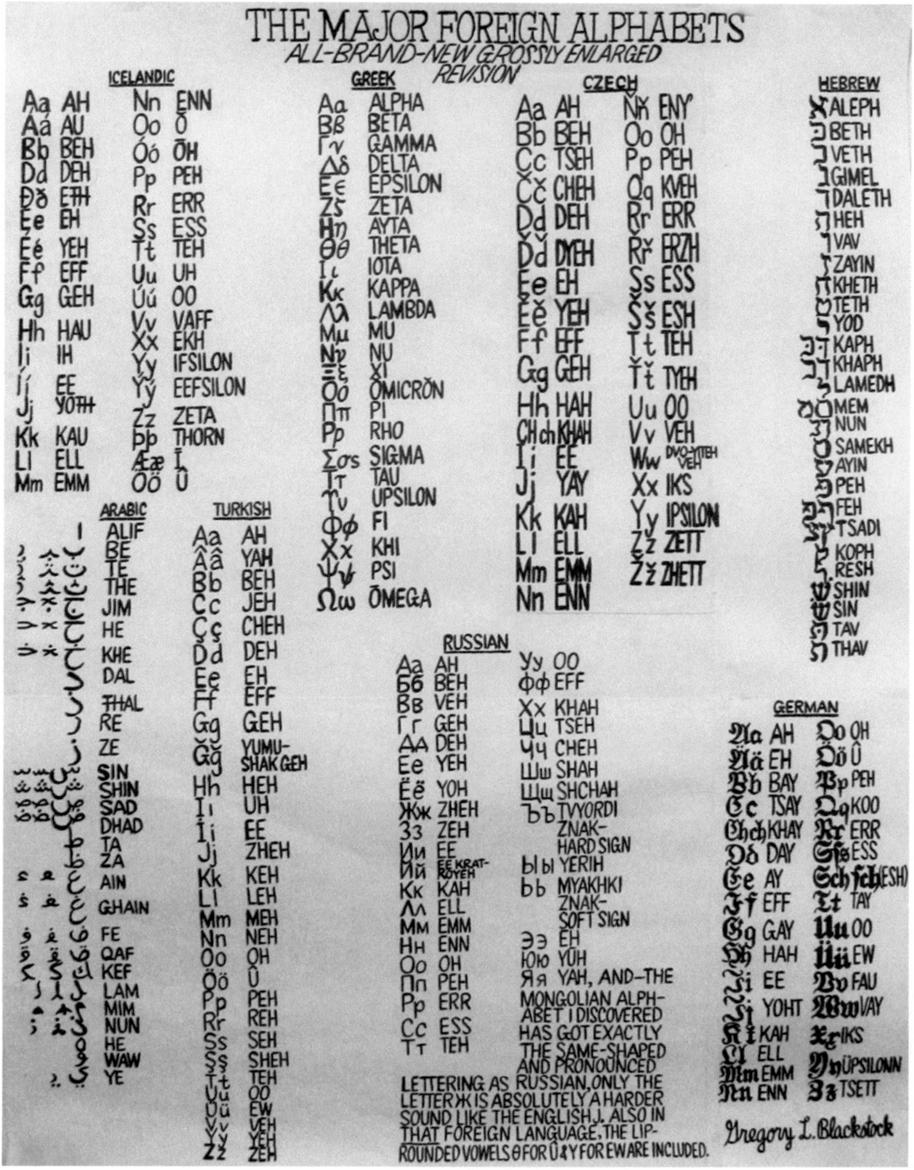

Figure 5.1 Gregory Blackstock: The Major Foreign Alphabets.

Photo courtesy of Gregory Blackstock and Dorothy Frisch.

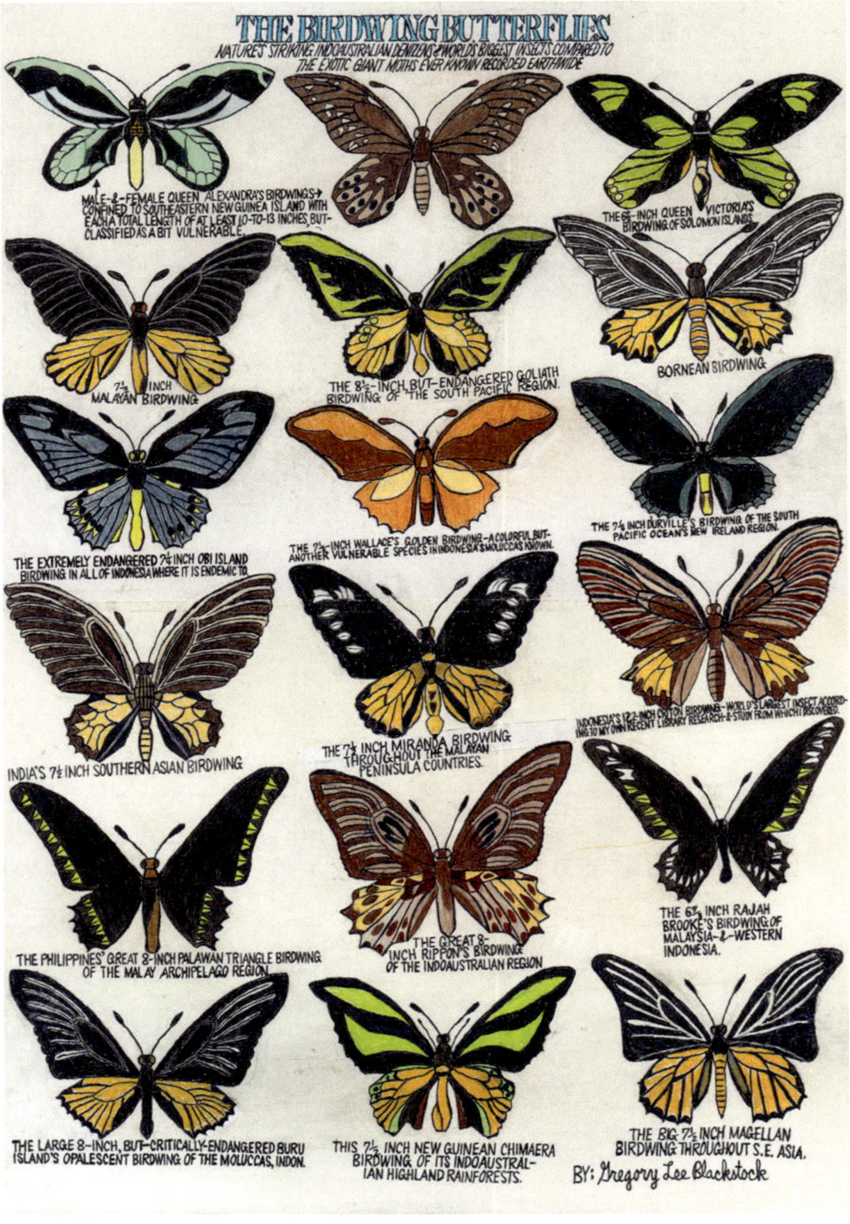

Figure 5.2 Gregory Blackstock: The Birdwing Butterflies.

Photo courtesy of Gregory Blackstock and Dorothy Frisch.

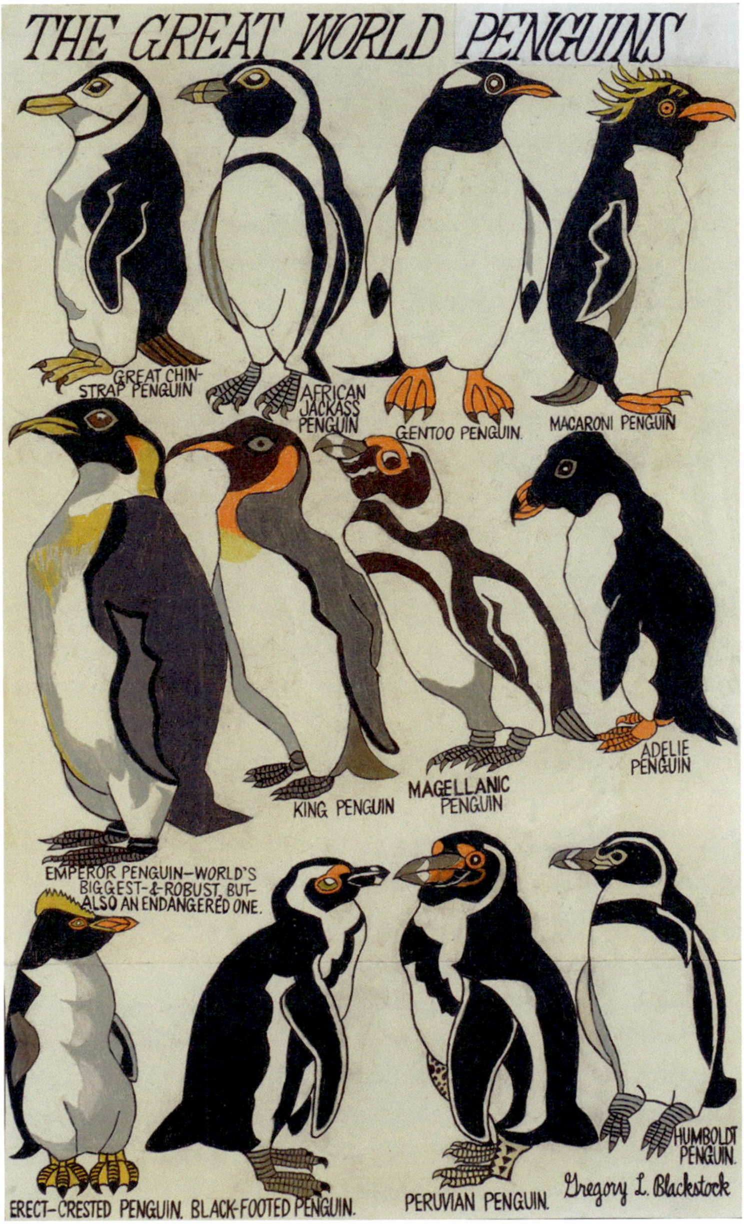

Figure 5.3 Gregory Blackstock: The Great World Penguins.

Photo courtesy of Gregory Blackstock and Dorothy Frisch.

however, until late 2003, when his work came to the attention of a gallery in Seattle, Washington, and was shown in a solo exhibit at the same gallery in February 2004. Blackstock also has a command of many languages. In fact, he can be considered a polyglot, able to speak and understand approximately around twelve languages (some only to a rudimentary extent) which he learned from listening to his coworkers from foreign countries, including Japanese, Mandarin Chinese, German, Tagalog, and Czech. He can read and write in the Cyrillic alphabet as well.

Blackstock is known for his large mixed-media drawings, which depict his unique taxonomies of the natural and man-made world, from animals and dictionary definitions to clothing, accordions, hydroplanes, Labrador retrievers, flags, cars and buildings. Most of the images he draws are taken from books, photos, or his own memory.

For Blackstock, who has socialization and communication problems, art is a powerful tool that enables him to bring people into his own world, where he feels comfortable communicating in his own way. "For him, the world is made up of things which need to be identified, ordered, and arranged – be they bugs, birds, vehicles or landmarks" (gregkucera.com).

Impairments: Autism. Socialization and communication problems. Blackstock spent five years in institutional schools.

Skills: Artist, draftsman, polyglot. Blackstock is known for his large mixed-media drawings, which depict his unique taxonomies of the natural and man-made world. Today, he is a renowned artist known for his taxonomist's acumen, artistic sensibility, and meticulous, obsessive drawings. Blackstock also handles approximately 12 languages which he has learned by himself, including Japanese, Mandarin Chinese, German, Tagalog, and Czech, and he can read and write in the Cyrillic alphabet as well.

Below are references, links to some videos, and additional reading about Gregory Blackstock.

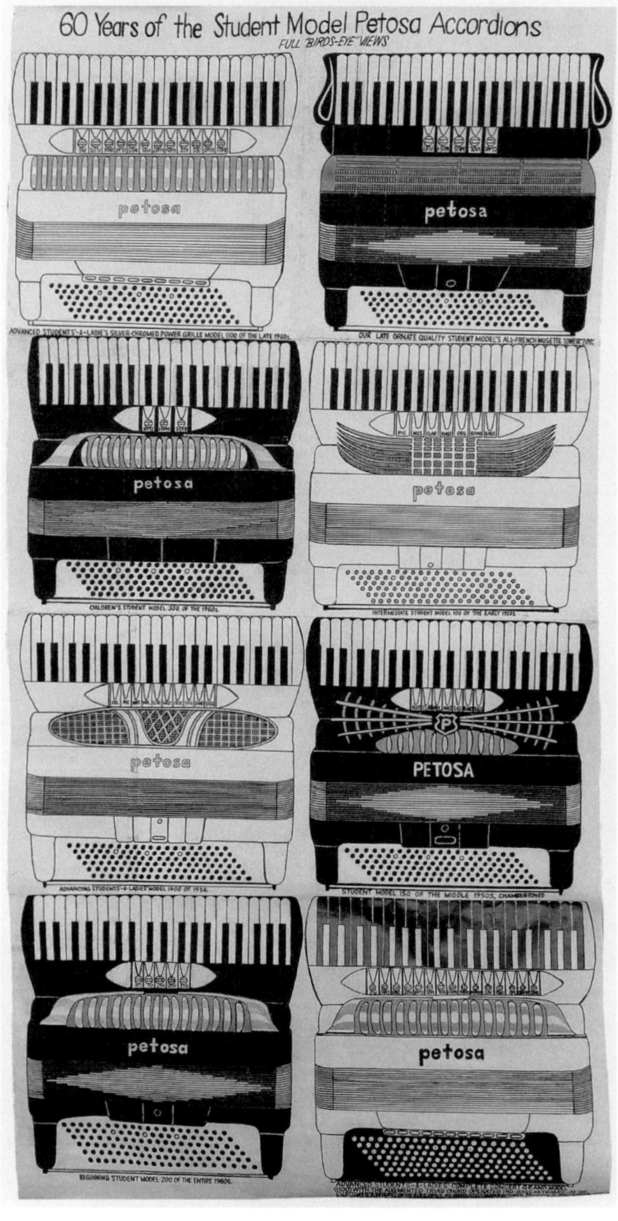

Figure 5.4 Gregory Blackstock: 60 Years of the Student Model Petosa. Accordions. Photo courtesy of Gregory Blackstock and Dorothy Frisch.

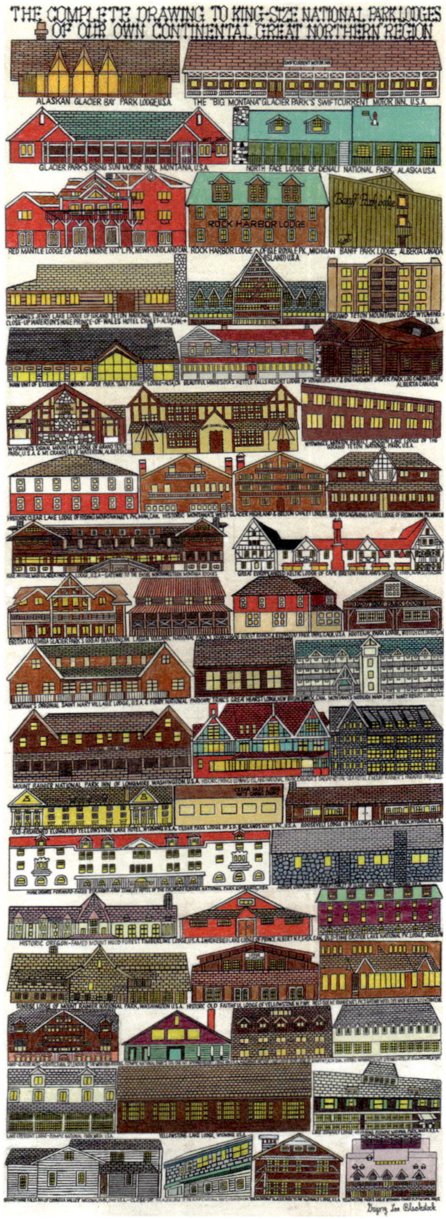

Figure 5.5 Gregory Blackstock: National Park Lodges.

Photo courtesy of Gregory Blackstock and Dorothy Frisch.

- Gregory Blackstock: *The Incomplete Historical World, Part I. Greg Kucera Gallery.* https://www.gregkucera.com/blackstock.htm
- Roth, I. (2020). Autism, Creativity and Aesthetics. *Qualitative Research in Psychology, 17*(4), 498-508.
- Mullin, J. (2014). *Drawing autism.* Akashic Books.
- Ayers, R. (2012). "Gregory Blackstock's intricate world is a charming one, too | Art review", The Seattle Times, December 14, 2012. https://www.seattletimes.com/entertainment/gregory-blackstockrsquos-intricate-world-is-a-charming-one-too-art-review/
- McKenzie, R. (2012). A different way to think about creativity: The case of autism and outsider art. In *Creative Engagements with Children: International Perspectives and Contexts* (pp. 107-119). Brill.
- Cardinal, R. (2009). Outsider Art and the autistic creator. *Philosophical Transactions of the Royal Society B: Biological Sciences, 364*(1522), 1459-1466.
- Piedmont-Palladino, S. (2007). *Tools of the imagination: Drawing tools and technologies from the eighteenth century to the present.* Princeton Architectural Press.
- Beeferman, L. (2006). Artists on Artists: Leah Beeferman on Gregory Blackstock. *Bomb,* (97), 32-33. https://bombmagazine.org/articles/gregory-blackstock/
- Blackstock, G. (2006). *Blackstock's Collections: The Drawings of an Artistic Savant.* Princeton Architectural Press.
- 2011, Gregory Blackstock: L'Encyclopediste, documentary film by Philippe Lespinasse, Collection de l'Art Brut & Lokomotiv Films, Lausanne/Le Tourne.
- Frisch, D. (2017). Wynn Newhouse Awards: Gregory Blackstock. https://www.wnewhouseawards.com/gregoryblackstock.html
- Gregory Blackstock. https://www.youtube.com/watch?v=-IMxt0DjWeA
- Gregory Blackstock's Infinite Possibilities. https://www.facebook.com/EricJohnsonKOMO/videos/gregory-blackstocks-infinite-possibilities/331827767448342/

5.4 Mary Temple Grandin (born 1947)

I am deeply indebted to Dr. Temple Grandin for her extensive assistance in the final revisions of this profile.

Mary Temple Grandin was born in Boston, Massachusetts, United States, on August 29,1947, to an educated and well-to-do family. She is an extraordinary savant, prominent author, and speaker on both autism and animal behavior, and is arguably the most famous autistic person in the world. She is a professor of ethology at Colorado State University and is recognized as a pioneer in improving the handling and welfare of farm animals.

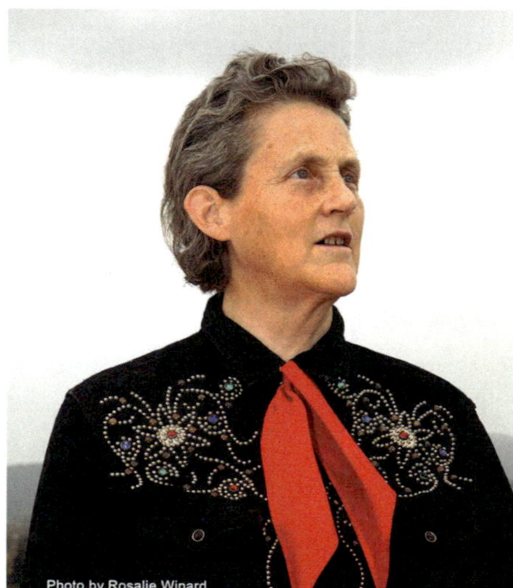

Figure 5.6 Temple Grandin.

Photo courtesy of Temple Grandin and Rosalie Winard.

Temple, as she was known to her family, did not speak a single word until she was three and a half years old. She showed great discomfort at being touched and sensitivity to loud noises and exhibited other behavior now known to be stereotypical of autism. This caused her to live in painful isolation for much of her early life, during which screaming was the only way she could communicate. When Grandin was two years old, doctors told her parents that she had brain damage (cerebellar abnormalities) and that the standard medical recommendation was institutionalization. Her father was willing to follow the advice, but her mother energetically refused (Plank, 2006), trying different types of therapy instead, which helped to create an environment that could accommodate Grandin's needs and sensitivities. As Grandin herself says, she was fortunate to receive early speech therapy. Grandin began talking and making progress at age four. Autism only began being treated as such in the 1980's, so Grandin lived through her childhood and youth without knowing and understanding exactly what was happening to her. Although her mother had sensed it, Grandin was not diagnosed with autism until she was in her forties. This diagnosis was corroborated through cerebral imaging conducted at the University of Utah in 2010, when she was 64 (Grandin and Panek, 2013).

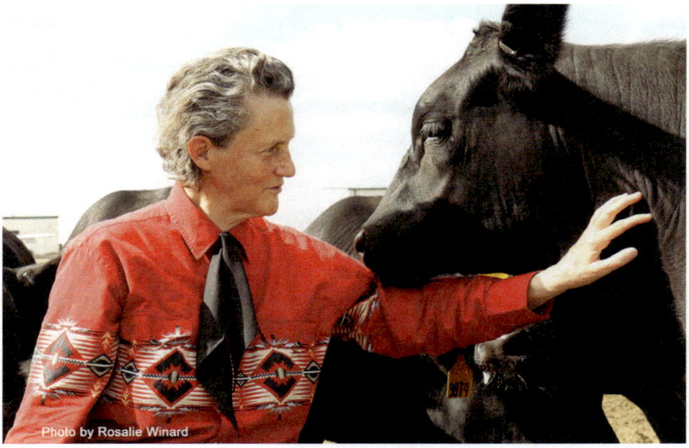

Figure 5.7 Temple Grandin with cow.

Photo courtesy of Temple Grandin and Rosalie Winard.

Grandin attended a normal school that did not recognize her special needs. Life was hard and she was teased incessantly. Grandin was expelled from middle school at the age of 14 for throwing a book at a schoolmate who ridiculed her. Shy and bookish, she was an easy target for bullying. Grandin (2012) says, "I could laugh about it now, but back then it really hurt." She was later enrolled in a school for children with behavior problems and there she met William Carlock, a science teacher who had worked for NASA. Carlock became her mentor, helping to significantly building her self-confidence, and encouraging her interest in science (Aspergers Test Site, 2013). She later earned her bachelor's degree in human psychology in 1970, a master's degree in animal science from Arizona State University in 1975, and a PhD in animal science from the University of Illinois at Urbana–Champaign in 1989.

While Grandin was attending high school, she invented the hug machine, or squeeze machine, a deep-pressure device designed to calm hypersensitive persons, usually individuals with autism spectrum disorders (Grandin, 2006). The idea to build this machine came up on a visit to her uncle's ranch in Arizona. She watched as animals were placed in a squeeze chute for inoculation and noticed that they calmed in that device. If it worked for animals, it could also be very helpful for hypersensitive individuals like herself. In fact, she had already noticed how a strong hug from a loved one helped her. The device was initially not approved by the school psychologists and was confiscated, but her science teacher helped her establish objective grounding for the device's ability to reduce anxiety by delivering comforting pressure to large areas of the body. For example, Lorna Wing has mentioned that some children with sleeping problems may do better in a mummy sleeping bag that fits their body perfectly (Grandin, 1992). Grandin wrote that "[a] high functioning autistic woman stated, 'I need heavy blankets on me to sleep well, or else my muscles won't calm down'" (Grandin, 1992). Different institutions in the United States use today the "hug machine" to reduce tension, nervousness, panic attacks and anxiety.

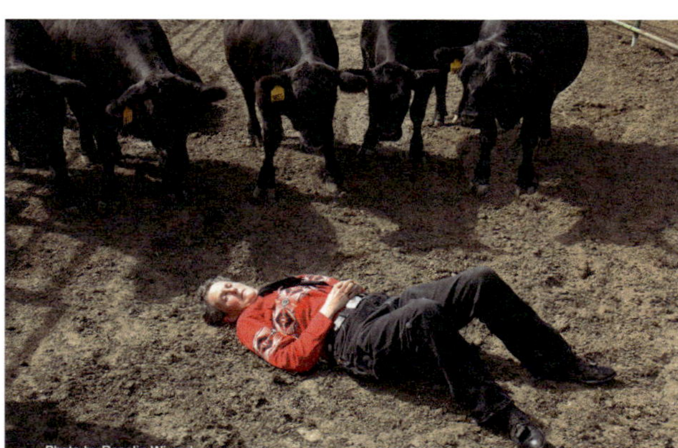

Figure 5.8 Temple Grandin on ground.

Photo courtesy: Temple Grandin and Rosalie Winard.

Grandin was the first person with autistic spectrum disorder who was able to self-examine and document the sensory and cognitive experience of being autistic. As she tells us, Grandin literally sees the world in in photo-realistic pictures—all of her thinking is visual, and she can then tell what she sees. This has been a formidable help for people within the autistic spectrum and their families, raising the hope that we may finally learn the causes of autism and treatments for it. Her comments and opinions should also be strongly taken into account by both educators and physicians of autistic children. No one better than she can describe all the frustrations of an autistic person who is not understood. Her comments, taken from her own experience, are a great learning opportunity that should not be wasted.

During a visit to Darold Treffert's autism center, Grandin said: "Some people diagnosed on the autism spectrum think in a way that would make them ideal for skilled trade and professional positions that may require complex visual thinking, precise mathematical thinking or patterned word thinking" (Minda, 2019).

Dr. Grandin (1992b) also wrote in one of her essays "teachers need to use fixations to motivate instead of trying to stamp them out" (p.115). In a subsequent interview with Medscape she was asked about this and she clarifies the subject perfectly:

> Let's say that a child loves trains—that's a very common fixation. Well, read a book about trains, do math problems with trains, read about the history of the railroad. In other words, if a kid loves trains, you can somehow drag a train into just about every subject in school to get him motivated to study it. Fixations are tremendous motivators (White, 2005).

In 2012, Grandin's brain was scanned using different imaging technologies: high-resolution magnetic resonance imaging (MRI), diffusion tensor imaging (DTI), and functional MRI. This gave scientists a window into her remarkable brain so that they could gain a better understanding of how savants' minds work. Jason Cooperrider (2011) of the University of Utah, who presented the work at the 2012 Society for Neuroscience annual meeting in New Orleans, reported that Grandin has greater volume in the right hemisphere, increased thickness of the entorhinal cortex, overall larger brain size, an enlarged amygdala, and a smaller cortical thickness in the fusiform gyrus. Grandin has also four times the typical number of connections in a brain area that controls the visual system. The images reveal an atypical neural scenery that reflects Grandin's deficits (as autistic) and talents (exceptional visual and spatial abilities). This also explains why she goes through life thinking in pictures.

Dr. Grandin has gained recognition as an outstanding researcher of animal behavior who has published more than ten books and 100 peer-reviewed scientific papers. She is also a prominent author and speaker on both autism and animal behavior. She was the subject of the 2010 HBO film *Temple Grandin*, winner of seven Emmy awards. The film, directed by Mick Jackson and starring Claire Danes as Temple Grandin, tells the story of an autistic woman whose innovations revolutionize practices for the humane handling of livestock, mainly on cattle ranches. In the same year, Grandin was included on the annual *Time 100* list of the most influential people in the world, in the "Heroes" category. In 2011, she was featured in an episode of the Science Channel documentary series *Ingenious Minds*. Temple has been featured on different TV and radio programs, among them the BBC Special "The Woman who thinks like a Cow," *Larry King Live, 20/20, 60 Minutes, Fox and Friends,* and *Fresh Air* with Terry Gross. She has also appeared in publications such as *Time, The New York Times, Discover, People, Forbes* and *USA Today*.

She has also received honorary doctorates from many universities, including McGill University (1999), the University of Illinois (2004), the Swedish University of Agricultural Sciences (2009), Duke University (2010), Lakehead University (2010), Carnegie Mellon University (2012), Western College of Veterinary Medicine (2012), Franklin Pierce University

(2012), Arizona State University (2012), Washington University in St. Louis MO (2014), Texas A&M University (2014), Dalhousic University (2015), the University of Buenos Aires (2015), Emory University (2016), North Carolina State University (2018), and University of Pennsylvania (2019). Dr. Grandin was inducted to the Colorado Women's Hall of Fame in 2012, into the American Academy of Arts and Sciences in 2016, and into the National Women's Hall of Fame in 2017.

Impairments: Autism. Grandin did not speak a word until she was three and a half years old and showed great intolerance to being touched and loud noise. She exhibited behavior typical of autism and lived in painful isolation for much of her early life.

Skills: Perfect pitch. Expert in animal behavior. Visualization (all her thinking is visual). Seeing things from another perspective has allowed her to tackle and solve highly difficult problems.

Below are references, links to some videos, and additional reading about Dr. Temple Grandin.

- Temple Grandin's Official Autism Website: https://www.templegrandin.com/
- Temple Grandin inside ASD: https://www.autism.org/temple-grandin-inside-asd/
- Temple Grandin: Professional resume. https://www.grandin.com/professional.resume.html
- Publications about Grandin: https://en.wikipedia.org/wiki/Temple_Grandin#Publications
- Lion, V. (2020). Disrupting Temple Grandin. *Disability and Animality: Crip Perspectives in Critical Animal Studies.*
- Grandin, T. (Ed.). (2019). *Livestock handling and transport*. Cabi.
- Minda, J. (2019). Treffert autism center hosts author Temple Grandin. December 15, 2019. https://www.chausa.org/publications/catholic-health-

world/archives/issues/december-15-2019/treffert-autism-center-hosts-author-temple-grandin

- Wood, A. (2016). *Temple Grandin: Voice for the Voiceless*. Skyhorse.
- Grandin, T. (Ed.). (2015). *Improving animal welfare: a practical approach*. Cabi.
- Grandin, T. and Panek, R. (2013). *The autistic brain: Thinking across the spectrum*. Houghton Mifflin Harcourt.
- Wolfe, C. (2013). Learning from Temple Grandin, or, animal studies, disability studies, and who comes after the subject. *Re-Imagining Nature: Environmental Humanities and Ecosemiotics*, 91-107.
- Aspergers Test Site (2013). How the squeeze machine came to be. June 6, 2013. https://www.aspergerstestsite.com/1095/squeeze-machine-by-temple-grandi/
- Sacks, O. (2012). *An anthropologist on Mars: Seven paradoxical tales*. Vintage.
- Montgomery, S. and Grandin, T. (2012). *Temple Grandin: How the girl who loved cows embraced autism and changed the world*. Houghton Mifflin Harcourt.
- Grandin, T. (2012). Temple Grandin Inducted into Colorado Women's Hall of Fame. March 8, 2012. https://web.archive.org/web/20131228000859if_/http://www.wherefoodcomesfrom.com/article/2281/Temple-Grandin-Inducted-into-Colorado-Womens-Hall-of-Fame#.Ur4Wmyj7TIU
- Grandin, T. (2011). *The way I see it: A personal look at autism & Asperger's*. Future Horizons.
- Cooperrider, J. (2011). Dr. Temple Grandin: a neuroimaging case study. In *Poster Presented at the International Meeting for Autism Research (IMFAR), San Diego, CA, USA*.
- Grandin, T. (2009). How does visual thinking work in the mind of a person with autism? A personal account. *Philosophical Transactions of the Royal Society B: Biological Sciences, 364*(1522), 1437-1442.
- Grandin, T. and Johnson, C. (2009). *Animals in translation: Using the mysteries of autism to decode animal behavior*. SUNY Press.
- Grandin, T. (2008). *Thinking in pictures, expanded edition: My life with autism*. Vintage.

- Plank, A. (2006). Interview with Temple Grandin. WrongPlanet.net. January 2, 2006. https://wrongplanet.net/interview-with-temple-grandin/
- White, R. (2005). Autism First-Hand: An Expert Interview with Temple Grandin. *Medscape Psychiatry.* https://www.medscape.org/viewarticle/498153
- The 2010 Time 100: Temple Grandin. http://content.time.com/time/specials/packages/article/0,28804,1984685_1984949_1985222,00.html
- Grandin, T. (2008). *Thinking in pictures, expanded edition: My life with autism*. Vintage.
- Edelson, S., Edelson, M., Kerr, D. and Grandin, T. (1999). Behavioral and physiological effects of deep pressure on children with autism: A pilot study evaluating the efficacy of Grandin's Hug Machine. *American Journal of Occupational Therapy*, 53(2), 145-152.
- Grandin, T. (1992). Calming effects of deep touch pressure in patients with autistic disorder, college students, and animals. *Journal of child and adolescent psychopharmacology*, 2(1), 63-72.
- Ratey, J., Grandin, T. and Miller, A. (1992). Defense behavior and coping in an autistic savant: the story of Temple Grandin, PhD. *Psychiatry*, 55(4), 382-391.
- Grandin, T. (1992b). An inside view of autism. In *High-functioning individuals with autism* (pp. 105-126). Springer, Boston, MA.
- The world needs all kinds of minds | Temple Grandin. https://www.youtube.com/watch?v=fn_9f5x0f1Q
- Temple Grandin (Trailer). https://www.youtube.com/watch?v=cpkN0JdXRpM
- Dr. Temple Grandin: "The Autistic Brain: Thinking Across the Spectrum" | Talks at Google. https://www.youtube.com/watch?v=IA4tE3_2qmI
- Temple Grandin on Mark Zuckerberg and Overcoming Autism. https://www.youtube.com/watch?v=nwnlWX4iyj4
- What it feels like to be autistic. https://www.youtube.com/watch?v=1qPFAT4p8Lc
- Dr. Temple Grandin on Autism. https://www.youtube.com/watch?v=51zNRn62um0

5.5 Tommy McHugh (1949-2012)

I greatly appreciate the contributions of Dr. Alice Flaherty of Harvard Medical School in writing and reviewing this profile.

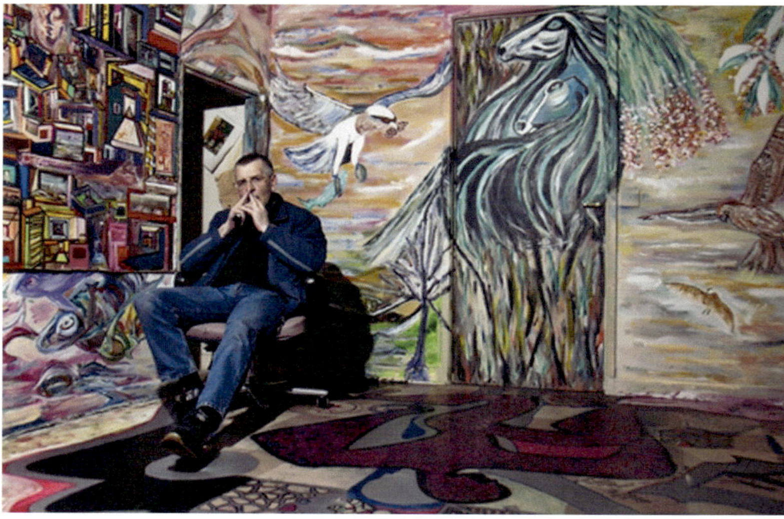

Figure 5.9 Tommy McHugh.

Photo courtesy of Frances Passman and Gianni Bianchini.

Tommy McHugh was born in England in 1949 and passed away from liver cancer in the same country on September 19, 2012. He was an acquired savant, artist, poet and sculptor. Tommy grew up in Birkenhead, a suburb of the post-industrial city of Liverpool, with eight brothers and three sisters. He left school at 14, and although he found work as a builder, he also became a juvenile delinquent, best known for street fights that landed him in correctional institutions where he spent much of his life between the ages of 15 and 21.

When Tommy was 51, a blood vessel burst in his brain. This caused a massive (or bilateral) stroke that put him in a coma for a week, and permanently changed his perception and personality. Tommy described the moment when he had the stroke:

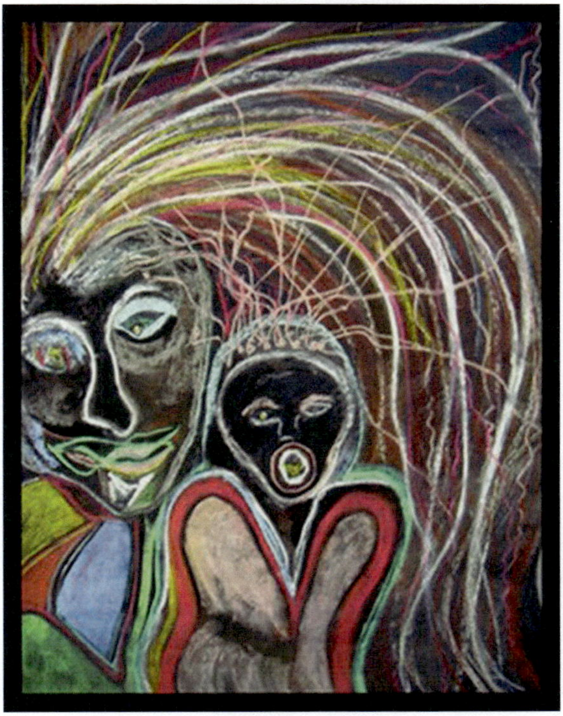

Figure 5.10 Tommy McHugh: Untitled.

Photo courtesy of Frances Passman and Gianni Bianchini.

> I was sitting on the toilet. I suddenly felt an explosion in the left side of my head and ended up on the floor. I think the only thing that kept me conscious was that I didn't want to be found with my pants down. Then the other side of my head went bang! I woke up in hospital and looked out of the window to see the tree was sprouting numbers. 3, 6, 9. Then I started talking in rhyme... (Thomson, 2013).

Until that moment, Tommy had had no experience with art, except with the tattoos that covered his arms. While relearning after the stroke, he suddenly experienced an overwhelming need to express himself. He found he had a strong desire to speak in rhyme and began to write down

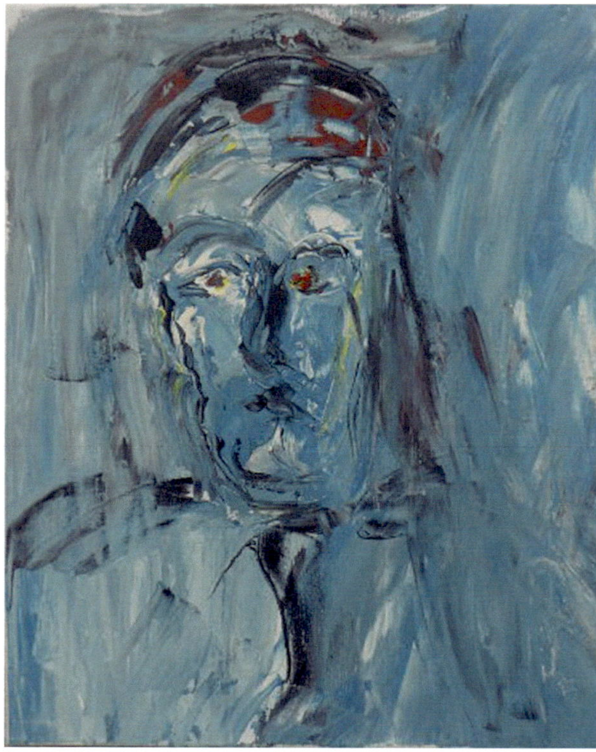

Figure 5.11 Tommy McHugh: Tasting understanding a stroke.

Photo courtesy of Frances Passman and Gianni Bianchini.

his thoughts as poems. He also began to paint, sculpt, carve, and create passionately in his home for up to 19 hours a day. Since he had little money for art materials, he turned everything nearby into art. He painted directly on all surfaces of his house, made sculptures out of everything carvable, and even dripped wax sculptures onto the lid of his toilet. His habitual aggression changed to gentleness, and he felt sad even for accidentally killing an insect. At first, his new creativity baffled and frightened him. Gradually he came to terms with his new life. "I like what I'm being, what I am. I'm happy being the Tommy I am now, not the Tommy people remember. Whatever happened inside my brain I find it absolutely fantastic," he said (BBC News, 2004).

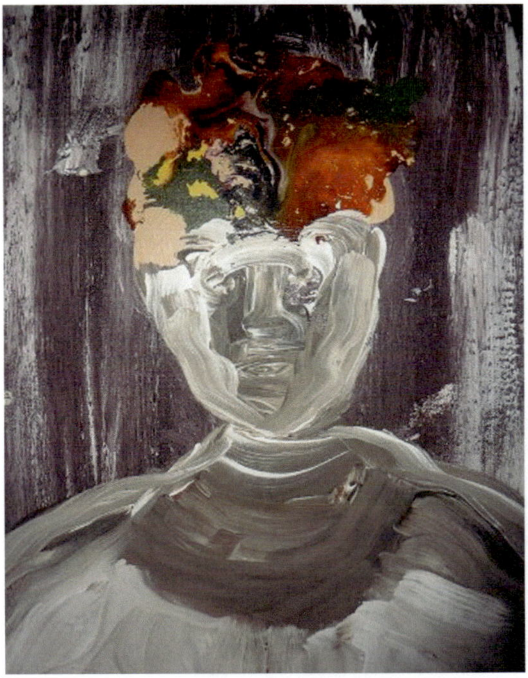

Figure 5.12 Tommy McHugh: 07S – Coming mind out.

Photo courtesy of Frances Passman and Gianni Bianchini.

The only possible explanation for Tommy's abrupt transformation is that the damage to some regions of his brain led to disinhibited activity in other brain areas. Dr Alice Flaherty, a Harvard neurologist who studied Tommy, described his stroke as "a crack that let the light in." Tommy is one of the known cases in the world of an individual becoming a savant following a cerebral hemorrhage.

> It is difficult to understand how terrifying it was for Tommy to find himself suddenly obsessed with making art, with philosophical ideas, with speculations about how the brain works and how we perceive our worlds. To find our body changed after an illness is shattering enough. What if your thoughts and even your temperament change too? How do you deal with that when 'you' no longer exist? (Alice Flaherty, June 2008, Tommy McHugh's official website).

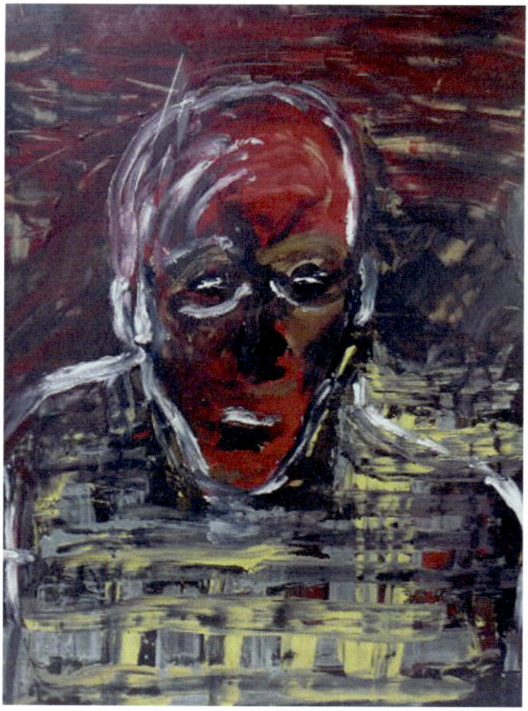

Figure 5.13 Tommy McHugh: 07S – Bewildered bewitched bothered.

Photo courtesy of Frances Passman and Gianni Bianchini.

Tommy's art has been exhibited at various Liverpool libraries and galleries. He also participated in several documentaries about the brain. Tommy donated his paintings and sculptures to English and American charity fundraisers and helped set up a free gallery allowing amateur artists suffering from some type of illness to display their work.

Impairments: A stroke on both sides of his brain that was caused by a ruptured artery, which nearly killed him.

Skills: Painter, poet, and sculptor. Following a cerebral hemorrhage, he suddenly began to write poetry and developed a strong urge to paint. He became a prolific artist.

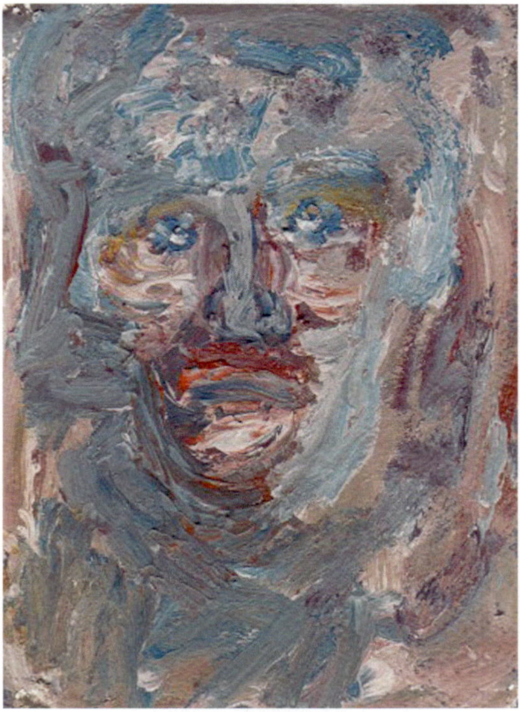

Figure 5.14 Tommy McHugh: 04S – 1 Assembly.

Photo courtesy of Frances Passman and Gianni Bianchini.

Below are references, links to some videos, and additional reading about Tommy McHugh.

- Tommy's website: http://www.tommymchugh.co.uk/
- Piechowski-Jozwiak, B. and Bogousslavsky, J. (2020). Painting in Neurology. In *Brain and Art* (pp. 41-52). Springer, Cham.
- Treffert, D. (2014c). Accidental genius. *Scientific American, 311*(2), 52-57.
- Horstkötter, D. and Snoek, A. (2013). The importance of the self for autonomous behavior. *AJOB Neuroscience*, *4*(4), 62-63.
- Thomson, H. (2013). Mindscapes: Stroke turned ex-con into rhyming painter. New Scientist. Health. May 10, 2013. https://www.newscientist.com/article/dn23523-mindscapes-stroke-turned-ex-con-into-rhyming-painter/

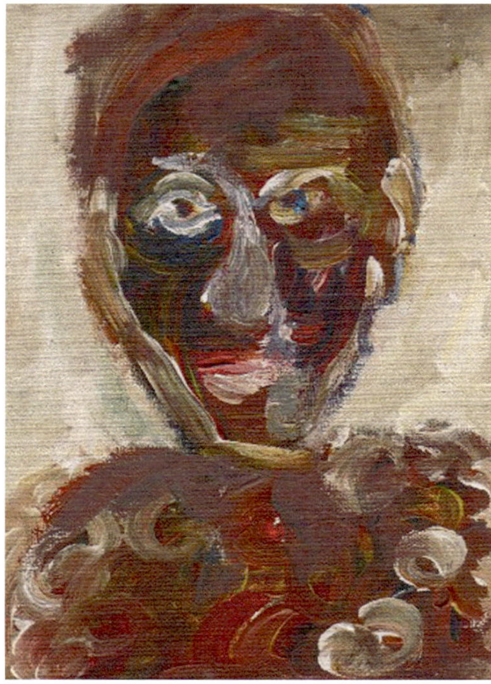

Figure 5.15 Tommy McHugh: 04S – 2 Confusion.

Photo courtesy of Frances Passman and Gianni Bianchini.

- Daily Mail Reporter (2010). Ex-street fighter, 60, turned into a fanatical artist by a brain haemorrhage that physically altered his mind. March 15, 2010. https://www.dailymail.co.uk/news/article-1256967/Man-survived-brain-haemorrhage-transformed-fanatical-artist-paints-18-hours-day.html
- Bäzner, H. and Hennerici, M. (2006). Stroke in painters. *International review of neurobiology*, *74*, 165-191.
- Edelstyn, N. (2006). Creativity and the brain. *The Psychologist*, *19*(10), 616.
- Lythgoe, M., Pollak, T., Kalmus, M., De Haan, M. and Chong, W. (2005). Obsessive, prolific artistic output following subarachnoid hemorrhage. *Neurology*, 64(2), 397-398.
- BBC News (2004). Creative side unlocked by stroke. BBC News June 21, 2004. http://news.bbc.co.uk/2/hi/health/3826857.stm

- Giles, J. (2004). Change of mind.
- The Empty Chair. Filmed in August 2012 at Tommy's home in Birkenhead. http://www.tommymchugh.co.uk/the_empty_chair.html
- Bo Balderson: Savant – Tommy McHugh. https://www.youtube.com/watch?v=6Tmzh0swD1Q
- Tommy McHugh – Art Exhibition. https://www.youtube.com/watch?v=35GJqkO866g
- My Brilliant Brain. Episode 3 – Accidental Genius: Tommy McHugh http://www.windfallfilms.com/show/1034/episode-3-accidental-genius.aspx
- Tommy McHugh – Art Exhibition. https://www.youtube.com/watch?v=35GJqkO866g&t=59s
- The Incredible Story of Tommy McHugh on Vimeo. https://vimeo.com/85016040

5.6 Laurence Kim Peek (1951-2009)

Laurence Kim Peek was born in Salt Lake City, Utah on November 11, 1951, and died on December 19, 2009 in Murray, Utah, at the age of 58. Peek was an extraordinary American mega-savant and one of the world's most famous savants, best known for serving as the inspiration for the autistic savant character Raymond Babbitt in the 1988 film *Rain Man*. Peek was famous for his prodigious memory, possessing near-total recall in 14 or 15 different subject areas, according to his father (Burke, 2003). These topics ranged from history, literature, and geography to numbers, sports, music, and dates. His overall IQ score was 87, although this result should not be considered an objective indicator of his intellectual abilities (Treffert and Christensen, 2005). The IQ score was designed as a general measure of human intelligence, but is not suited to evaluate this class of geniuses (savants). Indeed, it generally fails in evaluating the capacities of this type of individuals.

Peek, who was known by his middle name, Kim, was born with severe brain damage, as well as various impairments: macrocephaly, damage to the cerebellum, agenesis of the corpus callosum (partial or complete absence of the transverse fibers that connect the left and right hemispheres), and FG syndrome (Opitz et al., 2008), a rare genetic syndrome caused by one or more recessive genes located on the X chromosome. FG syndrome produces intellectual disability, hyperactivity, hypotonia, and macrocephaly.

Kim had difficulty walking (he did not take his first steps until he was four) and generally poor motor skills. He could not dress or take a bath, brush his teeth, or button up his shirt unassisted, and he could not decide for himself what to eat. Kim was also initially diagnosed with autism, but his diagnosis was later changed to Pervasive Developmental Disorder – Not Otherwise Specified (PDD-NOS). His doctors suggested that he be institutionalized, since his parents would not be able to care for him with all his problems. His father refused, and Kim remained with his family.

Despite all these limitations, Kim was capable of feats that were virtually impossible for other human beings. At 16-20 months of age, Kim was able to memorize every book that was read to him. "Kimputer" (Treffert and Christensen, 2005), as he was lovingly known to many, was able to read with dizzying speed by absorbing two pages simultaneously, one with each eye, in about eight seconds. He could read a book in about an hour and remember almost everything he had read. In his lifetime, he was able to memorize more than 12,000 books (including the Bible) and could accurately recite the contents of each (Treffert, 2010). Since he also had perfect recall of all the maps of the United States, Kim was considered a human GPS. Kim knew the highways that go to each American city, town or county in the United States, along with their area codes and zip codes (Treffert and Wallace, 2002) and could identify hundreds of classical compositions, including the name of each piece's composer and their biographical details. As Dr. Darold Treffert (2010) said, "he became a living Google." There is speculation that due to their agenesis of the corpus callosum problem, neurons connected in an unusual way, generating an overwhelmingly enhanced memory (Treffert & Christensen, 2005).

After *Rain Man* (which won four Oscars, including Best Picture, Best Actor, Best Screenplay and Best Director), Kim toured United States and Canada with his father, during which time he became more sociable and calmer, and began to find it easier speak before a crowd. He was awarded his high school equivalency certificate, which "he had been denied for many years" (Allen, 2009). Kim appeared on numerous television shows, among them *20/20* and *Good Morning America*. When he was at home in Utah, Kim spent many afternoons at the city's public library, reading and memorizing books, one of his passions. Referring to Kim in an interview, Treffert remarked that Kim "was the Mount Everest of memory." Kim Peek's parents divorced in 1981 (Weber, 2009), and his father provided the supervision his son required until Kim's death of a heart attack on December 19, 2009.

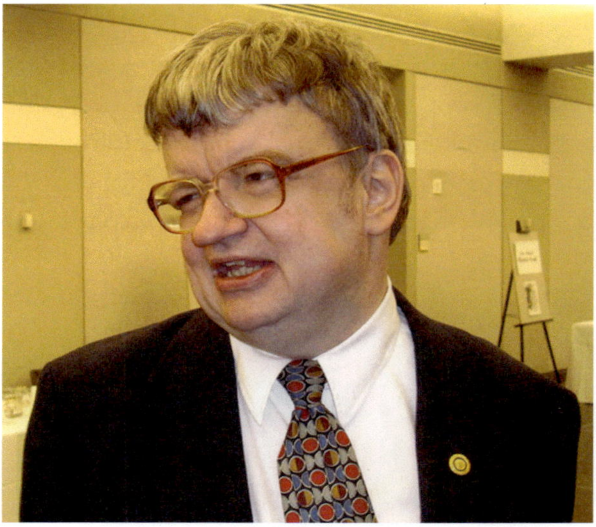

Figure 5.16 Kim Peek. Jan 16, 2007. Author: Dmadeo. Source: Own work.

https://en.wikipedia.org/wiki/Kim_Peek#/media/File:Kim_Peek_on_Jan_16,_2007.png
Creative Commons Attribution-Share Alike 3.0 Unported license. (CC BY-SA 3.0)

Impairments: PDD-NOS, macrocephaly, damage to the cerebellum, agenesis of the corpus callosum, and FG syndrome. His overall IQ score was 87. Peek had difficulty walking and generally poor motor skills.

Skills: Mnemonist. One of the world's best-known mega-savants. Kim's memory extended to at least 15 subjects. He was able to read extremely fast, two pages simultaneously, one with each eye, in about eight seconds. During his life, he memorized approximately 12,000 books and could accurately recite the content of each one. Because he perfectly recalled all the maps of the United States, Kim was considered a human GPS. He could also identify hundreds of classical compositions, including the name of each piece's composer and their biographical details.

Below are references, links to some videos, and additional reading about Laurence Kim Peek.

- Charuchandra, S. (2020). Savant in the Limelight, 1988-2009. The Scientist. May 1, 2020. https://www.the-scientist.com/foundations/savant-in-the-limelight-19882009-67446
- Feldman, D. and Morelock, M. (2011). Prodigies and savants. *The Cambridge handbook of intelligence*, 210-234.
- Treffert, D. (2010). *Islands of genius: The bountiful mind of the autistic, acquired, and sudden savant.* Jessica Kingsley Publishers.
- Treffert, D. (2010b). Kim Peek 1951-2009. *Wisconsin Medical Journal*, 109(2), 61.
- Hughes, J. (2010). A review of Savant Syndrome and its possible relationship to epilepsy. *Epilepsy & behavior*, *17*(2), 147-152.
- Allen, N. (2009). Kim Peek: The 'RealRainMan' dies. The Telegraph. December 22, 2009. https://www.telegraph.co.uk/news/obituaries/medicine-obituaries/6867567/Kim-Peek.html
- Weber, B. (2009). *Kim Peek, Inspiration for 'Rain Man,' Dies at 58*. December 26, 2009. The New York Times. https://www.nytimes.com/2009/12/27/us/27peek.html
- Pilkington, E. (2009). The real Rain Man dies of heart attack in home town of Salt Lake City, aged 58. The Guardian. December 22, 2009. https://www.theguardian.com/world/2009/dec/22/kim-peek-rain-man-dies
- Stephenson, K. (2009). Kim Peek, Murray man who inspired 'Rain Man', dies. The Salt Lake Tribune. December 21, 2009. https://archive.sltrib.com/story.php?ref=/ci_14043625

- Peek, F. and Hanson, L. (2008). *The life and message of the real Rain Man: The journey of a mega-savant*. Port Chester, N.Y: Dude Pub.
- Opitz, J., Smith, J. and Santoro, L. (2008). The FG syndromes (online mendelian inheritance in man 305450): Perspective in 2008. *Advances in pediatrics*, 55(1), 123-170.
- Normann, C. and Berger, M. (2008). Neuroenhancement: status quo and perspectives. *European archives of psychiatry and clinical neuroscience*, 258(5), 110-114.
- Tammet, D. (2007). *Born on a blue day: Inside the extraordinary mind of an autistic savant*. Simon and Schuster.
- Baron-Cohen, S., Bor, D., Billington, J., Asher, J., Wheelwright, S. and Ashwin, C. (2007). Savant memory in a man with colour form-number synaesthesia and asperger. *Journal of consciousness studies*, 14(9-10), 237-251.
- Treffert, D. and Christensen, D. (2005). Inside the mind of a savant. *Scientific American*, 293(6), 108-113.
- Burke, B. (2003). 'Rain Man' reigns in Casper. Casper Star Tribune. March 13, 2003. https://trib.com/news/local/rain-man-reigns-in-casper/article_0c374fd8-9737-51b8-87e8-f896ad30d317.html
- Treffert, D. and Wallace, G. (2002). Islands of genius. *Scientific American Mind*, 14(1), 14-23.
- Peek, F. (1996). *The real rain man, Kim Peek*. Salt Lake City, Utah: Harkness Pub. Consultants.
- Peek, F. (1996). *The real rain man, Kim Peek*. Harkness Pub. Consultants.
- Kim Peek: savant who was the inspiration for the film Rain Man. December 23, 2009. https://www.thetimes.co.uk/article/kim-peek-savant-who-was-the-inspiration-for-the-film-rain-man-29n3jpp5hpw
- NASA studies mega-savant Peek's brain. USA Today. https://usatoday30.usatoday.com/news/science/2004-11-08-nasa-rain-man_x.htm
- Kim Peek – The Real Rain Man [1/5]. https://www.youtube.com/watch?v=k2T45r5G3kA
- Kim Peek – The Real Rain Man [Full Film]. https://www.youtube.com/watch?v=DLpCfHH1OVU
- Kim Peek – el autentico "Rain Man." https://www.youtube.com/watch?v=-zt0sWrLIUg

- 2019 Peek Award – Kim Peek Tribute Video. https://www.youtube.com/watch?v=-w-bfdLHjSU
- Kim Peek videos: https://www.wisconsinmedicalsociety.org/professional/savant-syndrome/profiles-and-videos/videos/kim-peek-videos/

5.7 Richard Wawro (1952-2006)

Richard Wawro was born on April 14, 1952 in Newport-on-Tay in Fife, Scotland, and passed away in the same country on February 22, 2006. He was an autistic savant who was a gifted artist. At the age of three, with an IQ of 30, Richard was diagnosed as moderate to severely mentally retarded (a condition later recognized as autism). Wawro never went to regular school, did not learn how to write, and did not learn to speak until he was 11. Cataract surgery on both eyes during his childhood left him legally blind. Wawro's behavior was similar to that of almost any autistic child: walking in circles, spinning objects incessantly, and striking the same note on the piano for hours at a time.

Despite all these difficulties, Wawro began to show his impressive artistic gifts at the age of six. His family protected, loved, and supported him, and he went on to enjoy an outstanding career as a painter. Wawro's experience with painting began one day with his special instructor, Molly Leishman. Wawro was absorbed in playing with some crayons and his teacher went to see what he was doing. As she tells it:

> I went to see how his drawing was progressing and to give the usual praise and encouragement. What I saw was magic. It was impressionism and I couldn't believe my eyes. I was afraid to believe them and said nothing to anyone. It would not do to raise false hopes, but I had difficulty in suppressing my excitement. To look at his next drawing was agony, wondering if the first had been a fluke, but no! There was another picture. When I had several examples of Richard's work, I took them for professional advice, without mentioning handicaps. To my great joy my hopes were confirmed – here was a talent beyond that of a normal child of his age (Molly Leishman: Richard Wawro's official website).

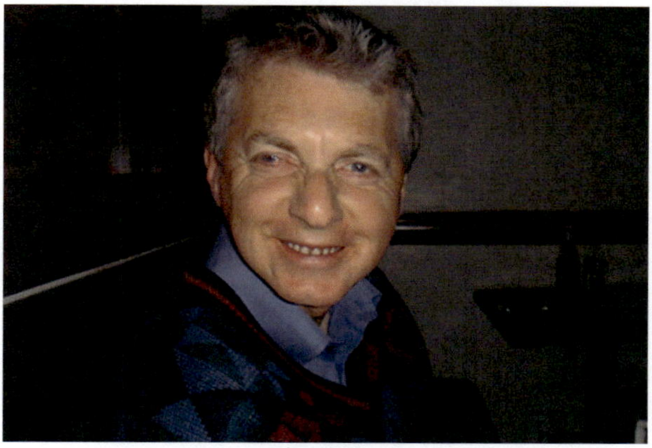

Figure 5.17 Richard Wawro, Artist.

Photo courtesy of Mike Wawro.

Wawro was known for his exceedingly detailed landscapes and seascapes of intense depth and color in wax oil crayon. He never used models to paint. He would generally take in a very blurred image from television documentaries or from travel guides viewed at one of the bookshops he loved to visit, record it perfectly in his mind, and then paint it superbly without missing the smallest detail. Professor Marian Bohusz-Szyszko (Richard Wawro's official website) of the Polish School of Art in London said he was "thunderstruck" by Wawro's drawings, describing them as "an incredible phenomenon rendered with the precision of a mechanic and the vision of a poet" (Treffert, 2006).

Wawro had his first exhibition in Edinburgh when he was 17 and became known in the UK when the BBC made a television show about him, and Richard Demarco exhibited Wawro's works in his gallery. Margaret Thatcher, then Education Minister and Prime Minister of the United Kingdom opened one of his exhibitions in 1970. Notable owners of Richard Wawro originals included Thatcher herself, as well as Pope John Paul II (Richard Wawro's official website). In 1983, the American autism expert Dr. Laurence Becker produced an award-winning documentary film about Wawro's life and art. In the movie, Becker explores this obvious contradiction, typical of savants: how can a person like Wawro, presumed to be mentally retarded and legally blind, create such wonderful art works? Wawro sold more than 1,000 pieces (for amounts of up to $10,000) in around 100 exhibitions throughout Europe and North America.

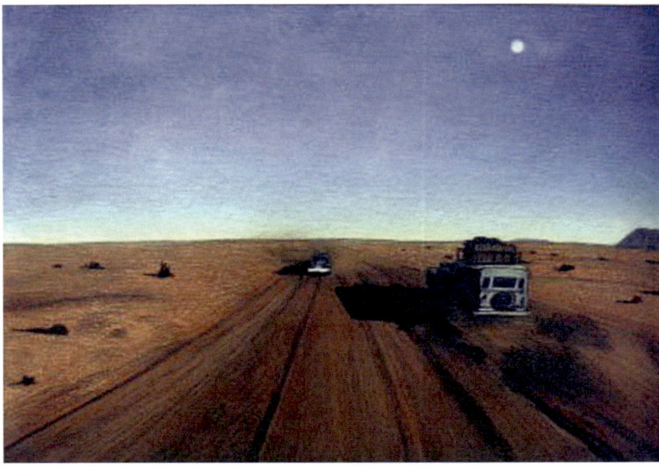

Figure 5.18 Richard Wawro, Artist (1754).

Photo courtesy of Mike Wawro.

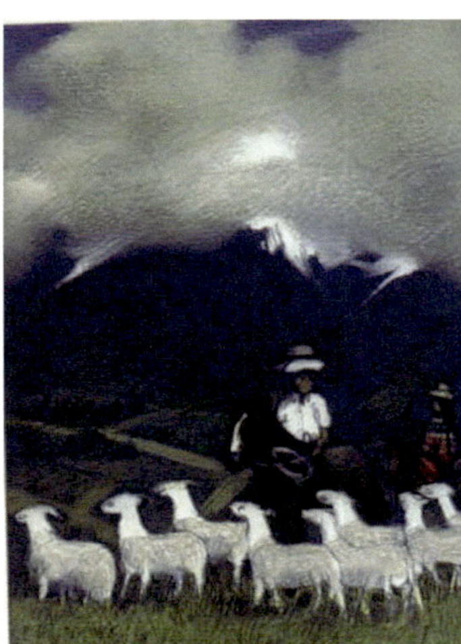

Figure 5.19 Richard Wawro, Artist (2253).

Photo courtesy of Mike Wawro.

For his entire life, Wawro had difficulty speaking as well as poor social skills. There was something special about him, however, which allowed him to connect with and charm almost everyone he met. Throughout his career as a painter, Wawro participated in countless television programs and studies, showing an unflaggingly cheerful and optimistic demeanor. Having survived cancer once, Richard Wawro died on February 22, 2006, at the age of 53, after a brave battle against lung cancer.

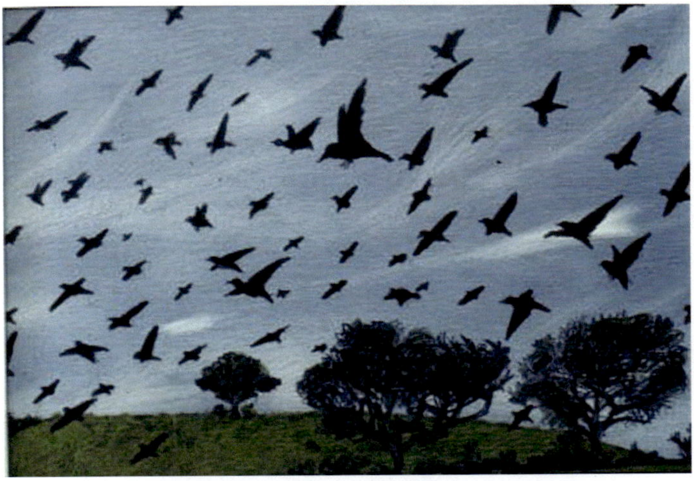

Figure 5.20 Richard Wawro, Artist (1745).

Photo courtesy: Mike Wawro.

Impairment: Autism, behavior rating moderately to severely retarded, obsessed with walking in circles, endlessly spinning objects, and a striking a single key of piano for hours. IQ of 30. Legally blind and virtually mute until the age of 11.

Skills: Art, phenomenal photographic memory, extraordinary painter. He was known for his vibrant landscapes and seascapes, created with the unusual medium of wax oil crayons. The tones he used to capture lights and shadows were considered masterful. He created more than 2,500 drawings and sold more than 1,000 paintings over the course of his lifetime.

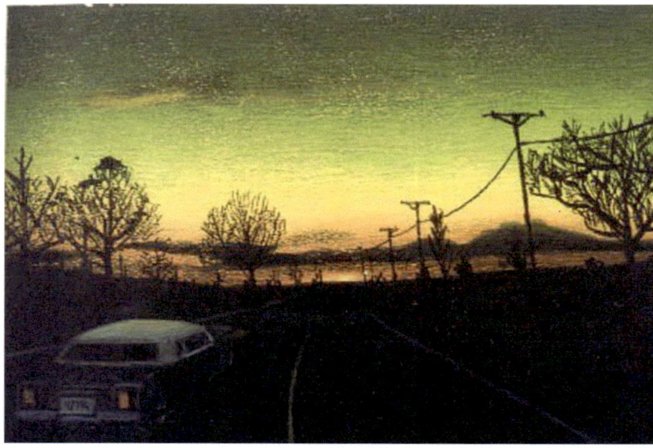

Figure 5.21 Richard Wawro, Artist (1945).

Photo courtesy of Mike Wawro

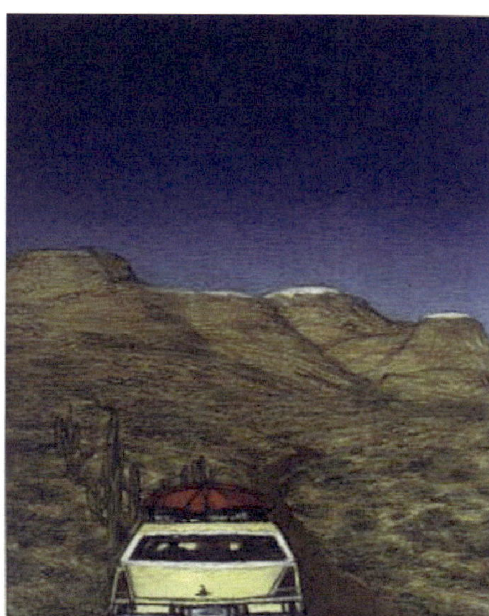

Figure 5.22 Richard Wawro, Artist (2205).

Photo courtesy of Mike Wawro.

Below are references, links to some videos, and additional reading about Laurence Richard Wawro.

- Richard Wawro's official website: www.wawro.net
- Wallace, G. (2008). Neuropsychological studies of savant skills: Can they inform the neuroscience of giftedness? *Roeper Review, 30*(4), 229-246.
- Treffert, D. (2006). "Richard Wawro – An Amazing Artist." https://www.wisconsinmedicalsociety.org/professional/savant-syndrome/profiles-and-videos/profiles/richard-wawro-an-amazing-artist/
- Richard Wawro. The Telegraph. March 11, 2006. https://www.telegraph.co.uk/news/obituaries/1512657/Richard-Wawro.html
- Richard Wawro. The Newsroom. The Scotsman. March 9, 2006. https://www.scotsman.com/news/obituaries/richard-wawro-2469518
- Treffert, D. and Wallace, G. (2004). Islands of genius. *Scientific American Mind, 14*(1), 14-23.
- Heaton, P. and Wallace, G. (2004). Annotation: The savant syndrome. *Journal of child psychology and psychiatry, 45*(5), 899-911.
- Treffert, D. and Wallace, G. (2002). Islands of genius. *Scientific American, 286*(6), 76-85.
- Treffert, D. (1999). The savant syndrome and autistic disorder. *CNS spectrums, 4*(12), 57-60.
- Hermelin, B., Pring, L., Buhler, M., Wolff, S. and Heaton, P. (1999). A visually impaired savant artist: Interacting perceptual and memory representations. *Journal of Child Psychology and Psychiatry, 40*(7), 1129-1139.
- Kellman, J. (1996). Making sense of seeing: Autism and David Marr. *Visual Arts Research*, 76-89.
- Pring, L. and Hermelin, B. (1993). Bottle, tulip and wineglass: semantic and structural picture processing by savant artists. *Journal of Child Psychology and Psychiatry, 34*(8), 1365-1385.
- With eyes wide open: the life and art of Richard Wawro. http://www.interactingwithautism.com/section/understanding/media/representations/details/23
- A selection of Richard's pictures can be seen in his website. http://www.wawro.net/Richard_Wawro/Gallery.html

- Richard Wawro videos: http://www.wawro.net/Richard_Wawro/Videos.html
- Richard Wawro – Autistic Savant (Scottish Artist). https://www.youtube.com/watch?v=53LovF4kEtE&t=7s

5.8 Leslie Lemke (born 1952)

I am deeply indebted to Dr. Darold Treffert for his extensive assistance in the final revision of this profile.

Leslie was born prematurely on January 31, 1952 in Milwaukee, Wisconsin, in the United States. He was born with cerebral palsy and moderately severe mental retardation. Furthermore, as a consequence of his premature birth, he developed retinal problems in the first months of life, then glaucoma, and finally his eyes had to be surgically removed (Treffert, 2015). His birth mother gave him up for adoption to May Lemke, a nurse-governess, who at the time was 52 and was raising five children of her own. May was warned that Leslie would surely die, but she claimed that under her care he would survive. When Leslie was four years old, he developed spasticity and echolalia. He learned to stand at 12, and was 15 when he began to walk, thanks to his mother, who taught him how to step by step. His verbal IQ was 58 (Treffert, 1988). Up until this time, Leslie had been always silent, distant, and unemotional.

> Lemke's verbal IQ is fifty-eight, which ranks him as mildly retarded. In recent tests for vocabulary, general information, arithmetic, comprehension, and similarities (How are a pear and a banana alike?), his scores were far below normal (Treffert, 1988).

Lemke was seven years old when his adoptive parents bought him a piano. Although he had a condition in which his muscles remained almost permanently contracted, Leslie learned to play the piano by himself merely by listening to songs. At age 16, after having heard Tchaikovsky's Piano Concerto No. 1 on television for the first time, his mother later found him at midnight performing the work with mastery. God's miracle, his mother said, came into full bloom that night. Thus Leslie began his musical career as a remarkable piano player, without ever having taken music lessons. "Due to his prodigious memory Leslie can also repeat music that he has heard on a single occasion: he has been able to exactly copy a 45 minute long opera" (Darius, 2007). As Treffert (2015) noted, "now he not only repeats a song accurately after hearing it only once, he improvises and, yes, even composes new songs with his own words and effects."

Lemke performs all styles of music, from ragtime to classical, and besides the piano, plays other musical instruments, including drums, accordion, xylophone, concertina, and chord organ. Leslie has given numerous concerts in music halls, churches, palaces, and prisons (Treffert, 1989) in Norway, Japan, and throughout the United States and has appeared on television shows including CBC's *Man Alive*, the *CBS Evening News* (where Walter Cronkite said "This is a season that celebrates a miracle, and this story belongs to the season. It's the story of a young man, a piano, and a miracle." (Treffert, 2015), *60 Minutes* (Morley Safer: "Leslie Lemke is a memorable man"), and *That's Incredible!*. Treffert has said that Dustin Hoffman watched the Morley Safer program and was "moved to tears" by Leslie. In 1983, the movie *The Woman Who Willed a Miracle* was released, which tells the story of May Lemke and her son.

Leslie Lemke currently lives with May's daughter, Mary Parker, who lovingly took over the difficulties of caring for him.

Impairments: Autism, cerebral palsy, moderately severe mental retardation, atonic diplegia, scoliosis, echolalia, spasticity, blindness. Lemke made no movements or sounds and showed no emotions for almost the first seven years of life. He was unable to stand on his own until 12 years of age, and it took another three years before he could walk unassisted. "His overall learning-ability was at the level of a normal 7-8-year-old child" (Darius, 2007). Verbal IQ: 58.

Skills: Musician and composer. Remarkable memory. He plays the piano, drums, accordion, xylophone, concertina and chord organ. He also sings with a baritone voice. Leslie may sit for hours listening to radio or records. He can recall and play a piece of music of any length flawlessly after hearing it just once.

Below are references, links to some videos, and additional reading about Leslie Lemke.

- Treffert, D. (2015). Leslie Lemke: An Inspirational Performance. https://www.wisconsinmedicalsociety.org/professional/savant-syndrome/profiles-and-videos/profiles/leslie-lemke-an-inspirational-performance/
- Treffert, D. (2014). Savant syndrome: Realities, myths and misconceptions. *Journal of Autism and Developmental Disorders, 44*(3), 564-571.
- Treffert, D. (2014b). *Whatever Happened to Leslie Lemke?* Scientific American. June 17, 2014. https://blogs.scientificamerican.com/guest-blog/whatever-happened-to-leslielemke/#:~:text=I%20am%20asked%20so%20often,whatever%20happened%20to%20Leslie%20Lemke%3F&text=Leslie%20is%20alive%20and%20well,after%20May%20died%20in%201993.
- Straus, J. (2014). Idiots Savants, Retarded Savants, Talented Aments, Mono-Savants, Autistic Savants, Just Plain Savants, People with Savant Syndrome, and Autistic People Who Are Good at Things: A View from Disability Studies.
- Monty, S. (2013). *May's boy: The rest of the history.* CreateSpace Independent Publishing Platform (February 13, 2013). Amazon.
- Treffert, D. (2010). *Islands of genius: The bountiful mind of the autistic, acquired, and sudden savant.* Jessica Kingsley Publishers.
- Treffert, D. (2009). The savant syndrome: an extraordinary condition. A synopsis: past, present, future. *Philosophical Transactions of the Royal Society B: Biological Sciences*, 364(1522), 1351-1357.
- Darius, H. (2007). Savant syndrome-theories and empirical findings. http://www.diva-portal.org/smash/get/diva2:2901/FULLTEXT01.pdf
- Treffert, D. (1989). An unlikely virtuoso: Leslie Lemke and the story of savant syndrome. *The sciences*, 29(1), 28-35.
- Lauerman, C. (1988). *Extraordinary People.* Chicago Tribune. https://www.chicagotribune.com/news/ct-xpm-1988-08-28-8801250943-story.html
- Monty, S. (1981). *May's boy: an incredible story of love.* Thomas Nelson Publishers.

- The Story of a Savant: Leslie Lemke: https://www.youtube.com/watch?v=tdqpp4IZI6E
- May's Miracle: https://www.youtube.com/watch?v=RuO0B56evT0&t=36s
- Leslie Lemke – ABC's That's Incredible 1981: https://www.youtube.com/watch?v=ZwtZA-ZmOAM
- Leslie Lords Prayer: https://www.youtube.com/watch?v=RuO0B56evT0
- Leslie Lemke videos: https://www.wisconsinmedicalsociety.org/professional/savant-syndrome/profiles-and-videos/videos/leslie-lemke-videos/
- Darold Treffert: To Creation and Beyond: The Remarkable Life of Leslie Lemke. https://www.wisconsinacademy.org/magazine/creation-and-beyond-remarkable-life-leslie-lemke

5.9 Anthony Cicoria (born 1952)

I am deeply indebted to Dr. Anthony Cicoria for his extensive assistance in the final revisions of this profile.

Anthony Cicoria was born in the United States in 1952. He is an acquired savant, physician, and orthopedic surgeon. Cicoria was chief of Orthopedics at Chenango Memorial Hospital and was Assistant Professor of Orthopedics at SUNY Upstate Medical School, in Syracuse, New York. He received his BS in Biology from The Citadel and is a graduate of the Medical University of South Carolina (MD, PhD) and the University of Virginia Orthopedic Surgery Residency.

In 1994, Anthony, who was 42 years old, was calling his mother on a public telephone booth when he was struck by a lightning, an event that in one electrifying instant changed his life forever. He still remembers every second of the near-death experience:

> I was calling my mother. There was a little bit of rain, thunder in the distance. My mother did not answer so I started to hang up. The phone was a foot away from where I was standing when I got struck. I remember a flash of light coming out of the phone. It hit me in the face. Next thing I remember, I was flying backwards (Sacks, 2007b).

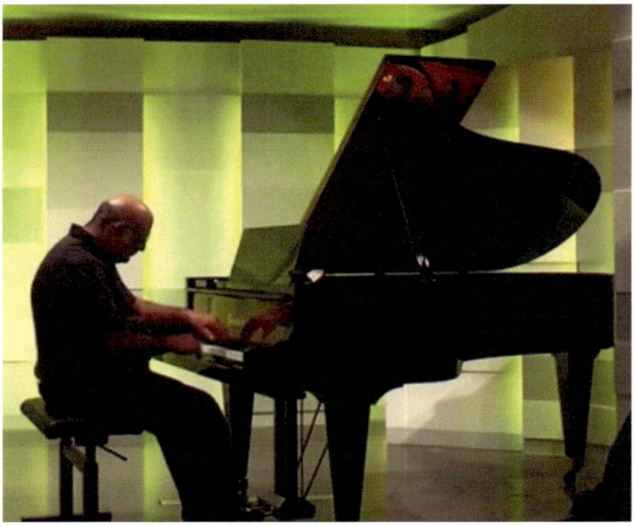

Figure 5.23 Tony Cicoria in concert at Mozart's home basement theater.

Photo courtesy of Anthony Cicoria.

Cicoria's heart apparently stopped, but an intensive-care-unit nurse, who had been waiting to use the phone, resuscitated Tony by giving him CPR. "After a minute or two, when he could speak, he said, 'It's O.K.—I'm a doctor!' The woman, who turned out to be an intensive-care-unit nurse, replied, 'A few minutes ago, you weren't'" (Sacks, 2007b).

Cicoria suffered burns on his face and left foot, where the electric current had entered and left his body. He also suffered from memory problems for a while. His neurologist, consulted shortly thereafter, found nothing unusual and, a couple of weeks later, Cicoria returned to work.

Shortly after this, however, Cicoria began to feel an insatiable desire to listen to classical music and to begin performing the piano (Cicoria, 2014). This would have not been as surprising if it weren't for the fact that he had never felt an affinity for much beyond classic rock. "When I walked into the music store, a CD of Vladimir Ashkenazy playing his favorite Chopin seemed to fly into my hands. I listened repeatedly throughout the day" (Cicoria, 2014).

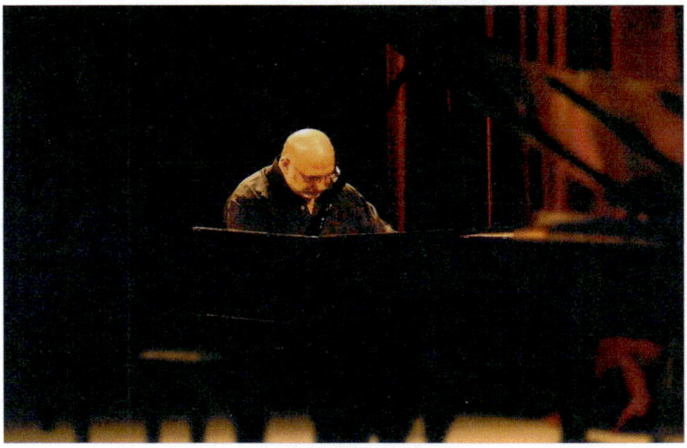

Figure 5.24 Tony Cicoria in in concert at Goodyear Theater SUNY Oneonta NY.

Photo courtesy of Anthony Cicoria.

Cicoria bought a piano and obtained the sheet music for the pieces on the CD he listened to daily, and began initially teaching himself how to play, realizing the futility of that, began formal lessons in 1998. Although he had never tried to write or notate music before, he composed dozens of themes that seemed to come from nowhere. The music was there, deep in his being. A few years later, he gave his first solo recital as a pianist and composer.

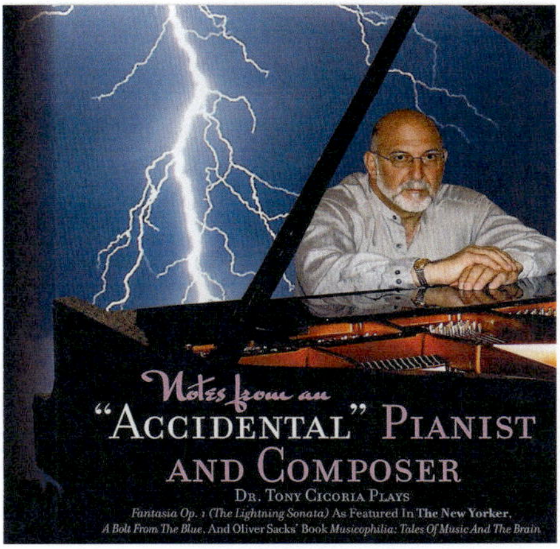

Figure 5.25 Album cover: Notes from an "Accidental" Pianist and Composer.

Photo courtesy of Anthony Cicoria.

The year 2008 marks an important milestone in Cicoria's musical career, when he gave his first public concert at the Goodyear Performing Arts Theater at State University College at Oneonta in New York. The music was recorded live by Granada Media UK, BBC One, and German National Television. A CD on this concert is available at CDBaby.com. Since then, Cicoria has appeared in numerous magazines, including *The Week*, *SuperConsciousness Magazine*, and the *Financial Times*. He also has appeared in numerous television presentations such as BBC One's documentary series *Imagine*, CBC's *The Hour*, A&E's *Beyond and Back*, Discovery's *Expedition Unknown* with Josh Gates, and the *Nova* episode "Musical Minds." He was profiled by Oliver Sacks (2007) in Sacks' book *Musicophilia: Tales of Music and the Brain.* Cicoria currently continues to work part-time as a surgeon, but his heart and mind are now centered on music.

Impairment: Acquired savant. He was struck by lightning and his heart apparently stopped. An intensive care nurse who was nearby managed to resuscitate him.

Skills: Musician, composer. Shortly after his accident, he began to have an indomitable desire to play the piano. He bought a piano, learned to play, and became a competent concert performer and composer.

Below are references, links to some videos, and additional reading about Anthony Cicoria.

- Tony Cicoria channel on YouTube: https://www.youtube.com/channel/UCkBCBccOIH6UW0xCprbOI1A
- Gorvett, Z. (2018). The mystery of why some people become sudden geniuses. January 6, 2018. *BBC Future.* https://www.bbc.com/future/article/20180116-the-mystery-of-why-some-people-become-sudden-geniuses
- Cicoria, T. (2014). The electrifying story of the accidental pianist & composer. *Missouri medicine, 111*(4), 308-308.
- Treffert, D. (2014c). Accidental genius. *Scientific American, 311*(2), 52-57.

- De Bruijn, J. (2011). *Managing professionals*. Routledge
- Sacks, O. (2010). *Musicophilia: Tales of music and the brain*. Vintage Canada.
- Sacks, O. (2007). *Tales of music and the brain*. London, UK: Picador.
- Sacks, O. (2007b). A Bolt from the Blue. Where do sudden intense passions come from? The New Yorker, 23 July 2007. https://www.newyorker.com/magazine/2007/07/23/a-bolt-from-the-blue
- Gottlieb, A. (2007). Take Five, and Call Me. October 28, 2007. *The New York Times*. https://www.nytimes.com/2007/10/28/books/review/Gottlieb-t.html
- Duguid, S. (2007). First Person: Tony Cicoria. September 21, 2007. *Financial Times*. https://www.ft.com/content/c69f7968-6655-11dc-9fbb-0000779fd2ac
- 2013 Tony Cicoria is performing his "Lightning-Sonata" at Mozart House in Vienna. https://www.youtube.com/watch?v=tDtYkxSCV18
- Tony Cicoria. The lightning bolt that made me a music maestro. BBC. April 15, 2020. https://www.bbc.co.uk/sounds/play/p089jy89
- Part 7 – Tony Cicoria – ITTV Show. https://www.youtube.com/watch?v=L6CSbMqnQWg
- Notes fan Accidental Pianist and Composer. Classical style piano compositions following a Near Death Experience. https://store.cdbaby.com/cd/drtonycicoria
- The Profound Death Experience of Dr Anthony Cicoria I Anthony Cicoria and Lynn Fishman RN. https://www.youtube.com/watch?v=rK73CZKfWFE
- Struck by Lightning: What Is It Like? https://www.youtube.com/watch?v=JSeG8nchaNc

5.10 Jon Sarkin (born 1953)

Jon Sarkin was born in Newark, New Jersey, United States in 1953. He is an artist and an acquired savant. Jon's life was completely normal until he was 35 years old. He studied, got married, and had a child, as well as a successful profession as a chiropractor. Then, suddenly, he suffered a series of unusual health problems that changed his life forever. His brain was altered and rewired, and the effects generated a neurological condition known as "sudden artistic output" (according to Sarkin's official website) or, more commonly, acquired savantism. His case is exceptionally rare, as very few savants are known to have become so after a stroke.

Emerging from this bout of health problems, Jon began to draw and paint obsessively and compulsively, and made it such a priority that he became a wildly prolific artist. He is still doing so today. As Jon eloquently writes on his website:

> So he drew.
> All the time.
>
> And he painted.
> And made collage.
> And wrote poetry.
> And scribbled over.
> And rubbed dirt into things.
> And some people noticed and kinda liked it.
>
> And Jon drew some more.
>
> All the time.

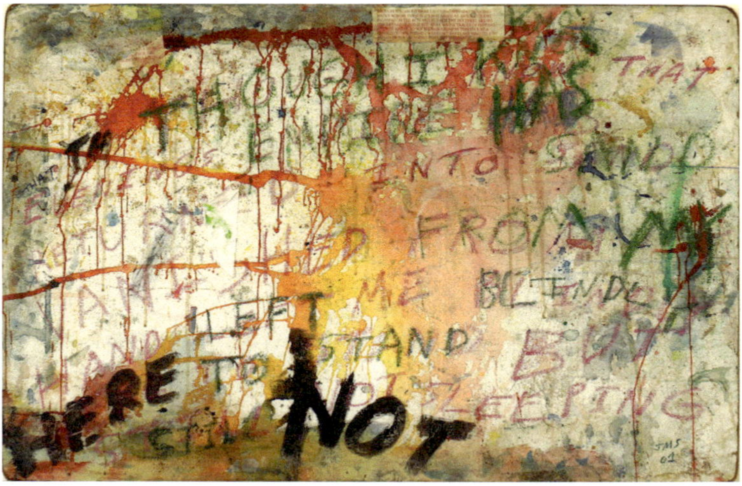

Figure 5.26 Jon Sarkin. Here Not.

Photo courtesy of Jon Sarkin.

Before he was a savant, Jon had a good life and was a good student. He graduated from the Pingry School in Elizabeth, New Jersey, earned his undergraduate degree in Biology from the University of Pennsylvania, an M.S. degree in Environmental Science from Rutgers University, and finally a D.C. (Doctor of Chiropractic) degree from Palmer College of Chiropractic in 1980 (Sarkin's website).

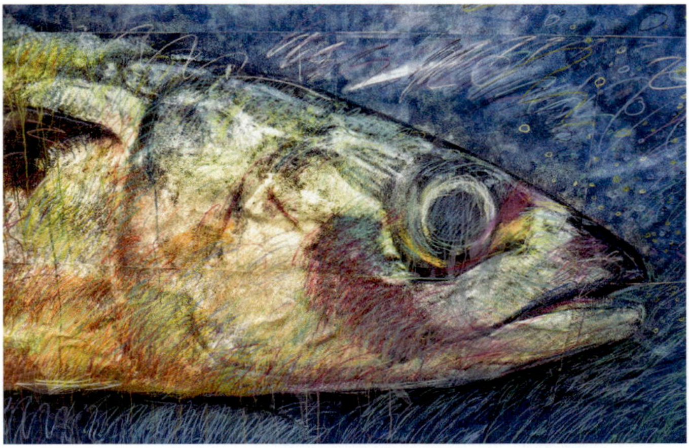

Figure 5.27 Large-scale collaborative work by Jon Sarkin and Paul Cary Goldberg.

Photo courtesy of Paul Cary Goldberg.

His life took a dramatic turn in 1988, when Jon suddenly developed tinnitus and hyperacusis. The problem was linked a blood vessel pressing on his acoustic nerve (Vitelli, 2013). Tinnitus is the perception of sound such as clicking, buzzing, roaring, or ringing, with no external source (Levin and Oron, 2015). "The sound may be soft or loud, low or high pitched, and may interfere with concentration or increase feelings of anxiety or depression" (NIH, Tinnitus). This symptom signals a problem in the auditory system, head or neck. It is not usually considered serious—sometimes it can be caused by a buildup of wax in the ears, or simply by aging. But it can also be an indication that there is an underlying problem which requires diagnosis. Hyperacusis, on the other hand, which often coincides with tinnitus, is a rare hearing disorder characterized by an increased sensitivity to certain frequencies and volume ranges of sound (Knipper et al., 2013).

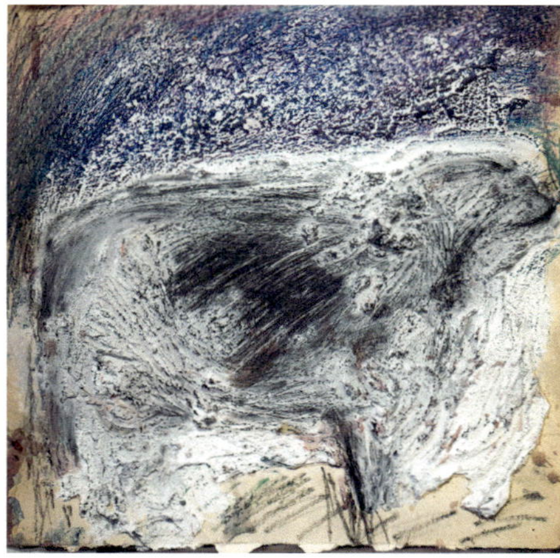

Figure 5.28 Jon Sarkin. Crop.

Photo courtesy of Jon Sarkin.

In 1989, Sarkin underwent surgery to alleviate the condition, after which he suffered a cerebellar hemorrhage, which led to a subsequent stroke. The procedure was directed by Dr. Peter Jannetta, a neurosurgeon at Presbyterian University Hospital with extensive experience in this condition, having performed hundreds of microvascular decompressions, none of whom had suffered serious complications. Dr. Janetta believe that the surgery would have an 80% chance of success at calming Jon's annoying buzzing sounds, and Jon was convinced, eager to once and for all put an end to the maddening noise in his ears. But his problems were just beginning:

> Shortly after surgery, a swollen blood clot at the base of his brain caused him to suffer the massive stroke. Near death and in a semi coma, he had life-saving emergency surgery to remove part of his brain on the left side of his cerebellum which had been compressed and killed by the blood clot (Spencer, 2011).

The main damage was in the left hemisphere and in particular to the left side of the cerebellum (Nutt, 2011). "Jon awoke deaf forced in one ear, his vision splintered, and his balance permanently skewed. Parts of his brain had been sliced and removed" (Sarkin's website). An impaired sense of balance forced him to walk with a cane for the rest of his life.

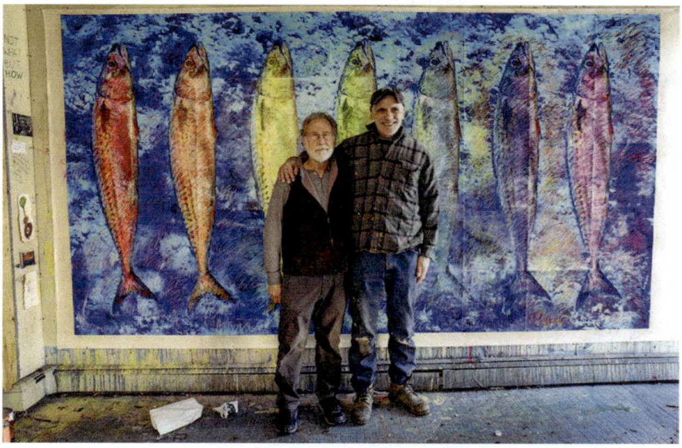

Figure 5.29 Large-scale collaborative work by Jon Sarkin and Paul Cary Goldberg.

Photo courtesy of Paul Cary Goldberg.

After further emergency surgery, Jon lingered for weeks in a semi-coma (Nutt, 2011b) and was later moved to a rehabilitation hospital, where he stayed for another month, slowly recovering. Finally, in December 1989, he returned home.

> He quickly moved from a wheelchair to a walker, but it would take another six months to make the transition to a cane, and he would depend on it for the rest of his life (Nutt, 2011b).

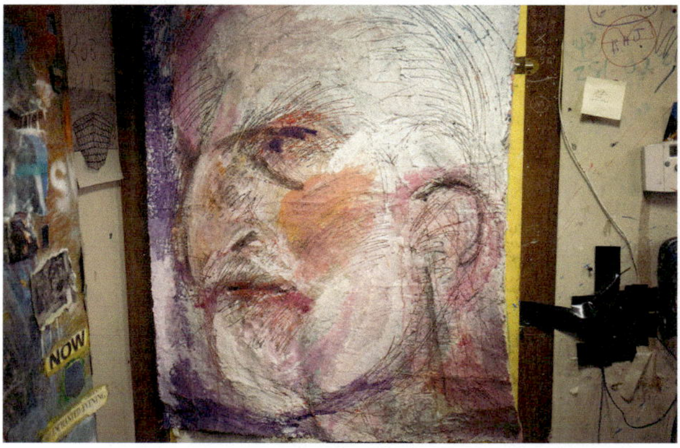

Figure 5.30 Jon Sarkin.

Photo courtesy of Jon Sarkin.

After months of slow recovery, Sarkin returned to his office as a chiropractor, but nothing would be the same again. His brain had changed: he was a new man. What most attracted him was painting and drawing, which he had an insatiable appetite for. This is how his new life as an artist began.

Jon's works are simply extraordinary. "These basically have an origin in popular culture, comics, literature, and music" (Sarkin website). Sarking himself defines his work as "frenetic, bouncy, a stream of consciousness, a short-attention span" (Bradford, 2020).

Sarkin has been featured in different media outlets, including *The New Yorker*, *The New York Times*, ABC's Primetime, *This American Life*, *GQ*, and *ARTNews*, as well as in galleries in New York City, Los Angeles, and elsewhere in the world (Sarkin website). In 2010, Sarkin created the cover for the album *Easy Wonderful* by the American alternative rock band Guster. In 2011, science writer Amy Nutt, a Pulitzer Prize-winning author, published *Shadows Bright as Glass*, a book about Sarkin's life (Nutt, 2011).

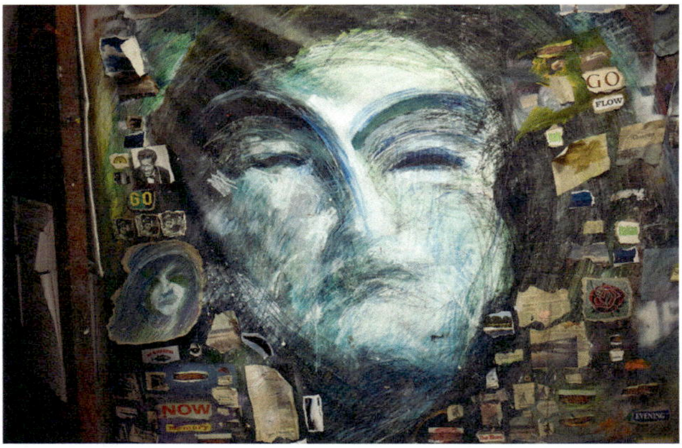

Figure 5.31 Jon Sarkin.

Photo courtesy of Jon Sarkin.

Sarkin currently lives in Cape Ann, Massachusetts, with his wife and children. He continues to paint and draw with great passion.

Impairments: Acquired savantism. Jon developed tinnitus and hyperacusis when he was 35 years old. He underwent surgery to alleviate the condition, after which he suffered a cerebellar hemorrhage, which led to a subsequent stroke.

Skills: Artist, painter, and draftsman. Jon became a brilliant painter following a massive stroke.

Below are references, links to some videos, and additional reading about Jon Sarkin.

- Jon Sarkin's official website: https://www.jsarkin.com/
- Jon Sarkin on Facebook: https://www.facebook.com/jon.sarkin.5
- Jon Sarkin on Instagram: https://www.instagram.com/jonsarkin/
- Jon Sarkin on Twitter: https://twitter.com/jonsarkin
- Bradford, T. (2020). Renowned North Shore artist to show work at Princeton. The Salem News. January 2, 2020. https://www.salemnews.com/news/north_of_boston/renowned-north-shore-artist-to-show-work-at-princeton/article_67bdb742-4286-5d6b-8fb0-6a7035f3ec73.html
- McCarthy, G. (2019). Around Cape Ann: Celebrating art on the working waterfront. Gloucester Daily Tomes. January 10, 2019. https://www.gloucestertimes.com/news/the_catch/around-cape-ann-celebrating-art-on-the-working-waterfront/article_30b85cdb-be96-5f95-908e-a8cff4ba55e5.html
- Levine, R. and Oron, Y. (2015). Tinnitus. In *Handbook of clinical neurology* (Vol. 129, pp. 409-431). Elsevier.
- Knipper, M., Van Dijk, P., Nunes, I., Rüttiger, L. and Zimmermann, U. (2013). Advances in the neurobiology of hearing disorders: recent developments regarding the basis of tinnitus and hyperacusis. *Progress in neurobiology, 111*, 17-33.
- Vitelli, R. (2013). Creativity and the Healey Brain. Psychology Today. April 29, 2013. https://www.psychologytoday.com/us/blog/media-spotlight/201304/creativity-and-the-healing-brain
- Hill, E. (2011). Altered mind: creation of an artist. *The Lancet Neurology, 10*(11), 957-958.

- Spencer, K. (2011). My stroke turned me into an artist. Express. August 23, 2011. https://www.express.co.uk/life-style/health/266585/My-stroke-turned-me-into-an-artist
- Nutt, A. (2011). *Shadows bright as glass: The remarkable story of one man's journey from brain trauma to artistic triumph.* Simon and Schuster.
- Nutt, A. (2011b). The man who couldn´t stop drawing. The Guardian. July 29, 2011. https://www.theguardian.com/artanddesign/2011/jul/29/jon-sarkin-couldnt-stop-drawing
- Klappholz, A. (2008). Jon Sarkin: A Medical mystery and artist savant. Vanity Fair. December 18, 2008. https://www.vanityfair.com/news/2008/12/jon-sarkin-artist-savant
- Bäzner, H. and Hennerici, M. (2006). Stroke in painters. *International review of neurobiology, 74,* 165-191.
- Edgers, G. A changed man. The Boston Globe. June 11, 2006. http://archive.boston.com/ae/theater_arts/articles/2006/06/11/a_changed_man/
- NIH, Tinnitus. National Institutes of Health. https://www.nidcd.nih.gov/health/tinnitus
- Guster – Do You Love Me featuring Gloucester artist Jon Sarkin. July 11, 2019. https://www.gloucestertimes.com/multimedia/guster---do-you-love-me-featuring-gloucester-artist-jon-sarkin/video_df43a5da-a3e6-11e9-89b7-9f9b405a3bac.html
- An Evening With Guster and Jon Sarkin. https://www.youtube.com/watch?v=7g837CY9xN4
- Jon Sarkin – Compulsive Artist. https://www.youtube.com/watch?v=lgL3lgLRBBE
- Jon Sarkin's journey from brain trauma to artistic triumph. https://www.youtube.com/watch?v=WNq4WKSSZuU

5.11 Gloria Lenhoff (born 1955)

I greatly appreciate the contributions of Sylvia Lenhoff, Gloria's mother, in writing and reviewing this profile.

Gloria Lenhoff was born prematurely in the United States in 1955. She is a musical savant who excels at performing on the accordion. She is also a lyric soprano singer. Lenhoff has Williams syndrome and faces multiple difficulties with the simplest of mental and physical tasks, to the extent that she requires assistance with most tasks in her day-to-day living. Shortly after birth, her parents realized that their daughter had learning difficulties. The problems became more evident as Lenhoff grew. She could not walk, talk, or perform simple activities. Psychologists and physicians diagnosed her with mental retardation after a battery of tests. It was not until Lenhoff turned 33, however, that her parents received the diagnosis of Williams syndrome. The delay in obtaining the correct diagnosis was partly due to the fact that the syndrome had not yet been identified when Lenhoff was born.

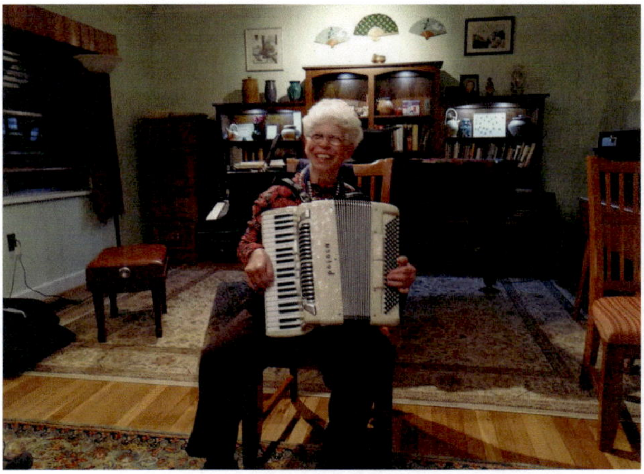

Figure 5.32 Gloria Lenhoff

Photo courtesy of Sylvia and Gloria Lenhoff.

Williams syndrome, which occurs in one out of every 7,500 births, is a multisystemic, genetic developmental disorder that is present at birth and is caused by the spontaneous deletion (mainly at the time of conception) of 26-28 genes on chromosome 7. The disorder is characterized by medical problems, including cardiovascular disease abnormalities (the most common being supravalvular aortic stenosis), developmental delays, and intellectual disabilities. Individuals with this syndrome are generally distinguished by their facial features, which include a broad forehead, short nose, and full cheeks with a poorly developed molar region. A Williams-afflicted person tends to have an outgoing personality (friendly and enthusiastic), strong emotional attachments, an easier time learning additional languages, and an affinity for music. Children with WS have a distinctive particularity: they turn the ordinary into extraordinary and the extraordinary into ordinary. "In the same way that you can look at a color and immediately know that it is blue, they can hear a note and know that it is a B flat" (Christian, 1990).

Lenhoff cannot add or subtract, give change for a dollar, cross the street alone, or distinguish right from left. Her IQ is 55 and her brain is 20% smaller than average. Lenhoff attended a special education program where she was schooled alongside children with Down syndrome, partly because there was still no precise classification for her disorder, although she was much more verbal than her classmates.

Though much of her world is not perfect, Lenhoff has been gifted with extraordinary musical talent. She has perfect pitch, a lyric soprano voice, a computer-like memory which allows her to remember and sing over 3,000 songs of different styles (religious, opera, folk, classical) in 30 foreign languages, and is able to "play the accordion as it were an extension of herself" (Christian, 1990). Although she is not able to read musical notation, music flows in her brain like water in a running river.

When she was twelve years old, Lenhoff's parents gave her an accordion. She loved music and singing, and this gift made her very happy. With the support of her parents from a young age and classes in both singing and accordion, Lenhoff grew up surrounded by music, developing skills which only some privileged individuals are able to acquire. Over the years, Lenhoff also began to show her linguistic talents. She can carry on conversations in half a dozen languages, including Spanish, Hebrew, French, and Japanese.

Lenhoff has performed concerts with some notable professional musical organizations. For example, under David Amos, director of the San Diego Symphony Orchestra, she met the challenges of singing the lead role in

Samuel Barber's opera *Knoxville: Summer of 1915*. After auditioning with Michael Ching, the Artistic Director of Opera Memphis, gloria was invited to sing with the Opera's soprano chorus for four different productions across the country. She has also collaborated with the San Diego Master Chorale and such popular groups as Aerosmith. In 1988, she was the subject of *Bravo Gloria*, a PBS documentary. She has also been featured on *60 Minutes*, *Nightline*, Discovery Health, The Learning Channel, and on various foreign TV specials. She has performed solo in England, Spain, Israel, and France. Gloria Lenhoff is important to the world not only for what she has accomplished as a musician with an intellectual impairment, but also as a peer model for other children with WS. Together with her father, Howard Lenhoff, Gloria has motivated hundreds of parents to provide an advanced musical education for their children.

Impairments: Williams syndrome. She has multiple difficulties with the simplest of mental and physical tasks. Her IQ is 55 and her brain is 20% smaller than average.

Skills: Perfect pitch. Soprano voice. She can sing nearly 3,000 songs of different genres (religious, opera, folk, classical) in 30 foreign languages. She can carry on conversations in half a dozen languages, including Spanish, Hebrew, French, and Japanese.

Below are references, links to some videos, and additional reading about Gloria Lenhoff.

- Broadus, V. (2011). For woman with Williams Syndrome, music was the key. Lexington Herald Leader. May 11, 2011. https://www.kentucky.com/news/local/community/article44095050.html
- Sforza, T. (2010). *The (Strangest) Song: One Father's Quest to Help His Daughter Find Her Voice*. Prometheus Books.
- Morris, C., Lenhoff, H. and Wang, P. (Eds.). (2006). *Williams-Beuren syndrome: Research, evaluation, and treatment*. JHU Press.
- Leung, R. (2004). A very special brain. 60 Minutes. CBS News. https://www.cbsnews.com/news/a-very-special-brain-06-01-2004/

- Lenhoff, H., Perales, O. and Hickok, G. (2001). Absolute pitch in Williams syndrome. *Music Perception: An Interdisciplinary Journal, 18*(4), 491-503.
- Maher, B. (2001). Music, the brain, and Williams syndrome: rare disorder offers insight into the genetic basis of cognition.(focus on Genes and Genomics). *The Scientist, 15*(23), 20-22.
- Sforza, T. (1998). Williams Syndrome. Chicago Tribune. September 18, 1998. https://www.chicagotribune.com/news/ct-xpm-1998-09-18-9809190188-story.html
- Lenhoff, H., Wang, P., Greenberg, F. and Bellugi, U. (1997). Williams syndrome and the brain. *Scientific American, 277*(6), 68-73.
- Stambaugh, L. (1996). Special Learners with Special Abilities: Developing the special musical abilities of children and adults with Williams syndrome can be a rewarding experience that requires specialized teaching strategies. *Music Educators Journal, 83*(3), 19-23.
- Christian, S. (1990). Perfect Pitch: Gloria Lenhoff Is a 'Musical Savant' Who Sings and Plays Beautifully but Can't Understand Mathematics. https://www.latimes.com/archives/la-xpm-1990-12-23-vw-9838-story.html
- Lenhoff, G. (2006). Religious Classics for Soprano. https://www.amazon.com.mx/Religious-Classics-Soprano-Gloria-Lenhoff/dp/1596155248
- Williams Syndrome Music Savant Gloria Lenhoff performs the classic "Summertime" beautifully! https://www.youtube.com/watch?v=68HCOj6z0Mw
- Williams Syndrome 1. https://www.youtube.com/watch?v=xC2j4HoWimE
- Williams Syndrome Music Savant Gloria Lenhoff covers many favorite tunes with her accordion! https://www.youtube.com/watch?v=7Zf-C2tSKq8

5.12 Ellen Boudreaux (born 1957)

Ellen Boudreaux was born in the United States in 1957. She is blind, autistic, and a very special musical savant with a pervasive sense of rhythm. Ellen was born prematurely, which caused her to develop a disease of the eye known as retrolental fibroplasia, or Terry syndrome. This condition affects mainly infants who receive oxygen therapy for lack of lung development. It may lead to blindness in serious cases, as it did with Ellen.

Ellen's parents noticed her extraordinary musical abilities when she was only six months old. Her sister ran to tell her mother that baby Ellen was singing (Treffert, 2010). When she was seven, her teacher was so impressed by Ellen's musical skills that she urged Ellen's parents to buy their daughter a piano. Ellen also learned to play the guitar by herself. Her musical ability, talent for improvisation and her memory are impressive. She is able to hear a piece of music in one form, like jazz, and transform it in a different genre, like classical. She can memorize a song, no matter how complex, after hearing it just once. Boudreaux's mental repertoire is so large that her mind is said to store hundreds or thousands of songs. Her favorite childhood singers were Frankie Avalon, Chubby Checker, and Elvis Presley, who she always listened to with her sister.

Ellen grew slowly and did not learn to walk until she was four years old. After that, her parents soon observed her incredible sense of spatial location when she walked, despite her blindness: she was, and still is, able to navigate her way around without colliding with objects in her path, making little chirping sounds as she walked that seemed to act as a human sonar. This apparently allowed her to detect objects, fences, and walls in her environment by sensing echoes from those objects and to navigate around them without complications, a process commonly known as biosonar, or echolocation.

Echolocation is a biological sonar used by humans and several animal species, including bats. In the case of humans, someone using echolocation might emit sounds towards their surroundings—lightly stamping their foot, snapping their fingers, or making clicking noises with their mouths—and listen for the echoes of those calls that return from various objects near them. These echoes make it possible to identify objects, determine their size and location, and adapt to one's environment accordingly. The technique is useful mainly for navigation, but in the case of animals it can also be used to search for food and to hunt (White et al., 1970; Griffin 1958; Griffin, 1944). Bats, toothed whales, dolphins, shrews, and cave-dwelling birds frequently use these sonars. Many blind individuals also use it almost automatically. Other notable examples of human users of echolocation are Daniel Kish (Thaler et al., 2017; Arnott et al., 2013; Kish, 2009), Thomas Tajo, Ben Underwood (Henshaw, 2012; Rojas et al., 2009), Tom De Witte (Schulze,

2016), and Lawrence Scadden (Arnott and Alain, 2014). It seems that this ability, like various others typical of savants, is latent in the human brain and is activated or developed spontaneously when the need for it arises.

Ellen herself undoubtedly has multiple skills. At about the age of eight, she developed the extraordinary ability to tell time without looking at the watch. Ellen always knows the hour, the minute, and the second of the day, and when tested she is perfectly accurate. This is truly extraordinary given that no one ever explained to her how time goes by or how a clock works. Even those of us who understand these concepts do not have the ability to state the time of day with such accuracy.

She currently plays with her rock and roll band, the Diremakers, which she is the lead soloist of. She has also had opportunities to perform solo in different venues around the world. For Ellen, music is without a doubt her bridge and connection to the world.

Impairment: Autism, blindness. She was born prematurely and developed retrolental fibroplasias as a result. Ellen did not learn to walk until she was four years old. Her IQ is estimated at 30-50.

Skills: Musician. Astonishing spatial sense. Remarkable memory. Extraordinary ability to tell time without looking at a watch: she knows the hour, minute, and second of the day without seeing a clock, with perfect precision when tested. She can play music perfectly after hearing it just once. Ellen has hundreds or thousands of songs stored in her head.

Below are references, links to some videos, and additional reading about Ellen Boudreaux.

- Thaler, L., Reich, G. M., Zhang, X., Wang, D., Smith, G., Tao, Z., ... and Antoniou, M. (2017). Mouth-clicks used by blind expert human echolocators–signal description and model based signal synthesis. *PLoS computational biology, 13*(8), e1005670.

- Marqués, M. and González, P. (2016). Savants músicos y oído absoluto. http://revistadigital2.csmvalencia.es/wp-content/uploads/2016/05/Savants-m%C3%BAsicos-y-o%C3%ADdo-absoluto.pdf
- Schulze, H. (2016). 10 Sonic Epistemology. *Sound as Popular Culture: A Research Companion*, 111.
- Arnott, S. and Alain, C. (2014). A brain guide to Sound Galleries. *The Multisensory Museum, Cross-Disciplinary Perspectives on Touch, Sound, Smell, Memory, and Space*, 85-108.
- Arnott, S., Thaler, L., Milne, J., Kish, D. and Goodale, M. (2013). Shape-specific activation of occipital cortex in an early blind echolocation expert. *Neuropsychologia*, *51*(5), 938-949.
- Henshaw, J. (2012). *A tour of the senses: how your brain interprets the world.* JHU Press.
- Treffert, D. (2010). *Islands of genius: The bountiful mind of the autistic, acquired, and sudden savant.* Jessica Kingsley Publishers.
- Kish, D. (2009). Human echolocation: How to "see" like a bat. *New Scientist*, *202*(2703), 31-33.
- Rojas, J., Hermosilla, J., Montero, R. and Espí, P. (2009). Physical analysis of several organic signals for human echolocation: oral vacuum pulses. *Acta acustica united with acustica*, *95*(2), 325-330.
- Allen, J. (2005). Perfect. Diremakers. News Review. https://www.newsreview.com/sacramento/diremakers/content?oid=35264
- White, B., Saunders, F., Scadden, L., Bach-Y-Rita, P. and Collins, C. C. (1970). Seeing with the skin. *Perception & Psychophysics*, *7*(1), 23-27.
- Griffin, D. (1958). Listening in the dark: the acoustic orientation of bats and men.
- Griffin, D. (1944). Echolocation by blind men, bats and radar. *Science*, 100(2609), 589-590.
- What is musical savant syndrome? Piano Report. https://pianoreport.com/musical-savant-syndrome/
- Ellen Boudreaux. The savant syndrome. http://thesavantsyndrome.blogspot.com/2014/01/ellen-boudreaux.html
- Autism and Artistic Talent. Study. https://study.com/academy/lesson/autism-artistic-talent.html

- Ellen Boudreaux: https://the-genius-of-autism.fandom.com/wiki/Ellen_Boudreaux
- Ellen Boudreaux performing "The price is right" song: https://www.youtube.com/watch?v=x0CZjefkvxc
- Ellen Boudreaux – The Question Community. https://www.youtube.com/watch?v=ffiK_pM3A8k

5.13 Alonzo Clemons (born 1958)

Alonzo Clemons was born in Colorado in 1958. He is an acquired savant and animal sculptor. He was a normal child, but at age of three, Alonzo suffered a terrible accident that left him with severe brain damage, a learning disability and with an intelligence quotient in the range of 40-50. That moment irrevocably changed the way he could think, learn, communicate, and live. For years, Alonzo was unable to speak, tie his shoes, eat on his own, carry on a simple conversation, or dress himself.

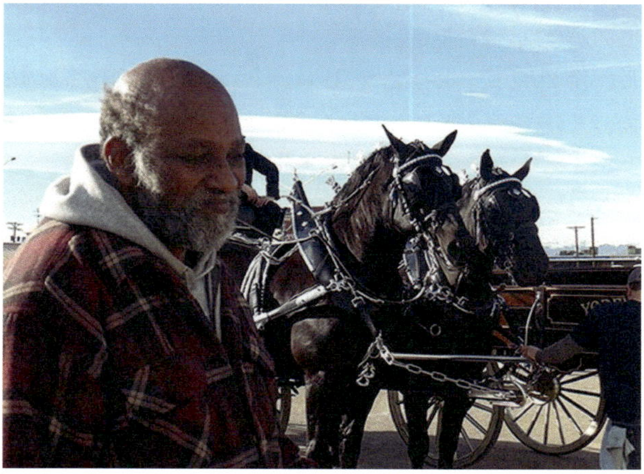

Figure 5.33 Alonzo Clemons.

Photo courtesy of Alonzo Clemons and Nancy Mason.

Alonzo was always good with his hands, but the accident enhanced his skills. He is now a genius at sculpture, particularly in clay, his preferred medium. He liked nothing more than sitting quietly for hours, molding the clay and shaping small animals. As Alonzo sometimes put it, "God gave a gift" (Alonzo Clemons' official website). Alonzo can see a fleeting image of an animal on a television screen only once and from that image he can build a perfect sculpture of an animal—preferably a horse, bull, or antelope—correct in every detail, every fiber and muscle and proportion (Treffert and Wallace, 2002), in less than one hour. His works are generally small in size.

> He has difficulty speaking, and if you ask him how he is able to shape such wonderfully exact figures of animals, without the benefit of models or photographs, he just smiles broadly and slowly taps the side of his head with his forefinger (Schmidt, 1983).

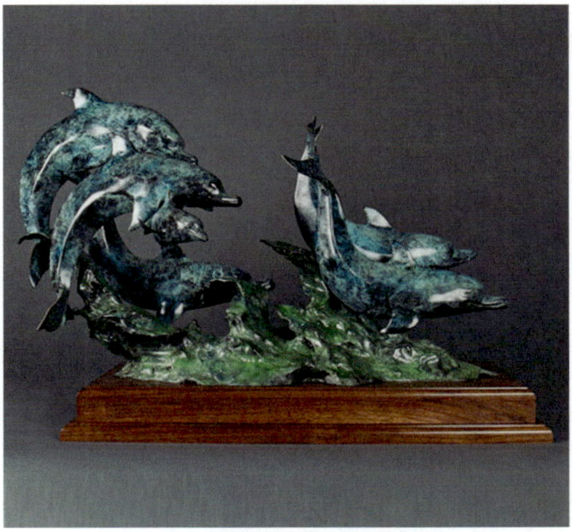

Figure 5.34 Alonzo Clemons. Family Gathering. 26" x 18" x 11".

Photo courtesy of Alonzo Clemons and Nancy Mason.

The starting point of Alonzo's career as a professional sculptor was a premiere exhibit featuring 30 of his bronze sculptures in Aspen, Colorado, in 1986. Pam Driscol, owner of the Driscol Gallery in Aspen remarked that "in a relatively short period of time there has been phenomenal growth. It just doesn't happen that way." One life-size bronze, *Three Frolicking Foals* was recently purchased for display at a building outside Chicago. Alonzo's works

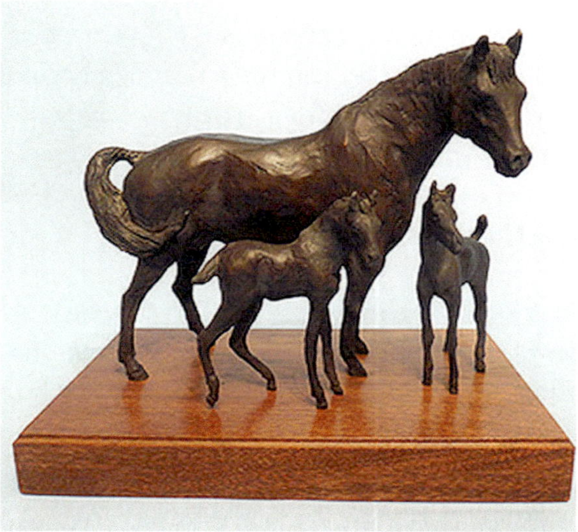

Figure 5.35 Alonzo Clemons. Mare and Two Foals.

Photo courtesy of Alonzo Clemons and Nancy Mason.

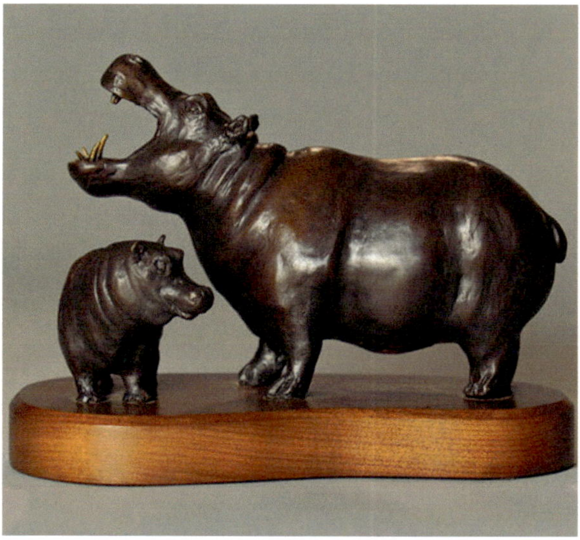

Figure 5.36 Alonzo Clemons. Hippo Momma. 7.5" high x 10" wide x 5.75" deep.

Photo courtesy of Alonzo Clemons and Nancy Mason.

have sold for as much as $45,000. Recently Alonzo has been doing some drawings, which are as impressive as his sculptures.

Alonzo is now considered to be one of the world's most talented sculptors. He is also recognized as a prodigious savant and has been featured on well-known TV programs such as *60 Minutes*, *Geraldo*, and the Discovery Channel's *World of Wonder*. He currently lives in in his own home, with some assistance, in Boulder, Colorado.

Impairment: Acquired savant. At age three, Alonzo suffered severe brain damage from a terrible accident, which left him practically disabled and with an intelligent quotient in the range of 40-50.

Skills: Artistic, photographic memory, sculptor. He has an extraordinary ability for sculpting animals that are full of life, with extraordinary formal accuracy and aesthetic beauty. Alonzo can sculpt an animal in three dimensions from clay or wax simply from seeing a two-dimensional photo, although he likes observing the animals in motion.

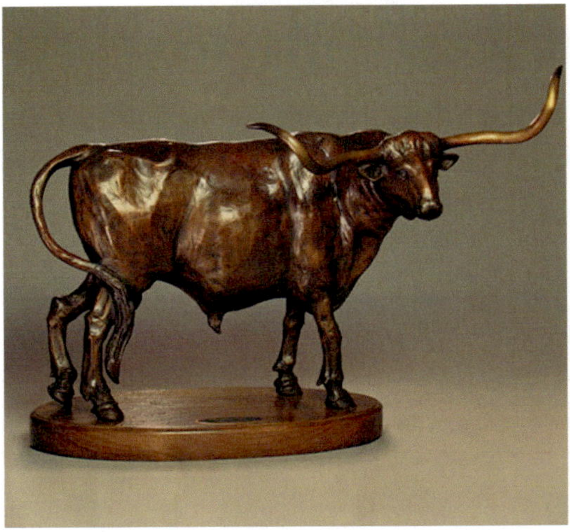

Figure 5.37 Alonzo Clemons. Dollar Bill. 26" long x 19.5" high x 12" deep.

Photo courtesy of Alonzo Clemons and Nancy Mason

Below are references, links to some videos, and additional reading about Alonzo Clemons.

- Alonzo Clemons' official site: https://www.alonzoclemons.com/
- Alonzo Clemons's Facebook: https://www.facebook.com/pg/AlonzoClemmonsA/about/?ref=page_internal
- Alonzo Clemons videos: https://www.alonzoclemons.com/videos
- Inspiration Matters (2017). Alonzo Clemons Interview. https://www.inspirationmatters.org/interviewshow.aspx?name=alonzo%20clemons&id=58&totalrec=8&alpha=a
- Treffert, D. and Rebedew, D. L. (2015). The savant syndrome registry: a preliminary report. *WMJ, 114*(4), 158-162.
- Treffert, D. (2014c). Accidental genius. *Scientific American, 311*(2), 52-57.
- Treffert, D. (2010). *Islands of genius: The bountiful mind of the autistic, acquired, and sudden savant*. Jessica Kingsley Publishers.
- Treffert, D. and Wallace, G. (2002). Islands of genius. *Scientific American, 286*(6), 76-85.
- Barry, A. (1997). *Visual intelligence: Perception, image, and manipulation in visual communication*. SUNY Press.
- Haensly, P. and Reynolds, C. (1989). Creativity and intelligence. In *Handbook of creativity* (pp. 111-132). Springer, Boston, MA.
- Schmidt, W. (1983). *Gifted Retardates: The Search for Clues to Mysterious Talent. The New York Times.* July 12, 1983. https://www.nytimes.com/1983/07/12/science/gifted-retardates-the-search-for-clues-to-mysterious-talent.html
- Savants: A hands-on artist. CBS Sunday Morning. https://www.youtube.com/watch?v=RrW4upZoXHA
- Savant syndrome, Beautiful minds. https://www.youtube.com/watch?v=IkDMaJ-wZmQ
- Alonzo Clemons "Savant, Sculptor and Artist" 05/10/19 https://www.youtube.com/watch?v=HEc-_DNWQG4
- Boulder savant creates inspiring sculptures with national following. https://www.youtube.com/watch?v=8Im71yE9D_s

5.14 George Widener (born 1962)

I greatly appreciate the contributions of Henry Boxer (Henry Boxer Gallery, London) in reviewing this profile.

George Widener was born in Cincinnati, Ohio on February 8, 1962. He is an artist, mnemonist, and calendar savant who uses his mathematical and memory skills to create art ranging from complex calendars and numerical palindromes to Asian scrolls. George showed clear signs of autism as a child. However, autism was not commonly diagnosed at that time, so George lived in uncertainty and difficulty throughout his childhood and youth. He eventually became homeless, living rough on the streets for several years.

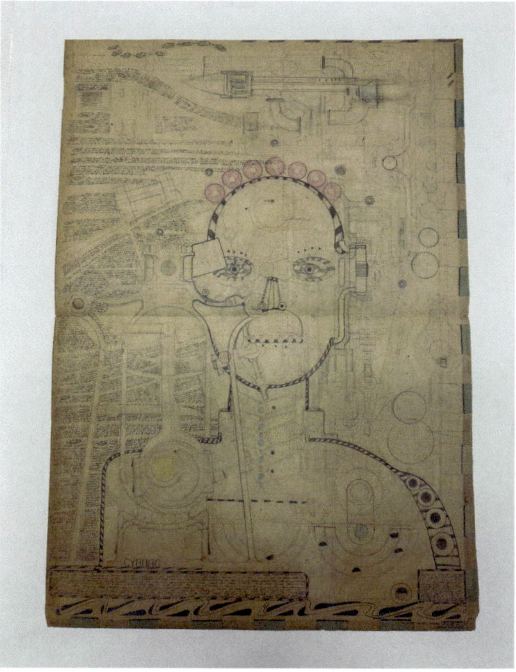

Figure 5.38 George Widener. Cyborg 1. Androgynous Portrait. Ink & crayon on found paper, 30x20 in.

Photo courtesy: Henry Boxer. Henry Boxer Gallery, London.

It was clear that something was definitely amiss, but no one could explain or diagnose what was happening to him. While displaying some autistic behaviors, he also showed skills typical of a gifted child which amazed everyone who knew him, making him something of an enigma. For some time, he was thought to be a depressive schizophrenic, and was wrongly treated for this in his late teenage years (Cardinal, 2009). It was not until George was in his thirties that he was finally diagnosed as suffering from Asperger syndrome, something he now accepts.

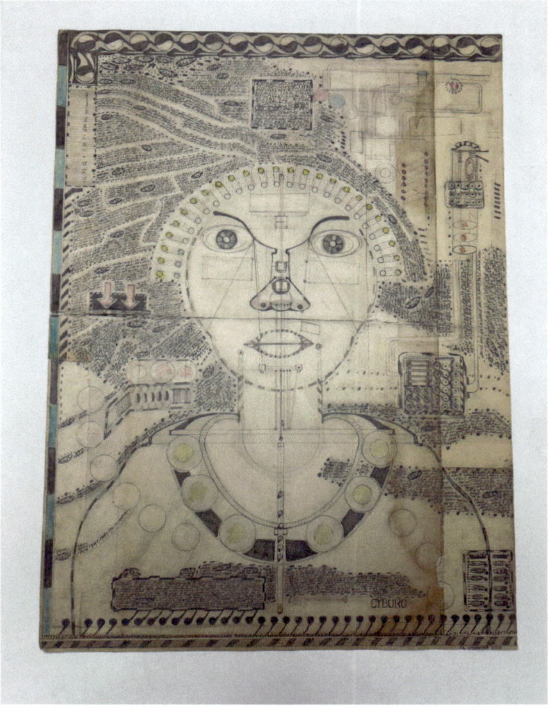

Figure 5.39 George Widener. Cyborg 2. Androgynous Portrait. Ink & crayon on found paper, 30x20 in.

Photo courtesy: Henry Boxer. Henry Boxer Gallery, London.

George wrote about these two pieces: *"This 'Androgynous Portrait' is a vision of a futuristic mechanical cyborg entity drawn on a rare 19th century paper used at Brooklyn iron works.* Hence my thoughts of a different time being superimposed on future time. *The dates are 1860/70's, then jump forward to 2260/70's – when cyborgs are real."*

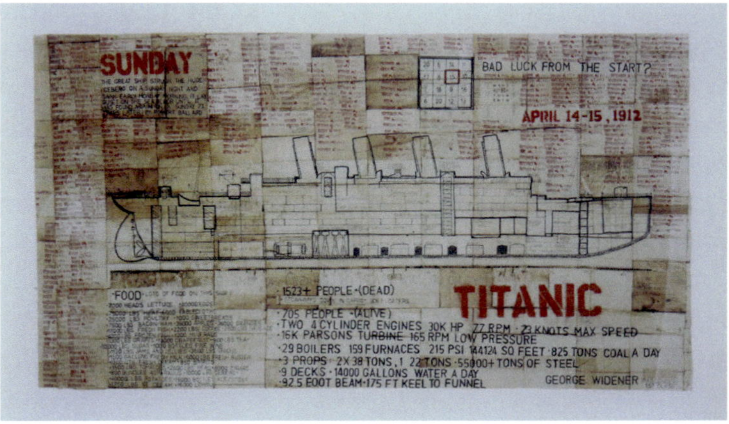

Figure 5.40 George Widener. Titanic' 2004. Ink on found paper. 25x42 in.

Photo courtesy: Henry Boxer. Henry Boxer Gallery, London.

George exhibited exceptional arithmetical skill and a phenomenal photographic memory. He developed a passion for calendars, numbers, and numerology. He could memorize the days and historical dates dating back to the year 180 AD and forward for the next 80,000 years. He was also a specialist in recalling statistical data from population censuses. George was definitely many things, but perhaps what best defined him was his compulsive drawing.

When he was 18 years old, George joined US military intelligence, where he worked analyzing photos from the Stasi and the KGB, drawing on his remarkable ability to recognize patterns. He also advised the British army during the Falklands War (Bellos, 2013). He was later accepted to study engineering at the University of Texas, but ended up abandoning this project because his head was so busy with numbers and calendars that he had no time for anything else. George's life was such a whirlwind that he ended up living on the street, until he was admitted to a hospital and diagnosed with Asperger syndrome. Suddenly, he had an explanation for what was happening to him, and for his obsession with dates. From that moment on, everything changed. Through painting, George found both a mode of expression and a meaning in life.

George paints numbers, cities, maps, machines, and magic squares that give aesthetic and visible form to highly complex, never-before-seen calculations, based mainly on dates and historical events, "usually those of catastrophic events, such as the sinking of the Titanic" (Cardinal, 2009). His world revolves around numbers, calendars date and magic squares that he calls "magic time squares." Everything is there. "Other kids lined toys up in a row," he has said. "I lined up dates" (Bellos, 2013).

Numbers and data are how George perceives the world. As a young man he created more than a thousand drawings, but did not share with others until he was in his thirties.

Today, George has exhibited in renowned art galleries all over the world, including the Jan Krugier Gallery in Geneva, Switzerland, famed for its relationship to the works of Pablo Picasso, the Kunsthaus Kannen in Münster, Germany, and the Salon du Dessins Contemporain in Paris, France. Art critic Roberta Smith proclaimed him to be "one of the Outsider Art Fair's most significant recent discoveries" (Henry Boxer Gallery). George has also been featured in Roger Cardinal's book *The Art of George Widener*. His work can be found in many private and public collections around the world, such us the ABCD Collection (Paris, France), the UC Davis M.I.N.D. Institute (California, USA), The Collection de l'Art Brut (Lausanne, Switzerland), The American Folk Art Museum (New York, USA), The Museum of Everything (London, UK), and The Kröller-Müller Museum (Hoge Veluwe National Park in Otterlo, Netherlands), which is also home to the world's second largest collection of paintings by Vincent van Gogh. He has also been featured on *Nova ScienceNow* ("How Smart Can We Get?"), and on the Science Channel's *Ingenious Minds* ("George Widener"). George was also a subject of the 2007 documentary film *My Brilliant Brain: Accidental Genius*. He is currently represented by the Henry Boxer Gallery in London and by the Ricco/Maresca Gallery in New York.

George Widener currently lives in Waynesville, in the mountains of North Carolina. He continues to create his unique artwork, much of which is based on preliminary sketches taken from notebooks and diaries which he carries with him everywhere. His drawings are to be found in numerous museum and public collections around the world, these include The Collection de l'Art Brut, Lausanne, The Museum of Everything, London, and The American Folk Art Museum in New York. He is happy to be able to draw daily and be in the company of his numbers. He is also developing codes for super-intelligent computers of the future.

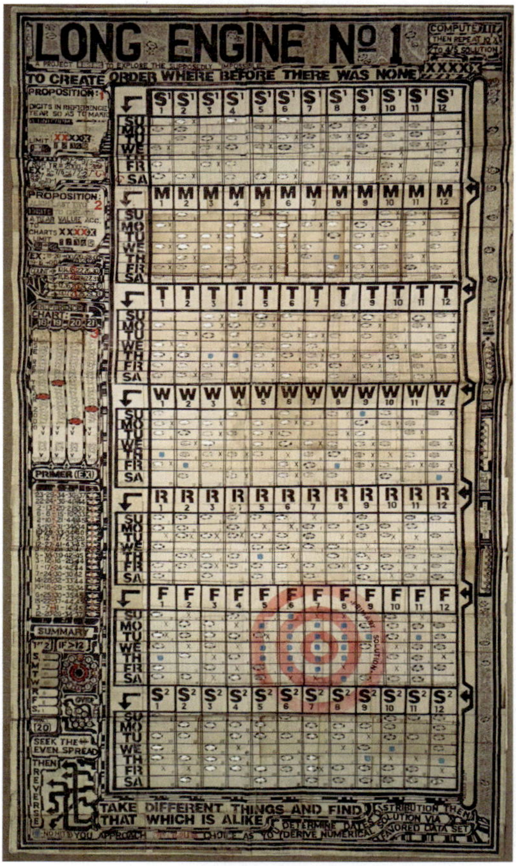

Figure 5.41 George Widener. Long Engine No. 1. Ink 65 x 40 in.

Photo courtesy: Henry Box. Henry Box Gallery, London.

> Influenced by the theories of Ray Kurzweil, a leading scientist in the field of artificial intelligence, Widener believes that in 2045, high-performance computers will fuse with the human brain and transform consciousness into software (Safarova, 2013).

George is considered by some to be the most important outsider artist the world has seen. He travels abroad whenever he can.

Impairments: Asperger syndrome. Permanently obsessed with numbers, dates, calendars, and patterns.

Skills: Artist, painter, mnemonist, photographic memory, calendar calculator, astonishing arithmetical skills. George can memorize the days and historical dates dating back to 180 AD and as far ahead as 80,000 years in the future. He is a specialist in recalling statistical data from population censuses. Compulsive draftsman.

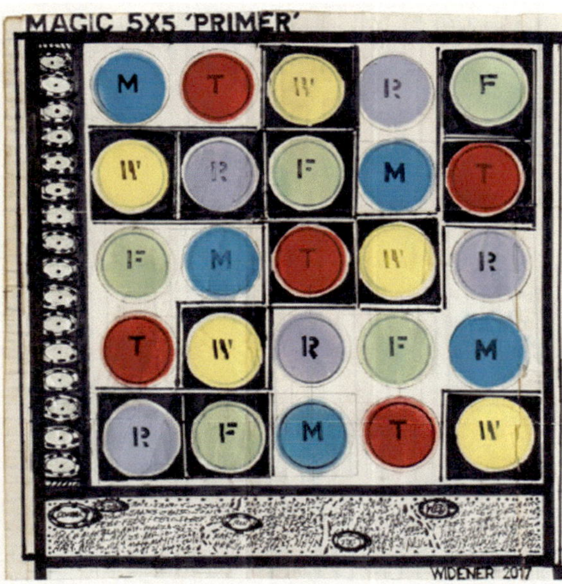

Figure 5.42 George Widener. Magic Circles 2017. Mixed media on paper. 24x25 in.

Photo courtesy: Henry Box. Henry Box Gallery, London.

Below are references, links to some videos, and additional reading about George Widener.

- Henry Boxer Gallery. https://www.outsiderart.co.uk/
- Wexler, A. (2020). Autism and outsiderism: The art of George Widener. *International Journal of Education Through Art, 16*(1), 83-99.
- Safarova, B. (2013). George Widener: Secret Universe IV Paperback. Walther König, Köln; Bilingual edition.
- Bellos, A. (2013). George Widener: the incredible life of the man who makes art for robots. https://www.theguardian.com/science/alexs-adventures-in-numberland/2013/jun/17/mathematics
- Treffert, D. (2010). *Islands of genius: The bountiful mind of the autistic, acquired, and sudden savant.* Jessica Kingsley Publishers.
- Cardinal, R. (2009). Outsider Art and the autistic creator. *Philosophical Transactions of the Royal Society B: Biological Sciences, 364*(1522), 1459-1466.
- Cardinal, R. and Rhodes, C. (2009). The art of George Widener. Oculeum. Henry Boxer Gallery. https://www.blurb.co.uk/b/570362-the-art-of-george-widener
- Gómez, E. (2009). On the Border. *Art & Antiques Magazine,* February Issue.
- Cardinal, R. (2005). The calendars of George Widener. *Raw Vision, 51,* 42-47.
- Smith, R. (2005). Untamed Art From the Fringes Is a Gust of Bracing Air. The New York Times. January 28, 2005. https://www.nytimes.com/2005/01/28/arts/design/untamed-art-from-the-fringes-is-a-gust-of-bracing-air.html
- Savants: Mark your calendar. https://www.youtube.com/watch?v=afrBJM0n12g
- George Widener's videos: http://bethanymissiongallery.org/george-widener/
- George Widener. https://www.youtube.com/watch?v=8xiOdRkTCeU
- Savants: Mark your calendar. https://www.youtube.com/watch?v=afrBJM0n12g
- Delmes & Zander – "George Widener" (2008/14') by Bruno Decharme. https://m.facebook.com/DelmesZander/videos/1860496471092/

5.15 Christopher (born 1962)

Christopher (henceforth C) was born in England on January 6, 1962. He is an autistic, hyper polyglot savant who developed proficiency to speak, write, and translate, between 15 and 20 languages with varying degrees of expertise. C was born with brain damage, possibly as a consequence of hydrocephaly. "His mother was 45 years old when he was born, the pregnancy was problematic, and (for reasons that are not clear) the parents were told when C was six months of age that he was brain damaged" (Bates, 1997).

Hydrocephalus is an abnormal buildup of cerebrospinal fluid in the ventricles of the brain. The fluid is under increased pressure inside the skull and can compress and damage the brain. Probably because of this, C has severe apraxia, a motor disorder that involves difficulty in carrying out tasks or movements when requested, even when the order is understood and there is the desire and the physical capacity to do it. An MRI scan taken in 1993 showed "a moderate cerebral atrophy with wide sulci over both hemispheres" (Bonatti, 1998). In other words, "there is no evidence for localized brain injury, although C's brain is unusual in size and shape" (Bates, 1997).

C was late in walking and talking, although this is compatible with both autism and hydrocephalus. He is also quite short-sighted. He has also deficits in key areas such as communication skills and visuo-spatial cognition (Morgan et al., 2002). C lives in an institution for the mentally disabled because he cannot properly communicate with others, is unable to take care of himself, and has severe difficulties in non-verbal cognitive domains (Morgan et al., 2007).

Despite all these difficulties, C is also brilliant in the domain of language, such much so that he is considered a hyper polyglot savant. Around the age of three, he began to show an extreme interest in language, an obsession with technical books and impressive reading ability. Around six or seven years old, he began to exhibit a fascination with foreign languages. This coincided with the 1968 Olympic Games in Mexico, which were shown on television. C was mesmerized by the images of athletes participating from all around the world, speaking in different languages.

Today he can speak, write, and translate more than twenty languages with varying degrees of expertise. These languages include Germanic languages such as Danish, Dutch, and German; Romance languages such as French, Italian, Portuguese, and Spanish; as well as Polish, Finnish, Greek, Hindi, Turkish, Welsh, Russian, Norwegian, and even Epun, an artificial language with peculiar properties that does not exist in the real world and thus could not be acquired by any normal child (Bates, 1997). Additionally, he can identify other languages from their spelling or alphabet, such as Bengali, Chinese, Czech, Arabic, Hebrew, Japanese, Icelandic, and Gujarati. C learned these languages mainly from native speakers who used them in his presence or through self-study materials, but without any formal training or education whatsoever.

C is clearly one of the most well-studied cases of linguistic savant syndrome. What makes linguistic savants in general, and C's case in particular, so rare is that the left hemisphere—the damaged hemisphere, in savants—is mainly responsible for language skills. Therefore, damage to the left hemisphere can be expected to cause a deficit in all language-related abilities. Thus, as Ammari (2011) stated, "the acquisition of languages would be out of question in the case of savants, since it is purely a left-brain function." Bates (1997) suggested that this characterization raises an important question: is C a linguistic savant, or simply a man with exceptional language skills who is at the same time severely impaired in visual and spatial terms? To date, although we can never underestimate the brain's plasticity or its ability to reorganize and adapt as a result of experience, we have no perfect answer to this question.

Whatever the case, there is no doubt that we have reached a temporary state in which we tend to group all individuals with intellectual impairments who also possess extraordinary abilities, under the same umbrella.

Impairment: Autistic, hydrocephalus, apraxic. Mentally retarded. Nonverbal IQ: 49-76. Verbal IQ: 89-102. Severe difficulties in his motor system and non-verbal cognitive domains. He was late in walking and talking.

Skills: Hyper polyglot savant. Can speak, write, and translate more than twenty languages with varying degrees of knowledge. These languages include Germanic languages such as Danish, Dutch, and German; Romance languages such as French, Italian, Portuguese, and Spanish; as well as Polish, Finnish, Greek, Hindi, Turkish, Welsh, Russian, Norwegian, and even Epun. Furthermore, he can identify other languages from their spelling or alphabet, such as Bengali, Chinese, Czech, Arabic, Hebrew, Japanese, Icelandic, and Gujarati.

Below are references, links to some videos, and additional reading about C.

- Hyltenstam, K. (2016b). The exceptional ability of polyglots to achieve high-level proficiency in numerous languages. *Advanced Proficiency and Exceptional Ability in Second Languages. Boston, MA: De Gruyter Mouton*, 241-272.
- Grover, V. (2015). Autistic Savants: Making Child Really Special. *International Journal of Science and Research*, *4*(1), 1824-1827.
- Ammari, E. (2011). Prodigious Polyglot Savants: The Enigmatic Adjoining of Language Acquisition and Emaciated Potentials. *International Journal of Business and Social Science*, 2(7).
- Smith, N., Tsimpli, I., Morgan, G. and Woll, B. (2010). *The signs of a savant: Language against the odds*. Cambridge University Press.
- Wallace, G. (2008). Neuropsychological studies of savant skills: Can they inform the neuroscience of giftedness? *Roeper Review*, *30*(4), 229-246.
- Morgan, G., Smith, N., Tsimpli, I. and Woll, B. (2007). Classifier learning and modality in a polyglot savant. *Lingua*, *117*(7), 1339-1353.
- Pring, L. (2005). Savant talent. *Developmental Medicine & Child Neurology*, *47*(7), 500-503.
- Morgan, G., Smith, N., Tsimpli, I. and Woll, B. (2002). Language against the odds: The learning of British Sign Language by a polyglot savant. *Journal of Linguistics*, 1-41.
- Pring, L. and Hermelin, B. (2002). Numbers and letters: exploring an autistic savant's unpractised ability. *Neurocase*, *8*(4), 330-337.
- Bonatti, L. (1998). Neil Smith and Ianthi-Maria Tsimpli, The mind of a savant: language learning and modularity. Oxford: Basil Blackwell, 1995. Pp. xviii+ 243. *Journal of Linguistics*, *34*(1), 227-297.

- Bates, E. (1997). On language savants and the structure of the mind. *International Journal of Bilingualism, 1*, 163-179.
- Smith, N. and Tsimpli, I. (1995). *The mind of a savant: Language learning and modularity*. Blackwell Publishing.
- O'Connor, N., Smith, N., Frith, C. and Tsimpli, I. M. (1994). Neuropsychology and linguistic talent. *Journal of Neurolinguistics, 8*(2), 95-107.
- Smith, N., Tsimpli, I. and Ouhalla, J. (1993). Learning the impossible: The acquisition of possible and impossible languages by a polyglot savant. *Lingua, 91*(4), 279-347.

5.16 Derek Amato (born 1966)

I greatly appreciate the contributions of Derek Amato in reviewing this profile.

Derek Amato was born in United States on November 19, 1966. He is an acquired savant and a prominent musician. Derek received a severe head injury on October 27, 2006, at the age of 40, and became a pianist and composer soon afterwards. He represents one of the very few cases of an acquired savant becoming a musician. Most acquired savants are artists, particularly painters.

Derek was a normal boy, without any special talents. In his youth, he played a number of sports, including baseball, football, basketball, wrestling, and even kung fu. Derek liked to play the guitar, which he had learned by ear. He learned a few chords to play AC/DC songs. He held some jobs. In an interview with NPR, Derek said:

> I was a pretty typical, aggressive businessperson. I was making great money by going to work and chasing the almighty dollar, and then I'd come home and go to bed and do it all over again the next day (NPR: Snap Judgement, 2014).

One day, Derek was enjoying a pool party with friends. He went running along the side of the pool, and he dove in towards the shallow end. That was the moment that changed his life. The severity of the blow to his head left him unconscious. He was diagnosed with a major concussion with no bleeding and

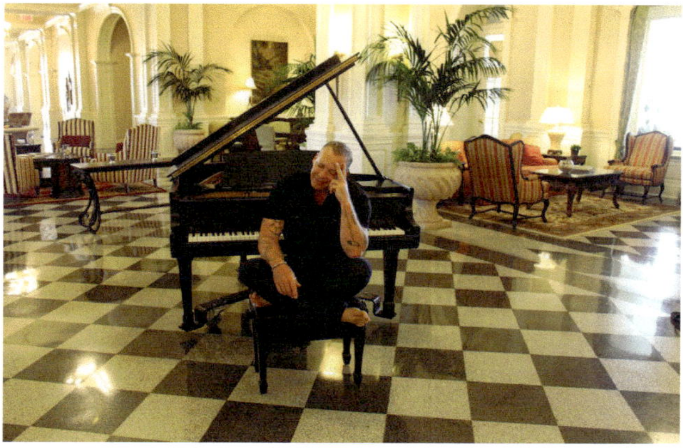

Figure 5.43 Derek Amato.

Photo courtesy of Derek Amato.

was sent to his mother's house to rest. The blow caused him to lose 35% of his hearing and gave him a form of synesthesia. Most importantly, it also gave him the ability to play the piano and become a composer.

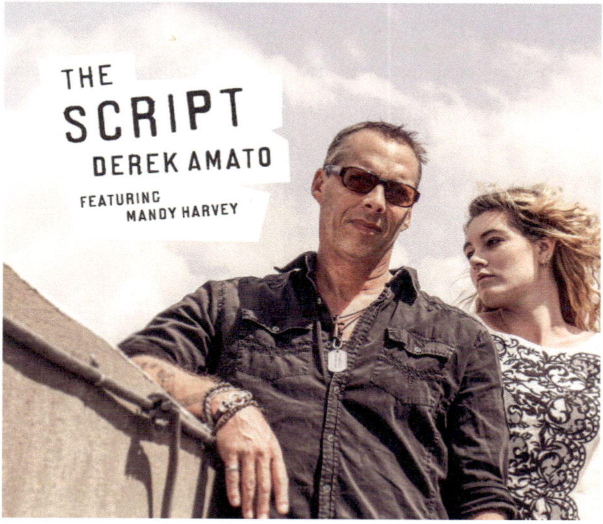

Figure 5.44 The Script (feat. Mandy Harvey). Derek Amato, January 2010.

Photo courtesy of Derek Amato.

A few days after his accident, Derek went to his best friend Rick's house. Rick is a musician who lives in an apartment full of musical instruments. Derek spied an electronic keyboard and sat down to play. The results were astonishing: in the blink of an eye, he had become a musical genius. Derek does not know exactly where the music is coming from, nor can he explain what key he should play to perform a song. He just knows that when he starts to play, his fingers begin to fly across the keys with ease. He has never had a single lesson. It just happened. "My hands took off like fire," Derek says (Rehagen, 2016). His mind basically creates a wave pattern of black and white squares which tell his hands where to go. The doctors refer to this as synesthesia, a combination of senses that allows Derek to see the music he is composing through the black and white squares. He sees it in his head, and his fingers do the rest. Derek went home and asked his mother to accompany him to a music store, where he sat down at a piano and began to play. His mother cried. It was a miracle.

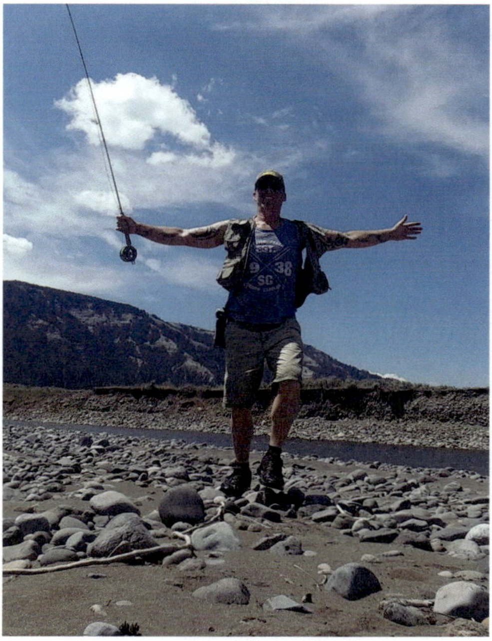

Figure 5.45 Fishing: Derek Amato.

Photo courtesy of Derek Amato.

Derek has performed on *The Today Show*, *The Steve Harvey Show*, The Discovery Channel, and NPR, and has been featured in articles in newspapers across the world. He currently lives in Colorado and is the father of three children. When he is not playing or composing, he loves fly fishing, and he advocates for several charitable organizations throughout the United States. Derek is today an accomplished professional musician and has recently released "The Script," a successful single you can download from iTunes or YouTube. Derek has a great gift, but somehow he perceives that just as it came upon him without explanation, it could leave him again without warning.

Impairments: Acquired savant. Synesthetic. Derek received a severe head injury and became a pianist and composer soon afterwards.

Skills: Musician, pianist, composer. His mind basically creates a wave pattern of black and white square, which tell his hands where to go. Amato sees the music in his head, and his fingers do the rest.

Below are references, links to some videos, and additional reading about Derek Amato.

- Derek Amato's official website: https://derekamato.wordpress.com/
- Derek Amato on Facebook: https://www.facebook.com/derekamatolive/
- Derek Amato on Instagram: https://www.instagram.com/derekamato/
- Derek Amato videos: https://derekamato.wordpress.com/media/

- Rehagen, T. (2016). Uncharted Waters. Southwest, pp56-59. October 2016. https://issuu.com/southwestmag/docs/oct2016/60?e=18825507%2F39247819
- Treffert, D. (2014c). Accidental genius. *Scientific American, 311*(2), 52-57.
- Wilkinson, D. (2014). A Half Deaf Guy Had a Head Injury and Now He's Amazing at Piano. March 6, 2014. https://www.vice.com/da/article/rnvpgx/youneedtohearthis-a-half-deaf-guy-had-a-head-injury-and-now-hes-amazing-at-piano-derek-amato

- NPR: Snap Judgement (2014). Sudden Savant. January 17, 2014. https://www.npr.org/2014/01/17/263364530/sudden-savant
- Amato. D. (2013). My Beautiful Disaster: My Brain Injury, My Gift, My Life. CreateSpace Independent Publishing Platform (January 1, 2014). Amazon.
- Brogaard, B. and Marlow, K. (2013). Hearing colours. *The Philosophers' Magazine*, (63), 28-35.
- Neal, M. (2012). 'Acquired savant' Derek Amato becomes musical prodigy after hitting his head hard diving into shallow end of pool. New York Daily News. June 7, 2012. https://www.nydailynews.com/news/national/acquired-savant-derek-amato-musical-prodigy-hitting-head-hard-diving-shallow-pool-article-1.1091812
- Amato, D. (2012). Experience: a head injury made me a musical prodigy. The Guardian. October 12, 2012. https://www.theguardian.com/lifeandstyle/2012/oct/12/experience-head-injury-musical-prodigy
- Derek Amato Featuring Mandy Harvey Perform "The Script" https://www.youtube.com/watch?v=rDDZMVaEwLE
- The Script (LIVE) | Mandy Harvey & Derek Amato (ft. Denver Philharmonic Orchestra). https://www.youtube.com/watch?v=hE5qaHsDJJ4
- Derek Amato, Sudden Musical Genius | HUMAN Limits. https://www.youtube.com/watch?v=GTHDuZo7G3Y
- Derek Amato: I Am Savant. https://www.youtube.com/watch?v=wgV5rcZtETg
- My Beautiful Disaster | Derek Amato | TEDxMiddlebury. https://www.youtube.com/watch?v=hxggorYIeWo
- Good News: Derek & Mandy. https://www.youtube.com/watch?v=-8U-TpnC
- 'Beautiful Disaster': Head Injury Reveals Hidden Talent. CVS Denver. February 10, 2019. https://denver.cbslocal.com/2019/02/10/derek-amato-acquired-savant-syndrome-piano/
- Amato musical savant: https://www.youtube.com/watch?v=0TpWerAMIxQ&t=8s
- Derek Amato: The Musical Savant. CBS. Radio. 8:13. https://www.cbc.ca/player/play/2314570947

5.17 Nadia Chomyn (1967-2015)

Nadia Chomyn was born on October 24, 1967, in Nottingham, England, and died in relative anonymity, following a brief illness at the age of 48, on October 28, 2015. She was autistic and an artistic savant with severe learning difficulties. Her parents were Ukrainian refugees, both with degrees in science, who moved to England in 1960. Nadia was never able to use language in a conventional way or live independently.

Nadia appeared healthy at birth, but after only a few months, her parents knew something was wrong. Nadia was a passive baby with poor muscle tone. She was unable to walk on her own until the age of two (Selfe, 2015). Although she began to pronounce single words at around nine months of age, she then stopped speaking until about the age of seven. She needed help getting dressed and feeding herself. She suffered uncontrollable episodes of screaming and destructive behavior. Nadia would often remain immobile, staring into the void, for extended periods of time.

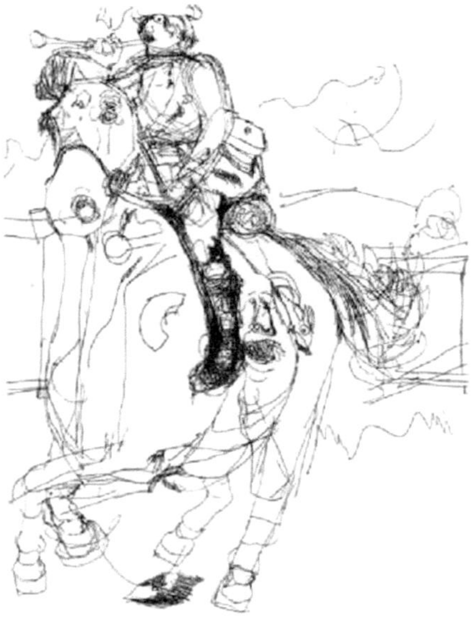

Figure 5.46 A horse and rider drawn by Nadia Chomyn when she was five.

Photo courtesy of Geoff Harrison Art.

Nadia's grandmother, herself described as introverted and sparing in her words, cared for Nadia when Nadia's mother went back to work and again when she was hospitalized for breast cancer. After Nadia's mother's operation and convalescence at home, mother and daughter spent many hours together, which is when her mother discovered Nadia's talent. At the age of five, Nadia was formally diagnosed with autism, echolalia, severe motor coordination disorder, and cognitive retardation. Around this time, Nadia's case was brought to the attention of Lorna Selfe at the University of Nottingham, who witnessed Nadia's remarkable painting abilities.

When Nadia was three years old, she began to draw animals, people, and objects with amazing mastery, incredible realism, proportion, and perspective, without any training and only from her photographic memory. Pariser (1981) said that "the most striking and unconventional feature of Nadia's work was her dexterous use of line and her sensitivity to optical detail."

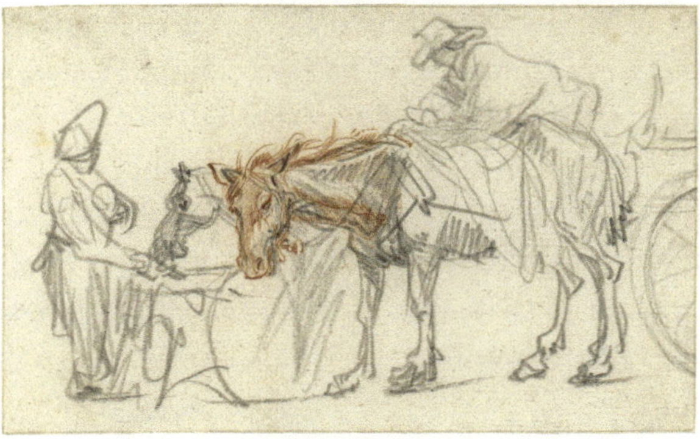

Figure 5.47 Two Horses at a Halting-place, Rembrandt van Rijn, c. 1637

Photo courtesy of Rijksmuseum. https://www.rijksmuseum.nl/en/collection/RP-T-1961-77

Nadia's work suffered a qualitative decline by age nine, which coincided with the period in which she began to improve her social skills and vocabulary. Her works became cartoon-like rather than naturalistic (Pariser, 1981). It seems that efforts to improve her autism came at the expense of her exceptional artistic ability. This leads one to wonder if an intervention in children with autism can provoke, in some cases, a parallel loss of other abilities. Nadia was moved to a residential care unit when was a young adult (Selfe, 2015).

Nadia's works surprised the art community because until that time there had been no reported cases of autism with a prodigious talent in painting at such a young age. That was what was so striking: a very young autistic child who could draw like Rembrandt. Psychologist Lorna Selfe (1977) first drew attention to Nadia's drawing in a case study, then in subsequent articles (Selfe, 1983; Selfe, 1995) and finally a book (Selfe, 2012). The psychiatrist Oliver Sacks and the psychologist Howard Gardner have discussed her work and written about her. Uta Frith commented that Nadia's case "is unique in the history of autism and in the history of outsider art" (Selfe, 2015). The Bethlehem Museum of the Mind in London holds over 200 of Nadia's works.

Impairment: Severe autism, mentally retarded. Nadia was unresponsive and withdrawn, showed impassivity, slow and poorly coordinated movements, and poor motor control. She was unable to dress herself or handle a knife and fork to eat, rarely made eye contact, and had no communicative speech or any form of social engagement until the age of seven.

Skills: Artist, painter. She developed an extraordinary ability to draw detailed depictions of horses and horsemen with a high degree of accuracy and style, marked by remarkable visual realism. Nadia never used an eraser, even to erase a tiny detail in a complex drawing.

Below are references, links to some videos, and additional reading about Nadia Chomyn.

- Dabell, J. (2019). Nadia's Drawings. January 5, 2019. https://johndabell.com/2019/01/05/nadias-drawings/
- Selfe, L. (2015). Nadia Chomyn obituary. The Guardian, December 9 2015. https://www.theguardian.com/artanddesign/2015/dec/09/nadia-chomyn
- Selfe, L. (2012). *Nadia revisited: A longitudinal study of an autistic savant.* Psychology Press.

- Pariser, D. and Zimmerman, E. (2004). Learning in the visual arts: Characteristics of gifted and talented individuals. *Handbook of research and policy in art education*, 379-405.
- Smolka, J. and Fox, D. (2002). The Inner Savant. Discover Magazine. February 1, 2002. https://www.discovermagazine.com/mind/the-inner-savant
- Selfe, L. (1995). Nadia reconsidered. *The development of artistically gifted children*, 197-237.
- Henley, D. (1989). Nadia revisited: A study into the nature of regression in the autistic savant syndrome. *Art Therapy*, 6(2), 43-56.
- Selfe, L. (1983). *Normal and anomalous representational drawing ability in children*. Academic Press, 1983.
- Pariser, D. (1981). Nadia's drawings: Theorizing about an autistic child's phenomenal ability. *Studies in Art Education*, 22(2), 20-31.
- Paine, S. (1981). *Six children draw*. Academic Press.
- Rayala, M. (1981). On "Nadia's Drawings: Theorizing about an Autistic Child's Phenomenal Ability". *Studies in Art Education*, 22(2), 70-72.
- Park, C. (1978). Review of Nadia: a case of extraordinary drawing ability in an autistic child. *Journal of Autism and Childhood Schizophrenia*, 8(4), 457-472.
- Selfe, L. (1977). *Nadia: A case of extraordinary drawing ability in an autistic child*. Academic Press.
- Nadia's Story Part 1 of 3 https://www.youtube.com/watch?v=MfaKeAUVcpg
- Nadia's Story Part 2 of 3 https://www.youtube.com/watch?v=txePA6kUskw

5.18 Patrick Fagerberg (born 1969)

I greatly appreciate the contributions of Patrick Fagerberg in reviewing this profile.

Patrick Fagerberg is an acquired savant and a passionate artist. He worked for 13 years as a successful attorney specializing in criminal law in Austin, Texas, never losing a case during his career. On March 19, 2011, Patrick went to see his favorite band, Orchestral Manoeuvres in the Dark (sometimes shortened to OMD), in concert at Stubbs Walter Creek Amphitheatre in Austin. There, a fluke accident happened: a 400-pound camera crane collapsed, crashing down onto Patrick's head (Patrick Fagerberg's official website). He suffered extensive injury to the left hemisphere of his brain, resulting in memory loss and language processing problems. "Two days later, I couldn't put sentences together. I knew I was in trouble," Patrick says (Tommaney, 2015).

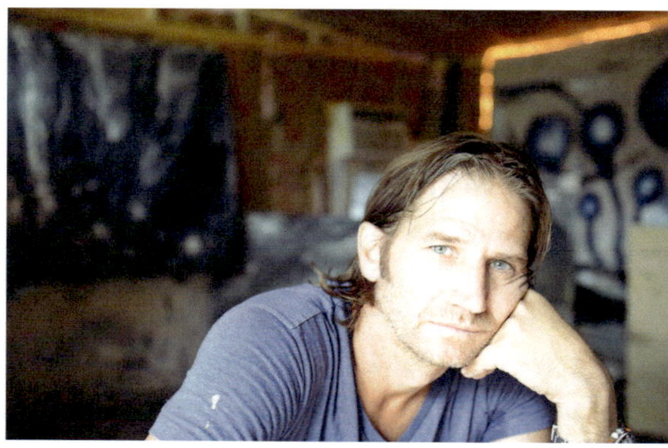

Figure 5.48 Patrick Fagerberg. Photo courtesy of Patrick Fagerberg.

When Patrick eventually regained consciousness, something had changed in his head. His life would never be the same: he could no longer work as a lawyer because he could not competently carry out the activities that his profession required, but his creative side had awoken in dramatic and unexpected ways.

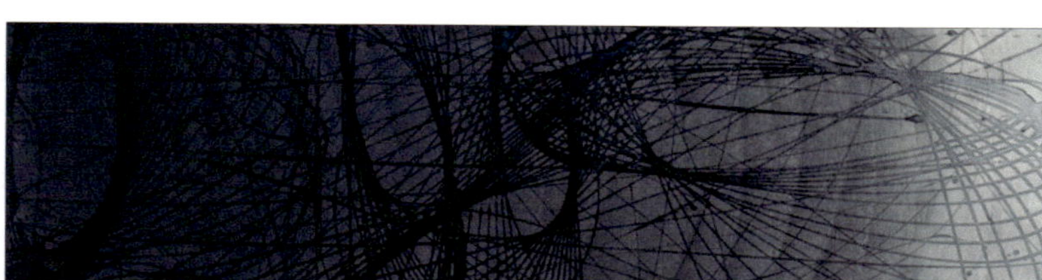

Figure 5.49 Patrick Fagerberg, 1200 x 322 in, 2014. (fagerbergart.com)

Photo courtesy of Patrick Fagerberg.

After a dark period that included problems with drugs and alcohol, Patrick began to attend a therapy class, and after the first class, he could not stop painting. He had no previous experience with or attraction to art, but he began to paint compulsively, 12 to 14 hours a day, and was making excellent copies of painters like Munch and Van Gogh. Soon, he was producing original works (Tommaney, 2015). Fine art had saved his life.

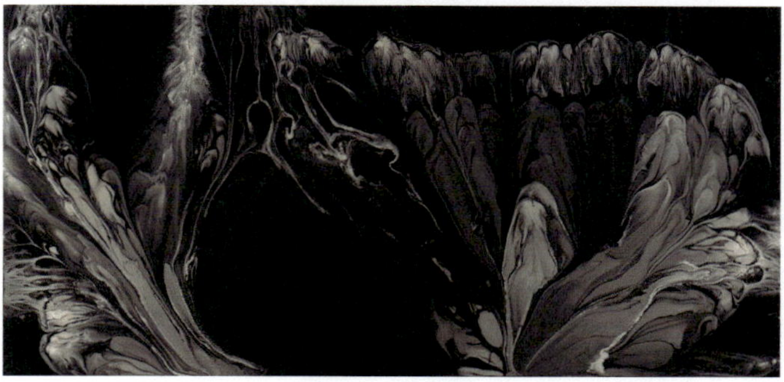

Figure 5.50 Patrick Fagerberg, 960 x 475 in, 2016. (fagerbergart.com)

Photo courtesy of Patrick Fagerberg.

Patrick's brilliant works, which always have mathematical connotations, have evolved to depict fractals and organic forms. His paintings are known for their magnificent abstraction in shades of whites and blacks, with infinite gradations in gray, an art of painting in which aesthetic elements seem to sing despite the somber palette. His works are exhibited at the Gremillon Gallery in Austin, Texas.

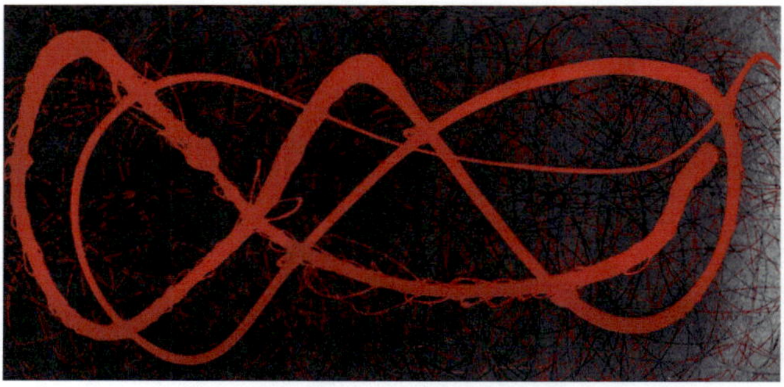

Figure 5.51 Patrick Fagerberg, 1200 x 594 in, 2014. (fagerbergart.com)

Photo courtesy of Patrick Fagerberg.

In recent years, Patrick has decided to pursue electric surfboarding, shifting his newfound creativity to e-transportation (rodasurf.com). He holds the patent for the first vehicle with asymmetrical wheel placement.

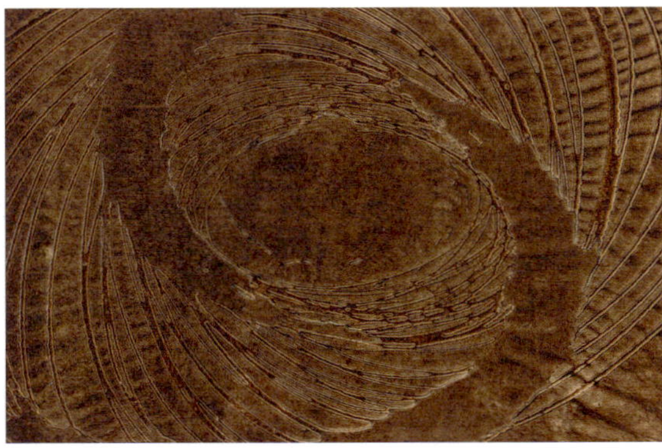

Figure 5.52 Patrick Fagerberg, 1200 x 895 in, 2014. (fagerbergart.com)

Photo courtesy of Patrick Fagerberg.

Impairments: Acquired savant. He suffered an extensive injury to the left hemisphere of his brain, resulting in memory loss and language processing problems.

Skills: Art, painting. His paintings are notable for their abstraction and mathematical connotations.

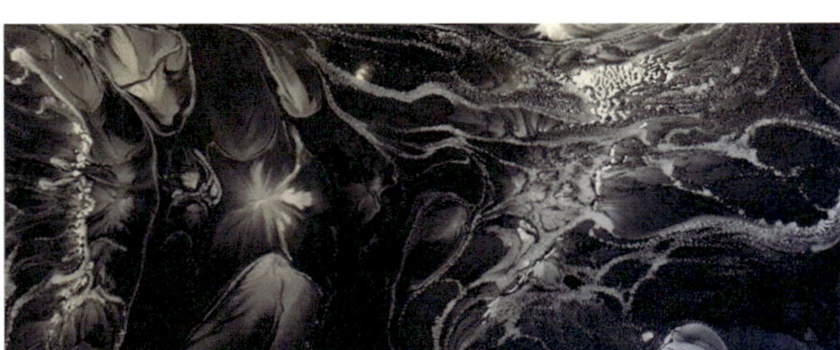

Figure 5.53 Patrick Fagerberg (fagerbergart.com)

Photo courtesy of Patrick Fagerberg.

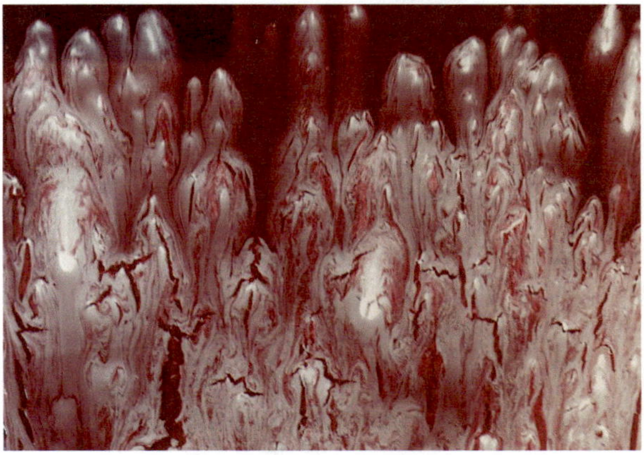

Figure 5.54 Patrick Fagerberg (Fagerberg's Facebook page)

Photo courtesy of Patrick Fagerberg.

Below are references, links to some videos, and additional reading about Patrick Fagerberg.

- Patrick Fagerberg's official website: https://www.patrickfagerberg.com/
- Patrick Fagerberg art: http://www.fagerbergart.com/WordPress/
- Facebook page: https://www.facebook.com/patrickfagerbergart/
- Roda Riders | Roda Surf. https://www.rodasurf.com/roda-riders
- Gremillion Gallery: https://www.gremillion.com/patrickfagerberg
- Nevins, T. (2017). Brain Injury Transforms Prominent Attorney into Impassioned Artist—Patrick Fagerberg. Medium. April 11, 2017. https://medium.com/@toddnevins/brain-injury-transforms-prominent-attorney-into-impassioned-artist-patrick-fagerberg-e243219493f4
- Brogaard, B. and Marlow, K. (2015). *The superhuman mind: Free the genius in your brain*. Penguin.
- Tommaney, S. (2015). A Lawyer's Head injury unveils artistic talents. Houston Press. February 23, 2015. http://www.houstonpress.com/arts/a-lawyers-head-injury-unveils-hidden-artistic-talents-6375112
- Bushak, L. (2015). Watch How A Traumatic Brain Injury Turned This Lawyer Into A Talented Artist. Medical Daily. February 20, 2015. https://www.medicaldaily.com/watch-how-traumatic-brain-injury-turned-lawyer-talented-artist-322972

- Brogaard, B: (2013). Hidden Talent Unleashed. Psychology Today. September 9, 2013. https://www.psychologytoday.com/intl/blog/the-superhuman-mind/201309/hidden-talent-unleashed
- Geighl, A. Texas Attorney Discovers Miraculous Painting Talent While Recovering from Head Injury (VIDEO). People. February 20, 2015. https://people.com/celebrity/patrick-fagerberg-texas-attorney-becomes-painter-after-head-injury/
- Vimeo Video: Embracing the Sublime
- 044 Brain Injury Transforms Prominent Attorney into Impassioned Artist – Patrick Fagerberg: https://www.youtube.com/watch?v=cZDUg-rDUK0
- Death and Rebirth after a Traumatic Brain Injury. https://www.youtube.com/watch?v=E_xeOLIRKDc

5.19 Anthony "Tony" DeBlois (born 1974)

Thanks are due to Janice DeBlois, Tony's mother, for her valuable contributions in reviewing this profile.

Tony DeBlois was born in Randolph, Massachusetts, United States, on January 22, 1974. He is a blind autistic savant and musician. Tony was born prematurely, weighing in at just 1 lb., ¾ oz., and barely breathing. He needed large amounts of pure oxygen to survive, which ended up causing blindness at just a few days old. As he began to grow up, his parents realized that his blindness was unfortunately not Tony's only disability. A few years later his parents learned that he was autistic. Tony was slow in verbal skills, and at 16 was unable to converse. "The only plus was his constant interest in sound and rhythm whether it came from the washing machine or the radio" (DeBlois and Felix, 2005). Tony began to play piano at the age of two.

Tony studied at the Texas School for the Blind in Austin, Texas, then the Perkins School for the Blind in Boston, Massachusetts, and finally at Berklee College of Music in Boston, where he was admitted as a full-time student. He graduated magna cum laude in 1996, a striking achievement for someone both blind and autistic, showing mastery of 22 instruments. In addition to being an excellent musician, Tony sings with perfect pitch and perfect enunciation in 11 languages.

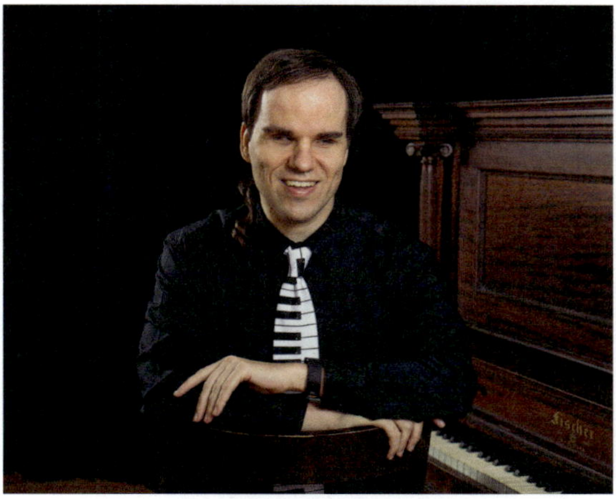

Figure 5.55 Tony DeBlois.

Photo courtesy of Janice and Toni DeBlois.

Although Tony is a tremendous jazz musician, he performs a wide range of musical styles, from country to classical. Tony knows more than 10,000 songs, all learned by ear since he cannot read sheet music. As if this were not enough, Tony is able to improvise magnificently. He plays with his own band, Goodnuf. Tony has five CDs available through the address on his website. His mother says that "when not playing musical instruments Tony enjoys swimming, exercise equipment, the computer, Mystery Tours and ballroom dancing" (DeBlois' official website).

He is the recipients of numerous awards. Tony has also appeared on various television programs, such as *The Today Show* and *CBS News Sunday Morning*. He was the subject of the 1997 CBS made-for-TV film *Journey of the Heart*. His story has been told in documentaries in Italy, England, Japan, Switzerland, and Australia. He has also given concerts in Singapore, Taiwan, Nigeria, and Ireland. Tony has produced a dozen albums. He proudly performed the musical score for two documentaries, *Purgatory* and *Love and Art*, and is working on a third, *Horse of a Different Color*.

Impairments: Autism, blindness. Tony was born prematurely and, because of his poorly developed lungs, needed large amounts of pure oxygen to survive.

This amount of oxygen resulted in blindness. He was slow in verbal skills and unable to converse at 16 years old.

Skills: Musician, composer, singer. He has learned to play over 20 musical instruments, including piano, organ, harmonica, guitar, harpsichord, violin, banjo, drums, and trumpet. He is now learning saxophone, clarinet, ukulele, mandolin, and flute. He can sing in German, French, and Spanish, among other languages.

Below are references, links to some videos, and additional reading about Tony DeBlois.

- Tony DeBlois official website: http://www.tonydeblois.com
- Tony Deblois Facebook: https://www.facebook.com/pg/Tony-DeBlois-8th-Wonder-of-Music-158749507486522/posts/
- Skudra, N. (2019). Journey Of The Heart: A Film About Blind, Autistic Musical Savant Tony DeBlois. The art of autism. https://the-art-of-autism.com/journey-of-the-heart-a-film-about-blind-autistic-musical-savant-tony-dublois/
- English, L. (2018). A Book Review on Musicophilia by Oliver Sacks. *Trent Notes on Linguistics, 1,* 89-92.
- Hanson, F. (2018). Tony DeBlois is on the move. The Patriot Ledger. https://www.patriotledger.com/news/20180517/tony-deblois-is-on-move
- Treffert, D. (2010). *Islands of genius: The bountiful mind of the autistic, acquired, and sudden savant.* Jessica Kingsley Publishers.
- DeBlois, J. and Felix, A. (2005). *Some kind of genius: The extraordinary journey of musical savant Tony DeBlois.* Rodale.
- Robertson, P. (2004). Music and the Brain: A Musicologist's Viewpoint. *Neurology of the Arts: Painting, Music, Literature,* 307.
- Darold Treffer: Tony DeDlois – A Prodigious Musical Savant: https://web.archive.org/web/20100626002913/http://www.wisconsinmedicalsociety.org/savant_syndrome/savant_profiles/tony_deblois
- Real People, Real Stories: Blind, Autistic, Musical Savant. https://www.youtube.com/watch?v=mE63EMou3dA

- Performance: Pianist Tony DeBlois at TEDxUMassBoston. https://www.youtube.com/watch?v=TzsA8ceXRbc
- Tony DeBlois. FIERCE LOVE & ART (trailer). https://www.youtube.com/watch?v=5W5gChg3rc0
- Tony DeBlois composes theme music for FIERCE LOVE and ART. https://www.facebook.com/FierceLoveArt/videos/140297569870309/

5.20 Stephen Wiltshire (born 1974)

I greatly appreciate the contributions of Annette Wiltshire, Stephen's sister and Art Director at The Stephen Wiltshire Gallery, in writing this profile.

Stephen Wiltshire was born in Greenwich, London, to Caribbean parents on April 24, 1974. His father was a native of Barbados and his mother was from Saint Lucia. Stephen is an autistic savant and a prodigious architectural artist. At the age of three, he was diagnosed as autistic. He was mute, distant, engaged in little or no eye contact, and lived locked in his own private world. At the age of five, he was sent to Queensmill, a school in London for children with special needs. Stephen soon developed a passion for painting, first animals and cars (especially American cars), then London buses and landmark buildings, then portraits of celebrities and close friends. Later, he would concentrate almost exclusively on architecture.

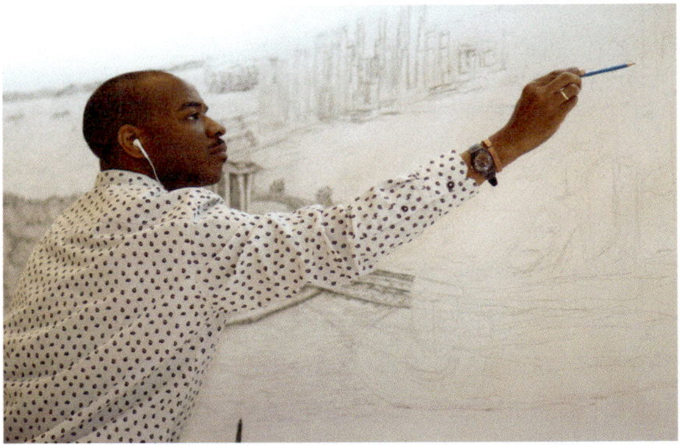

Figure 5.56 Stephen Wiltshire: Sketching Singapore skyline.

Photo courtesy of Stephen Wiltshire.

Stephen began communicating with the world through his paintings. His instructors encouraged him to speak, to voice his needs, and to request materials for his paintings. This was how he began to speak fully, at the age of nine. His first words were "paper" and "pen," both in relation to his drawings and painting. Stephen's artwork began to garner acclaim, and the press began publishing articles marveling at how such a young child could produce such masterful drawings. This brought him his first job at the age of eight, when he was commissioned by the late British Prime Minister Sir Edward Heath to create a drawing of Salisbury Cathedral (Ash, 2015).

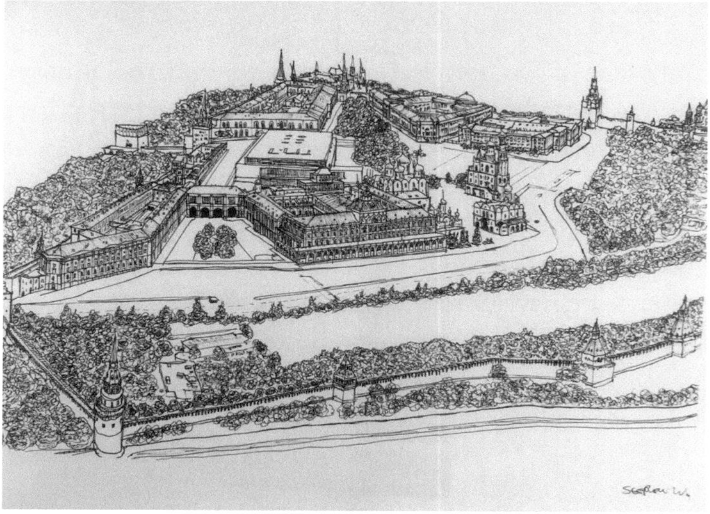

Figure 5.57 Stephen Wiltshire. Kremlin, 1991. Ink on paper. 14 x 19 in.

Photo courtesy of Henry Boxer. Henry Boxer Gallery, London.

In February 1987, a former president of London's Royal Academy of Arts, Sir Hugh Casson, referred to him as "possibly the best child artist in Britain" (Stephen Wiltshire's official website). The same year, at the age of 13, Stephen visited New York a city he loves and often visits, for the first time. After taking a short helicopter ride over the city, he was able to reproduce its skyline, including such legendary skyscrapers as the Empire State Building and the Chrysler Building, in just four days. He said he was truly inspired by the bird's eye view he got when flying over such an amazing metropolis. While in New York, Stephen met legendary neurologist Oliver Sacks.

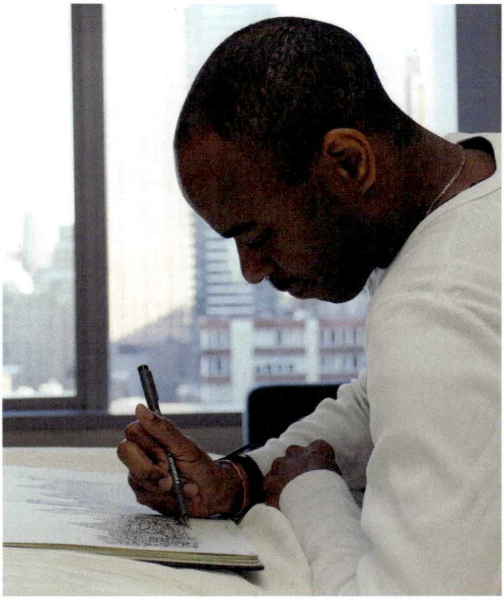

Figure 5.58 Stephen Wiltshire: Sketching New York in hotel room

Photo courtesy of Stephen Wiltshire.

Stephen published his first book, *Drawings* (Wiltshire, 1987), a volume of his early sketches, in 1987. In 1988, he published his second book, *Cities* (Wiltshire, 1988), which included some drawings of London, Docklands, Paris, and Edinburgh. His third book, *Floating Cities* (Wiltshire, 1992), contains the elaborate drawings he made on a tour of Venice, Amsterdam (Stephen said that this was the most challenging city to draw), Saint Petersburg, and Moscow. Stephen attracted crowds wherever he stopped to draw. *Floating Cities* book became a number one bestseller in England. In 1992, Stephen drew an accurate 10-meter-long panorama of Tokyo following a short helicopter ride over the city. He then traveled to the United States once again, a trip that resulted in the book *American Dream* (Wiltshire, 1993), which featured cityscapes of Chicago, San Francisco, and New York, as well as the desert landscape of Arizona. In 2001, he flew over London and produced a detailed aerial illustration with 12 historic landmarks and more than 200 other structures. In May 2005, he returned to Tokyo and took a helicopter ride over the city, after which he made the largest drawings of his career. In 2006, Stephen was made a Member of the Order of the British Empire (MBE) for services to the art world (Kirby, 2006). In July of the same year, he opened his own gallery in Pall Mall, central London (Jury, 2006), which is managed by his sister Annette. "He comes three days a week and he sits and does his drawings and sometimes paintings or commissioned work. He loves the fact that people come in and greet him and praise him", Annette said (Jury, 2006). In 2011, he drew an imposing (76 m) panoramic view of New York from memory after a helicopter ride, which is now on display at John F. Kennedy International Airport.

> In July 2014, Stephen was commissioned by Singapore PH to create a panoramic drawing of the city, which became part of the National Collection of Singapore to celebrate the nation's 50th birthday. 150,000 visitors attend his exhibition in just 5 days, setting an attendance record in the history of the country (Stephen Wiltshire's official website).

More recently, Stephen has visited cities across the globe, such as Hong Kong, Rome, Frankfurt, Madrid, Dubai, Jerusalem, Sydney, Shanghai, Brisbane, Doha, Mexico City, and Istanbul to undertake vast panoramic drawings after helicopter rides of no more than 45 minutes.

Oliver Sacks (2012) describes Stephen better than anyone else:

> It has often been said that savants have photographic or eidetic memories, but as I photocopied Stephen's drawings I thought how unlike a Xerox machine he was. His pictures in no sense resembled copies or photographs, something mechanical and impersonal – there were always additions, subtractions, revisions, and, of course, Stephen's unmistakable style. They were images and showed us some of the immensely complex neural processes that are needed to make a visual and graphic image. Stephen's drawings were individual constructions, but could they be seen, in a deeper sense, as creations?

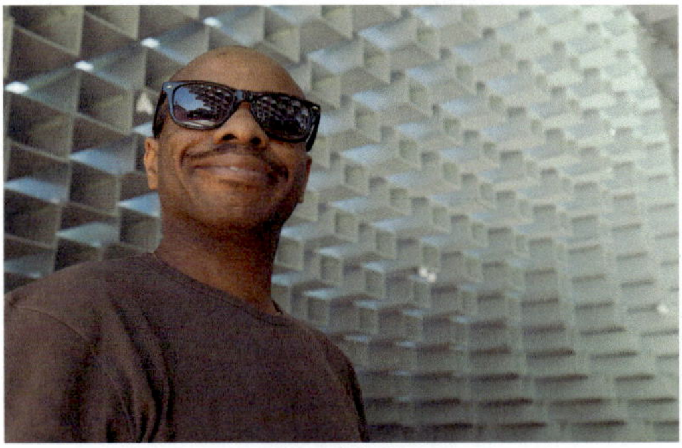

Figure 5.59 Stephen Wiltshire.

Photo courtesy of Stephen Wiltshire.

Stephen Wiltshire's work has been the subject of many TV documentaries in all over the world. Viewers across the globe have been astonished by his ability to draw masterfully detailed architectural drawings of cityscapes with mesmerizing accuracy after having observed them only briefly. His drawings are popular, exhibited frequently in venues all over the world, and sell for thousands of dollars. His success is continuously growing. Despite his condition and in addition to his resounding success in painting and drawing, Stephen also has a pitch-perfect voice, a natural talent for music, and is an accomplished pianist.

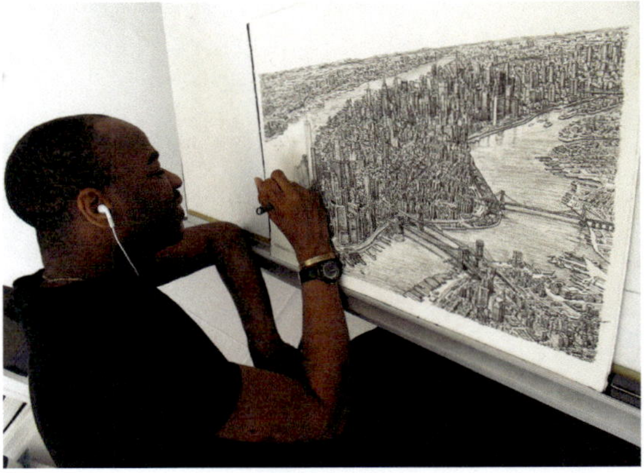

Figure 5.60 Stephen Wiltshire: Drawing Manhattan skyline.

Photo courtesy of Stephen Wiltshire.

"I am really good at playing 'Stand by me' by Ben E King and 'Wonderful World' by Sam Cooke. I also sang 'My Cherie Amour' by Stevie Wonder at my sister's wedding" (Philby, 2009). Music makes Stephen feel good and happy.

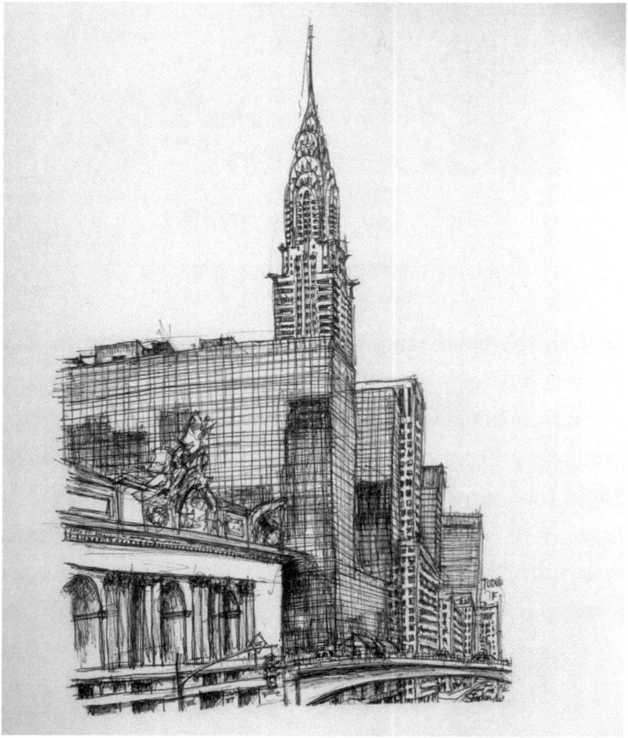

Figure 5.61 Stephen Wiltshire. Chrysler Building. 1991. Ink on paper. 18 x 13 in.

Photo courtesy of Henry Boxer. Henry Boxer Gallery, London.

Impairment: Autism. He was mute when young, did not relate to other people, and lived entirely in his own world, but enjoyed painting. He did not utter a word until age five and did not speak fully until he was nine years old.

Skills: Artistic ability, photographic memory, painting, musician, singer. He can draw a landscape with exceptional accuracy and in painstaking detail after seeing it just once.

Below are references, links to some videos, and additional reading about Stephen Wiltshire.

- Stephen Wiltshire's official website: https://www.stephenwiltshire.co.uk
- Stephen Wiltshire on YouTube: https://www.youtube.com/user/stephenwiltshire
- Stephen Wiltshire on Facebook: https://www.facebook.com/Stephen.Wiltshire.Artist/
- Henry Boxer Gallery, London. https://www.outsiderart.co.uk/
- Cosslett, R. (2017). This was my form of language: the artist who draws cities from memory. The Guardian. May 4, 2017. https://www.theguardian.com/cities/2017/may/04/artist-draws-cities-memory-stephen-wiltshire
- Ash, L. (2015). Drawing what our mouths cannot say. BBC News. June 12, 2015.
- Treffert, D. (2014). Savant syndrome: Realities, myths and misconceptions. *Journal of Autism and Developmental Disorders, 44*(3), 564-571.
- Pring, L., Ryder, N., Crane, L. and Hermelin, B. (2012). Creativity in savant artists with autism. *Autism, 16*(1), 45-57.
- Sacks, O. (2012). *An anthropologist on Mars: Seven paradoxical tales.* Vintage.
- Mottron, L. (2011). The power of autism. *Nature, 479*(7371), 33-35.
- Treffert, D. (2009). The savant syndrome: an extraordinary condition. A synopsis: past, present, future. *Philosophical Transactions of the Royal Society B: Biological Sciences, 364*(1522), 1351-1357.
- Philby, C. (2009). My secret life: Stephen Wiltshire, artist, 34. https://www.independent.co.uk/arts-entertainment/art/features/my-secret-life-stephen-wiltshire-artist-34-1488487.html
- Wansell, G. (2008). Revealed: How autistic genius Stephen Wiltshire drew his amazing picture of London's skyline. Daily Mail. April 8, 2008. https://www.dailymail.co.uk/news/article-557942/Revealed-How-autistic-genius-Stephen-Wiltshire-drew-amazing-picture-Londons-skyline.html
- Dwyer, J. (2009). Like a skyline is etched in his head. The New York Times. October 27, 2009. https://www.nytimes.com/2009/10/28/nyregion/28about.html

- Kirby, T. (2006). Honour for artistic man who speaks through art. Independent. January 4, 2006. https://www.independent.co.uk/news/uk/this-britain/honour-for-autistic-man-who-speaks-through-art-6112727.html
- Jury, L. (2006). Austistic man with prodigious eye for art opens own gallery. Independent. October 28, 2006. https://www.independent.co.uk/news/uk/this-britain/autistic-man-with-prodigious-eye-for-art-opens-own-gallery-421992.html
- Smith, D. (2004). *Introduction to special education: Teaching in an age of opportunity* (pp. 85-86). Pearson/A and B.
- Heaton, P. and Wallace, G. L. (2004). Annotation: The savant syndrome. *Journal of child psychology and psychiatry*, 45(5), 899-911.
- Hermelin, B., Pring, L., Buhler, M., Wolff, S. and Heaton, P. (1999). A visually impaired savant artist: Interacting perceptual and memory representations. *Journal of Child Psychology and Psychiatry, 40*(7), 1129-1139.
- Pring, L., Hermelin, B., Buhler, M., & Walker, I. (1997). Native savant talent and acquired skill. *Autism, 1*(2), 199-214.
- Wiltshire, S. (1993). *Stephen Wiltshire's American Dream*. Michael Joseph Ltd; 1st edition (April 29, 1993).
- Wiltshire, S. (1992). *Floating Cities: Venice, Amsterdam, Leningrad, and Moscow*. Summit Books; First Edition (January 1, 1992)
- Wiltshire, S. (1988). *Cities*. Orion Publishing Co; 1st Edition (1988).
- Wiltshire, S. (1987). *Drawings*. J. M. Dent & Sons (Canada).
- Oliver Sacks Scientist: The artist, Stephen Wiltshire. https://www.webofstories.com/play/oliver.sacks/247;jsessionid=3FC797163D551BA4F3F2CAEAD47CAFAE
- Stephen Wiltshire draws NYC for UBS. https://www.youtube.com/watch?v=bsJbApZ5GF0
- Stephen Wiltshire's Singapore Panorama. Full timelapse. https://www.youtube.com/watch?v=-73DQ1hLsDY
- Stephen Wiltshire: The autistic urban artist with the photographic memory | DW English. https://www.youtube.com/watch?v=CqKRfZHpYBs
- Wiltshire's NYC Matches Up. https://www.youtube.com/watch?v=ryQ0tfjXnkY

- The Human Camera (Autistic Savant Documentary) | Real Stories. https://www.youtube.com/watch?v=phkNgC8Vxj4

5.21 Ron Sandison (born 1975)

I greatly appreciate Ron Sandison's contributions in reviewing this profile.

Ron was born in Rochester Hills, Michigan on October 5, 1975. He is an author, speaker, the founder of Spectrum Inclusion, and an autistic savant with an extraordinary memory. Ron's birth and development were normal up until 18 months. At that point, however, he suffered a marked regression and began to show all the signs of an autistic child: he stopped talking, avoided eye contact, lapsed into repetitive behavior, and ceased practically all forms of communication. His parents received Ron's diagnosis of autism when he was seven years old. It was clear: Ron was an autistic child and would have to live with this impairment his entire life.

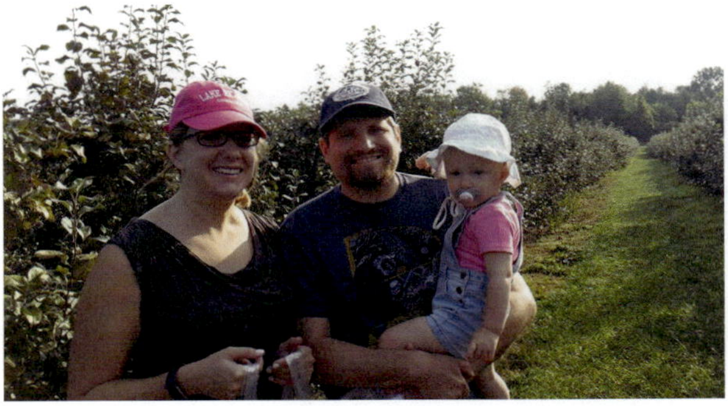

Figure 5.62 Ron Sandison and his family.

Photo courtesy of Ron Sandison.

> Educational specialists and doctors informed my parents that I would probably never read beyond a seventh grade level, attend college, or participate in athletics. Even so, my mom was determined to help me to excel in life. She empowered me to develop my unique gifts for independence, employment, and relationships (Ron Sandison's website).

His life as a child was obviously not easy. Although he experienced bullying in elementary and middle school, Ron persisted in his studies. He was able to graduate from college, obtain a master's degree, get married, and form a family.

Ron boasts an exceptional memory. He enjoys reading and has over 4,000 books in his personal library (Sandison, 2020). "During the last decade he has read over 950 books and he can recall over 80% of what he has read" (Sandison, 2020). Ron's skills are particularly evident in his mastery of biblical texts. As Ron describes it, "I can quote word perfect over 15,000 Scriptures including 22 complete books of the New Testament, the Gospel of Mark from Biblical Greek to my English translation, and over 5,000 quotes."

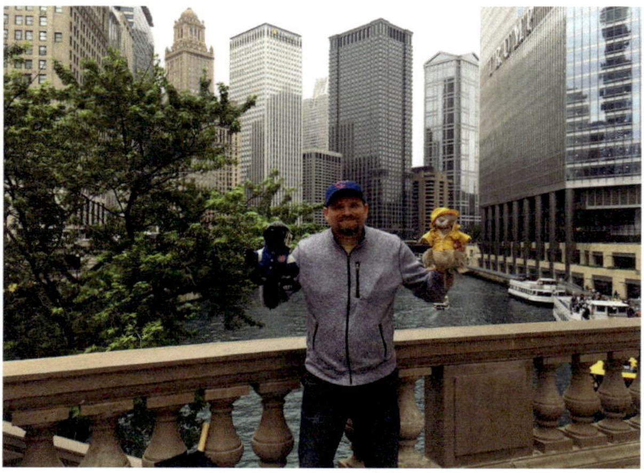

Figure 5.63 Ron Sandison in Chicago, USA.

Photo courtesy of Ron Sandison.

Ron works full-time in medicine and is also a professor of theology at the Destiny School of Ministry. He is a member of the advisory board of Autism Society of America's Faith Initiative (Sandison, 2020).

Ron's writing has been featured in major publications such as the *The Detroit News, The Oakland Press, Awana, The Autism Society of America blog, Autism*

Speaks' blog, Autism Parenting Magazine, The Mighty, Charisma Magazine, and many more (Ron Sandison's website).

"He has written three books, gives presentations all over the country and world, and is an adjunct professor and psychiatric care specialist" (Hirschberg, 2017). Ron is also now a very happy father: his daughter Makayla Marie arrived in 2016.

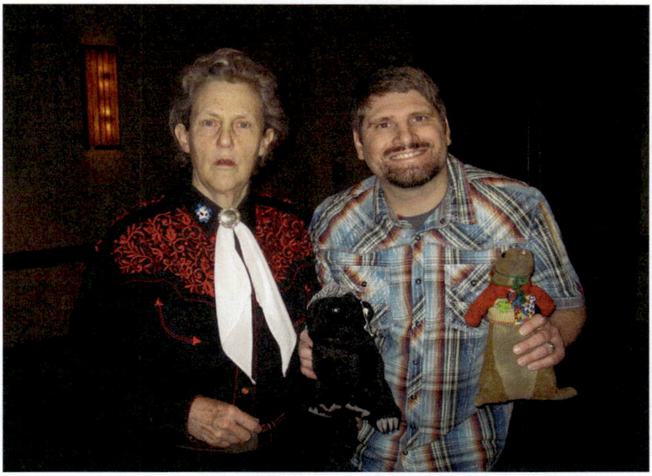

Figure 5.64 Ron Sandison and Temple Grandin.

Photo courtesy of Ron Sandison.

Impairments: Autism. He showed all the signs of autism as a child: he stopped talking, avoided eye contact, lapsed into repetitive behavior, and ceased practically all forms of communication.

Skills: Extraordinary memory. Author, speaker, founder of Inclusion Spectrum.

Below are references, links to some videos, and additional reading about Ron Sandison.

- Ron Sandison's official website: https://www.spectruminclusion.com/

- Ron Sandison on Facebook: https://www.facebook.com/ron.sandison
- Sandison, R. (2020). 5 Ways Autism Makes Me A Cool Dad. The Art of Autism. June 20, 2020. https://the-art-of-autism.com/5-ways-autism-makes-me-a-cool-dad/
- Holmes, S. (2017). How to Develop an Effective Support Ministry for Parents of Autistic and Special Needs Children. *The Struggle Is Real: How to Care for Mental and Relational Health Needs in the Church.*
- Hirschberg, E. (2017). The truth about autism: Ron's story. HS Insider. Los Angeles Times. August 10, 2017. https://highschool.latimes.com/san-dieguito-academy/the-truth-about-autism-rons-story/
- Sandison, R. (2016). *A Parent's Guide to Autism: Practical Advice. Biblical Wisdom.* Charisma Media.
- Sherman, B. (2015). ORU grad talks faith, autism. Tulsa World. August 15, 2015. https://tulsaworld.com/oru-grad-talks-faith-autism/article_93e068df-cef1-57ca-884d-2df78f98a588.html
- Different Brains. https://www.differentbrains.org/autism-and-the-power-of-memory-with-ron-sandison-exploring-different-brains-episode-11/
- Fierce, Love & Art documentary film by Dr. Laurence A. Becker share Ron's story. Temple Grandin narrated this film: https://www.youtube.com/watch?v=5W5gChg3rc0

5.22 Derek Paravicini (born 1979)

I greatly appreciate the contributions of Dr. Adam Ockelford of the University of Roehampton, London, in writing and reviewing this profile.

Derek Paravicini is autistic, blind, and an extraordinary musical savant. Paravicini, who lives in London, was born prematurely at 26 weeks, along with a twin sister who did not survive childbirth. Derek's blindness was caused by fluctuating levels of oxygen while he was in the neonatal intensive care unit. This also affected the development of his brain, resulting in severe learning difficulties. His life story is unique because no child who was born 14 weeks prematurely had survived at the Royal Berkshire Hospital, and because he has become a prodigious musician.

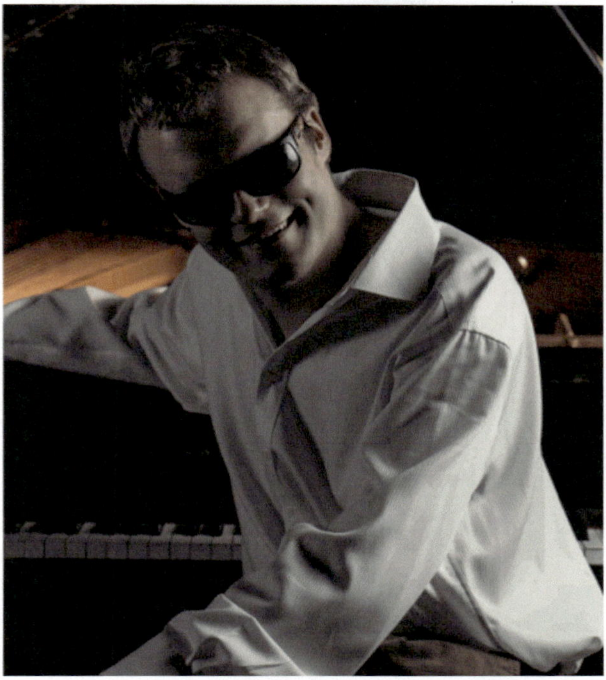

Figure 5.65 Derek Paravicini.

Photo courtesy of Derek Paravicini and Adam Ockelford.

Derek has absolute pitch and is a pianist of exceptional talent. He began playing the piano at age two and later mastered it under Adam Ockelford in London. He learns pieces merely by listening to them, and he has an exceptional long-term memory, with an instantly accessible catalogue of tens, maybe hundreds of thousands, of pieces. This amazing musical gift earned him the nickname "the human iPod" (Green, 2009). Music psychologist Dr. Adam Ockelford explains:

> His acute sense of absolute pitch means that he can accurately disaggregate chords and cluster of more than 10 notes played simultaneously. So when he hears an orchestral piece like 'The Swan', he can hear what every instrument in the orchestra is playing.

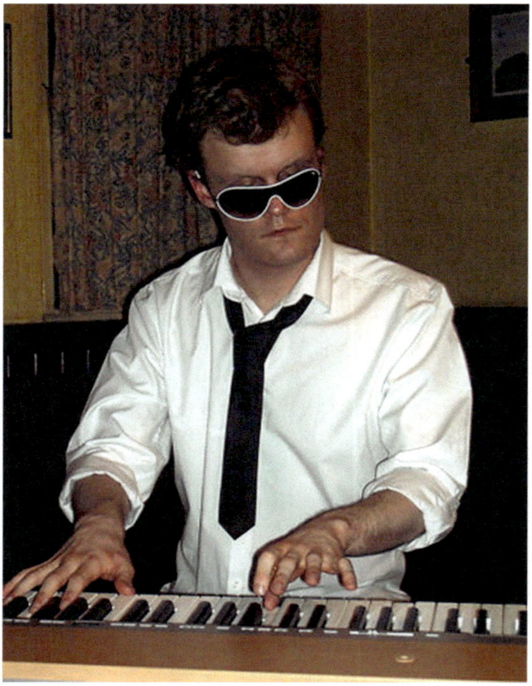

Figure 5.66 Derek Paravicini.

Photo of Derek Paravicini by Nick Wells, taken at the Station Hotel 20 of April 2008. Musical instrument is Yamaha P-140S. This file is licensed under the Creative Commons Attribution-Share Alike 3.0 Unported license.

At the age of nine, Derek performed in a public concert with the Royal Philharmonic Pops Orchestra at the Barbican Hall in London, "an event that launched a flurry of international media interest" (Ockelford, 2007). Diana, Princess of Wales, presented Derek with the Barnardo's Children's Champion Award for musical performance when he was 10. After this there was no turning back. He has appeared on numerous television shows in the UK and overseas and performed in different concerts with many other notable musicians. He played at Buckingham Palace for the Queen of England, and at 11 Downing Street for Chancellor of the Exchequer Alistair Darling. He has been interviewed three times by Lesley Stahl for CBS's *60 Minutes*. In 2010 Derek was featured on the History Channel's *Stan Lee's Superhumans*. He also participated, with the composer Matthew King, on a radio program for the BBC.

Impairments: Autism, severe learning difficulties, blindness. He was born 14 weeks prematurely and weighed just over half a kilogram. The lack of oxygen during his time in the neonatal intensive care unit caused him to become totally blind and led to severe learning difficulties and an autism spectrum disorder. This condition prevents Derek for performing even extremely simple tasks, such as dressing or washing himself.

Skills: Musician with absolute pitch. He began to learn to play the piano at the age of two. Just by listening to a song once, he can then reproduce it faithfully on the piano. His ability to process pitch is exceptional. He can disaggregate large clusters of notes with ease.

Below are references, links to some videos, and additional reading about Derek Paravicini.

- Derek website: http://www.derekparavicini.net/
- Derek Paravicini Quartet: https://www.derekparaviciniquartet.com/
- Derek's YouTube channel: https://www.youtube.com/user/derekparavicini
- Derek's Facebook page: https://www.facebook.com/derekparavicini/
- Twitter account: https://twitter.com/derekparavicini
- Treffert, D. (2014). Savant syndrome: Realities, myths and misconceptions. *Journal of Autism and Developmental Disorders, 44*(3), 564-571.
- Straus, J. (2014). Idiots Savants, Retarded Savants, Talented Aments, Mono-Savants, Autistic Savants, Just Plain Savants, People with Savant Syndrome, and Autistic People Who Are Good at Things: A View from Disability Studies.
- Ockelford, A. (2013). *Music, language and autism: Exceptional strategies for exceptional minds.* Jessica Kingsley Publishers.
- Green, C. (2013). The blind pianist who led our reporter to a closed courtroom. Independent. May 2, 2013. https://www.independent.co.uk/

news/uk/home-news/the-blind-pianist-who-led-our-reporter-to-a-closed-courtroom-8601774.html

- Ockelford, A. (2009). *In the key of genius: The extraordinary life of Derek Paravicini*. Random House.
- Ankan, J. (2011). Derek Paravicini: Musician or a Superhuman? EFI News. December 21, 2011. https://web.archive.org/web/20120509054943/http://www.efi-news.com/2011/12/derek-paravicini-musician-or-superhuman.html
- Allen, V. (2010). Family wins right to control future of piano prodigy known as 'Human iPod'. Daily Mail. May 14, 2010. https://www.dailymail.co.uk/news/article-1278253/Human-iPod-Derek-Paravicini-Family-win-right-control-piano-prodigys-future.html
- Sanderson, D. (2010). Autistic pianist's case heard in public after UK's last secret court opens. The Times. May 14, 2010. https://www.thetimes.co.uk/article/autistic-pianists-case-heard-in-public-after-uks-last-secret-court-opens-q72hrhdl92j
- Green, C. (2009). The human iPod: Meet the musical savant. Independent. May 28, 2009. https://www.independent.co.uk/arts-entertainment/music/news/the-human-ipod-meet-the-musical-savant-1691818.html
- Ockelford, A. (2008). *In the Key of Genius: The Extraordinary Life of Derek Paravicini*. Arrow, 2008.
- Ockelford, A. (2007). A music module in working memory? Evidence from the performance of a prodigious musical savant. *Musicae Scientiae, 11*(2_suppl), 5-36.
- Moss, S. (2007). He attacked the keyboard. The Guardian. April 30, 2007. https://www.theguardian.com/music/2007/apr/30/classicalmusicandopera.jazz
- Ockelford, A. and Pring, L. (2005, September). Learning and creativity in a prodigious musical savant. In *International Congress Series* (Vol. 1282, pp. 903-907). Elsevier.
- In the Key of Genius: Derek Paravicini and Adam Ockelford at TEDxWarwick 2013. https://www.youtube.com/watch?v=3S1HK7LQY2I
- Blind, Autistic Pianist Derek Paravicini Joins in at a Pub! https://www.youtube.com/watch?v=I5bS7dmkFFU

- Blind autistic man stuns the music world. BBC News. https://www.bbc.com/news/av/entertainment-arts-15086761/blind-autistic-man-stuns-the-music-world

5.23 Daniel Tammet (born 1979)

I am deeply indebted to Daniel Tammet for his extensive assistance in the final revisions of this profile.

Daniel Tammet was born in a working-class suburb in London, England, as the first of nine children on January 31, 1979. Tammet is an autistic and prodigious savant, novelist, poet and essayist. His childhood autism and epilepsy were inseparably related. Tammet, truly a beautiful mind, is one of the world's most famous and prolific savants. He is unique in part because, despite his autism and atypical background, Tammet is one of the few savants capable of living independently and being able to explain what is happening inside his head. Tammet was born Daniel Paul Corney, but went to court to change his name because it did not fit with the way he saw himself. He explains: "I first saw 'Tammet' online. It means oak tree in Estonian, and I liked that association" (Johnson, 2005).

Tammet has multiple abilities and is very successful with many of them. Tammet does face some limitations in his life, however. He could never work from 9 to 5; or go to the beach, because there are many pebbles to count; or to the supermarket because there are many shapes and textures, and he would not be able to buy a product because there would be dozens of them and thousands of cases to analyze before making a decision. These things, which tended to overwhelm and unnerve him, were especially difficult for Tammet growing up. His social skills, however, improved markedly as he matured. For instance, he occasionally goes to supermarkets now, although he is still unable to drive, a lasting difficulty. In 2004, Tammet finally had the opportunity to put a name to his difference, when he was diagnosed with Asperger syndrome by Professor Simon Baron-Cohen at the University of Cambridge's Autism Research Centre (Tammet, 2007).

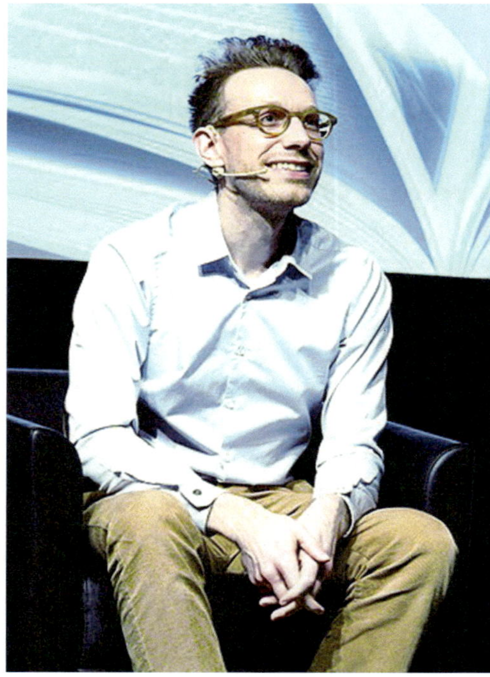

Figure 5.67 Daniel Tammet in Montréal, Canada.

Photo courtesy of Jérôme Tabet.

Tammet has numerical and word synesthesia, meaning that he sees numbers and worlds as shapes, colors, and textures, and he can perform extraordinary calculations in his head (Tammet, 2017). The number two, for instance, is a motion, and five is a thunderclap. 11 is a smooth number, whereas 37 is a lumpy number, like porridge. Nine is dark blue and one is a very bright white. Tammet says that each positive integer up to 10,000 has its own unique shape, color, texture, and feel. He also describes 289 as particularly ugly, 333 as particularly attractive, and pi as beautiful. Tammet says:

> When I multiply numbers together, I see two shapes. The image starts to change and evolve, and a third shape emerges. That's the answer. It's mental imagery. It's like maths without having to think (Johnson, 2005).

At school, Tammet always had an excellent performance. He was chosen best student during two different years. He was also bullied by other children, but says his teachers were always protective of him.

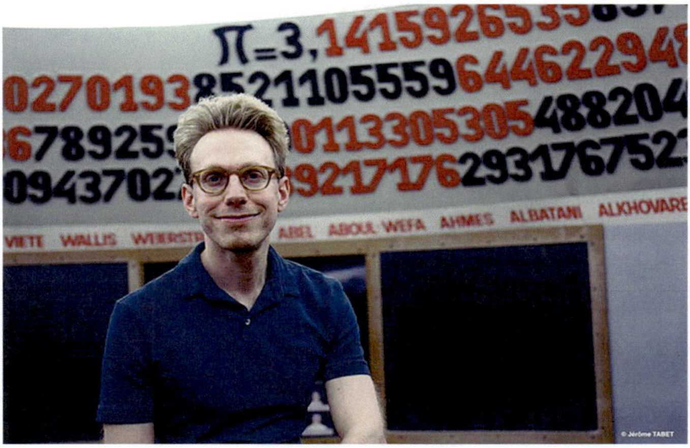

Figure 5.68 Daniel Tammet in Paris, France.

Photo courtesy of Jérôme Tabet.

In 2004, he set a new speed record for calculating decimals of pi, with an impressive 22,514 digits over the course of five hours and nine minutes. (The record for calculating the most decimals of pi is currently held by Suresh Kumar Sharma, a 21-year-old former vegetable vendor from Jaipur, India, with 70,030 decimals in 17 hours, 14 minutes on October 21, 2015). Tammet's achievement was recorded at the Museum of the History of Science in Oxford (it remains the European record today). In reviewing his profile, Tammet provided the following eloquent explanation:

> My recitation of Pi in 2004 was not a speed contest. Nor was it a matter of calculation. I wrote an essay about it in *Thinking in Numbers.* I experience Pi as a poem written in numbers and learned the digits by heart over several months before reciting it in public at the Museum of the History of Science in Oxford. It was like an artistic performance and helped me understand my vocation as a writer: I realised my gift

as a "contador" (counter) in both senses of the word, "contar" (count) numbers and "contar" (tell) stories.

As Johnson (2005) explained: "To him, pi isn't an abstract set of digits; it's a visual story, a film projected in front of his eyes." Bor et al. (2008) suggested that Tammet's abilities might be explained by hyperactivity in one brain region, the left prefrontal cortex, which results from his Asperger syndrome and synesthesia.

Tammet can also learn to speak new languages, from square one, in a week. To prove his incredible ability with languages, Tammet had an impressive challenge: he had to learn Icelandic, perhaps the most impenetrable language on earth, in just a week. "After just seven days of learning Icelandic, Tammet appeared live on an Icelandic television talk show and proved his gift to the world" (Watt et al., 2010). Daniel is humble about this gift:

> I learned conversational Icelandic in one week but could not use it fluently. I have studied or can use other languages but not all fluently. My French is fluent because I live in France. I have written several of my books in French. I have also used German, Icelandic and Esperanto with native speakers.

Tammet has also, over the years, become a prominent bestselling and award-winning writer. Nobel Prize laureate J.M. Coetzee, U.S Poet Laureate Billy Collins, Oliver Sacks, Rosa Montero, Amy Tan, and other major authors have publicly praised his work. His first book about his life with Asperger syndrome and savant syndrome, *Born on a Blue Day* (Tammet, 2007), was published in 2007. The book was named a Best Book for Young Adults by the American Library Association in 2008. In *Born on a Blue Day,* Tammet explores what it is like to be special and gives an insight into what makes us all human: our minds. The book has sold over 500,000 copies worldwide and been translated into more than 30 languages. His second book, *Embracing the Wide Sky* (Tammet, 2009), was one of France's best-selling books of 2009. In this book, he describes how his mind works to demonstrate the immense potential within us all. His third book, *Thinking in Numbers* (Tammet, 2013), a collection of essays, was published on August 16, 2012. In Tammet's world, numbers are beautiful, and mathematics illuminates our lives and minds. In his writings, he explores the way communication shapes reality. Tammet published his first novel, *Mishenka,* in 2016. One year later, he published *Every Word Is a Bird We Teach to Sing: Encounters with the Mysteries and Meanings of Language* (Tammet, 2017), a mesmerizing collection of essays about the world of words, letters, stories, and meanings. Most recently, Tammet published *Portraits,* a bilingual first poetry collection, in 2018. He has also published a fair number of essays.

Tammet has received awards and recognitions, mainly for his books, throughout his life. In 2000, he placed fourth in the World Memory Championships in London. In 2012, he was elected Fellow of the Royal Society of Arts (RSA) (Daniel Tammet's official website). In 2016, he graduated from the Open University with a Bachelor's degree in the Humanities, with First Class Honours. In 2020, Tammet was awarded an honorary doctorate by the same university for his "exceptional contribution to the arts and science." Tammet has appeared on several television and radio talk shows, including *60 Minutes* and *The Late Show with David Letterman* specials, and documentary films, including *Extraordinary People: The Boy with the Incredible Brain* on Channel 4. Tammet currently lives in Paris, France with his husband, Jérôme Tabet.

Impairment: Autism, synesthesia, epilepsy, and Asperger syndrome. He had some limitations and difficulties with social skills, although he has improved them over the years.

Skills: Mathematics, memory, language, polyglot, essayist, novelist, poet. He is one of few savants capable of living independently and being able to explain what is happening inside his head. He holds the European record for speed in calculating decimals of pi, with 22,514 digits over the course of five hours and nine minutes. His linguistic talent is laudable. Tammet can carry on conversations in English, French, German, Spanish, Lithuanian, Icelandic, Finnish, Romanian, Estonian, Welsh, and Esperanto. Tammet is the creator of Mänti, a constructed language of his own invention.

Below are references, links to some videos, and additional reading about Daniel Tammet.

- Daniel Tammet's official website: http://danieltammet.net/
- Daniel Tammet official Facebook page: https://www.facebook.com/DanielTammetAuthor
- Tammet, D. and Tabet, J. (2018. *Portraits.* http://www.danieltammet.net/portraits.php
- Tammet, D. (2017). *Every Word Is a Bird We Teach to Sing.* Little, Brown Spark.
- Tammet, D. (2017b). Languages Revealing Worlds and Selves. *The Times Literary Supplement.* TLS. https://www.the-tls.co.uk/articles/daniel-tammet-synaesthesia-languages/
- Hernando, S. (2017). Daniel Tammet: un talento incalculable. El País. May 30, 2017. https://elpais.com/elpais/2017/05/31/eps/1496181949_149618.html
- Tammet, D. (2016). *Mishenka.* ARENES. French Edition.
- Tammet, D. (2016b). Autism: a spectrum of speculation. *Brain, 139*(3), 999-1000.
- Tammet, D. (2014). *Je suis né un jour bleu.* Les arènes.
- Bouvet, L., Donnadieu, S., Valdois, S., Caron, C., Dawson, M. and Mottron, L. (2014). Veridical mapping in savant abilities, absolute pitch, and synesthesia: an autism case study. *Frontiers in psychology, 5,* 106.
- Tammet, D. (2013). *Thinking in Numbers: On Life, Love, Meaning, and Math.* Little, Brown Spark.
- Tammet, D. (2012). Olympics: Are the Fastest and Strongest Reaching Their Mathematical Limits. The Guardian. August 21, 2012. https://www.theguardian.com/sport/2012/aug/12/olympic-records-time-numbers-mathematics
- Tammet, D. (2012b). What I'm thinking about ... Tolstoy and maths. The Guardian. August 23, 2012. https://www.theguardian.com/books/booksblog/2012/aug/23/tolstoy-maths-daniel-tammet
- Watt, N., Strauss, E. and Rodrigues, A. (2010). Daniel Tammet: Mathematical Genius Visualizes Numbers, Solves Problems in Blink

of an Eye. ABC News. http://abcnews.go.com/2020/autistic-savant-daniel-tammet-solves-problems-blink-eye/story?id=10759598

- Hughes, J. R. (2010). A review of Savant Syndrome and its possible relationship to epilepsy. *Epilepsy & behavior, 17*(2), 147-152.
- Tammet, D. (2009). *Embracing the Wide Sky: A Tour Across the Horizons of the Mind.* Simon and Schuster.
- Wilson, P. (2009). A savvy savant finds his voice. The Australian. http://www.theaustralian.com.au/archive/news/a-savvy-savant-finds-his-voice/news-story/a44b6937e96177cba2e67f7f51b3f6ec
- Snyder, A. (2009). Explaining and inducing savant skills: privileged access to lower level, less-processed information. *Philosophical Transactions of the Royal Society B: Biological Sciences*, 364(1522), 1399-1405.
- Lehrer, J. (2009). Learn to Think Better: Tips from a Savant. Scientific American. April 2009. https://www.scientificamerican.com/article/think-better-tips-from-a-savant/
- Bor, D., Billington, J. and Baron-Cohen, S. (2008). Savant memory for digits in a case of synaesthesia and Asperger syndrome is related to hyperactivity in the lateral prefrontal cortex. *Neurocase, 13*(5-6), 311-319.
- Tammet, D. (2007). *Born on a Blue Day: Inside the Extraordinary Mind of an Autistic Savant.* Simon & Schuster/Free Press.
- Baron-Cohen, S., Bor, D., Billington, J., Asher, J., Wheelwright, S. and Ashwin, C. (2007). Savant memory in a man with colour form-number synaesthesia and asperger. *Journal of consciousness studies, 14*(9-10), 237-251
- Tammet, D. (2006). *Born on a blue day.* Hodder & Staughton.
- Johnson, R. (2005). A genius explains. The Guardian, February 12, 2005. https://www.theguardian.com/theguardian/2005/feb/12/weekend7.weekend2
- David Letterman: Math genius Worlds greatest math prodigy Mathematics savant Maths 3.14 Pi Day March 14 – Daniel Tammet. https://www.youtube.com/watch?v=t2uRuFgZSDc&t=5s
- Brain Man: The Boy With The Incredible Brain (Superhuman Documentary) | Real Stories. https://www.youtube.com/watch?v=PySn3slfXI
- Brainman. https://www.youtube.com/watch?v=Kf3-el-dJAw
- Autistic savant Daniel Tammet on 'the language of numbers' – BBC Newsnight. https://www.youtube.com/watch?v=j3Mecg8iuuE

- TED: Different ways of knowing | Daniel Tammet. https://www.youtube.com/watch?v=Pzd7ReqiQnE
- Math Genius Computes in the Blink of an Eye. https://www.youtube.com/watch?v=Xd1gywPOibg
- Daniel Tammet, un talento incalculable | Visionarios | El País Semanal. https://www.youtube.com/watch?v=fEVA-6qpymo
- Daniel Tammet – The Boy With The Incredible Brain [1/5] https://www.youtube.com/watch?v=AbASOcqc1Ss
- Daniel Tammet's colorful world of numbers. Brut. https://www.brut.media/us/international/daniel-tammet-s-colorful-world-of-numbers-832d4717-7c4a-423c-8354-3747e5895cfc

5.24 Seth Chwast (born 1983)

I am deeply indebted to Debra Chwast, Seth's mother, for her extensive assistance in the final revisions of this profile.

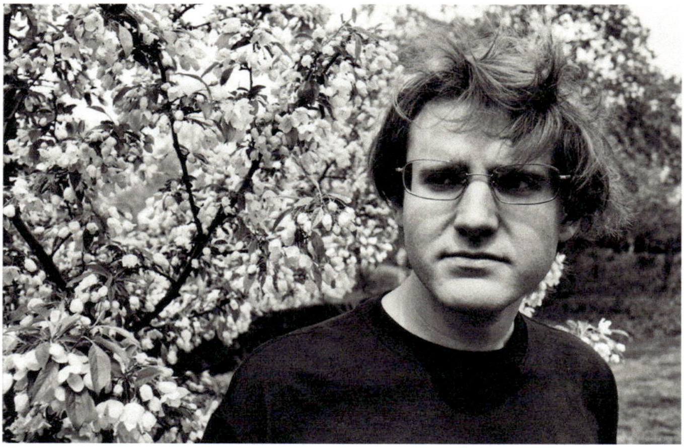

Figure 5.69 Seth Chwast.

Photo courtesy of Debra Chwast and Herb Ascherman.

Seth was born in Cleveland, Ohio in 1983. He is an American autistic savant and artist. He was diagnosed with severe autism when he was a toddler. Seth had all the features and difficulties of an autistic child. He is primarily non-verbal, cannot safely cross the street by himself and has always lived in his own insular world (Chwast and Chwast, 2011).

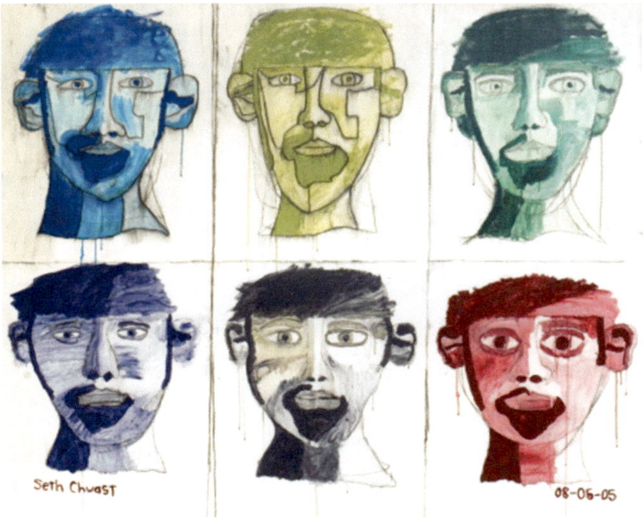

Figure 5.70 Seth Chwast: Six Self Studies. Acrylic spray paint on canvas, 70" x 44", 2005.

Photo courtesy of Seth and Debra Chwast.

He took his first art class when he was 20 years old at the Cleveland Museum of Art, which changed his life forever and gave him, for the first time, an uninhibited form and a voice with which he could communicate with the outside world (Treffert, agnesian.com). In three short years, he became a renowned artist. Seth has a raw talent for mixing colors and creating works of art that reflect his vision of the world he lives in. As an artist, he is difficult to classify. He is visionary, intuitive, extremely aware of his surroundings, and free in all things: lines, forms, technique, styles, and colors. Taking these details into account, we could say that his work might belong within what is called Art Brut, or Outsider Art. "No label can define Seth's work: Visionary art, Intuitive art, Marginal art, art Singulier; these are all ways to define, limit, and make this form of art comprehensible to us, the real outsiders," said Karen Lappon, an art critic (Lappon, International Confederations of Art Critics).

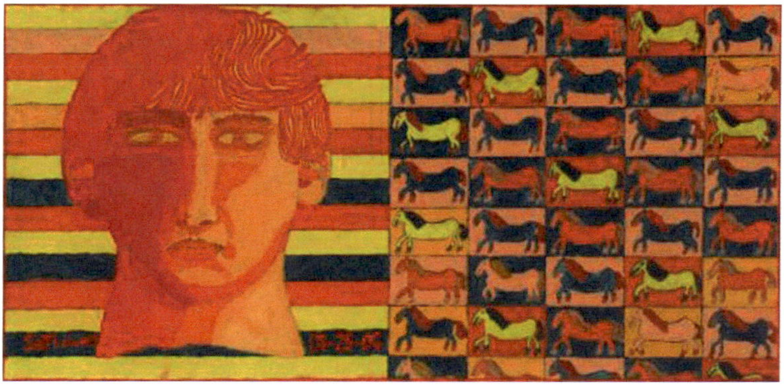

Figure 5.71 Seth Chwast: Red Orange Self Study with Horses and Striped Background. Acrylic on board, 15" x 30", 2006.

Photo courtesy of Seth and Debra Chwast.

Art Brut (a label created by French artist Jean Dubuffet) or Outsider Art (a term coined by art critic Roger Cardinal in 1972 as synonym for art brut) are the terms used to describe art which is created from solitude and is outside the boundaries of accepted cultural norms or the realm of "fine art," like that developed by the mentally ill, or patients in psychiatric hospitals. These artists are mainly self-taught or naïf art makers, who are typically unconnected with the mainstream art world, art institutions, or even any other forms of art other than their own. Their art is produced without regard to fame or fortune and illustrates extreme mental states, unconventional ideas, or elaborate fantasy worlds. Definition of terms has always been controversial. Jean Dubuffet characterized art brut as:

> Those works created from solitude and from pure and authentic creative impulses – where the worries of competition, acclaim and social promotion do not interfere – are, because of these very facts, more precious than the productions of professionals. After a certain familiarity with these flourishings of an exalted feverishness, lived so fully and so intensely by their authors, we cannot avoid the feeling that in relation to these works, cultural art in its entirety appears to be the game of a futile society, a fallacious parade (Dubuffet, 1988).

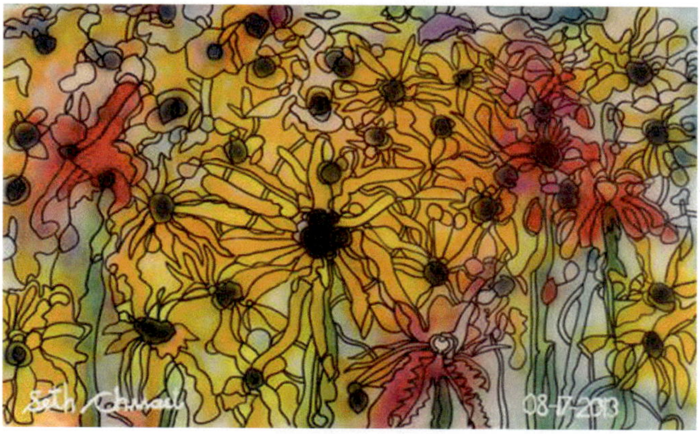

Figure 5.72 Seth Chwast: Many of Black-Eyed Susans with Red Cardinals. Acrylic spray paint on canvas, 30" x 48", 2013.

Photo courtesy of Seth and Debra Chwast.

Seth's work has been shown at numerous locations in the United States as well as in different countries around the world—Ecuador, Curacao, Costa Rica, Canada, Austria, the Cayman Islands, Ukraine, France, UK, Austria, and Italy, to name a few. "In 2011, Seth came in in first place in a world-wide United Nations competition and his art was placed on a postal stamp to promote autism awareness" (Seth Chwast's official website). He has been documented twice on NBC's *Today Show*. In 2017 and 2019, Seth was selected to participate in the London Art Biennale alongside 120 artists from 40 countries around the world, where he earned the European Confederation of Art Critics Award, Third Prize, and the Special Mention for Excellence Award. These awards were major milestones for Seth and his career.

Seth is unique in his ability to transform an impairment (autism) into an advantage. Most of us are never free of the social reality instilled in us; we live and behave in keeping with this reality. We can camouflage ourselves, but never completely escape. Seth, however, can: he is free to paint and say only what he wants and live life to its fullest, without caring what others have to say. "When we ask Seth why he loves to paint he says, 'My art will make people feel calm and comfort and tranquil. My art will be in books. My art will go to art shows'" (Debra Chwast, Seth's mother).

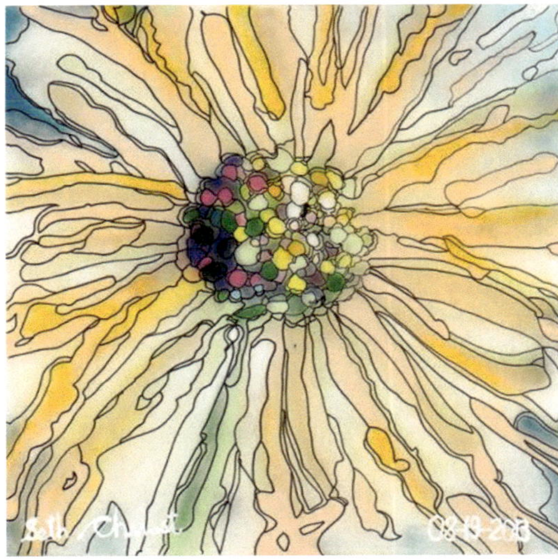

Figure 5.73 Seth Chwast: The Big Pink Flower. Acrylic spray paint on canvas, 36" x 36", 2013.

Photo courtesy of Seth and Debra Chwast.

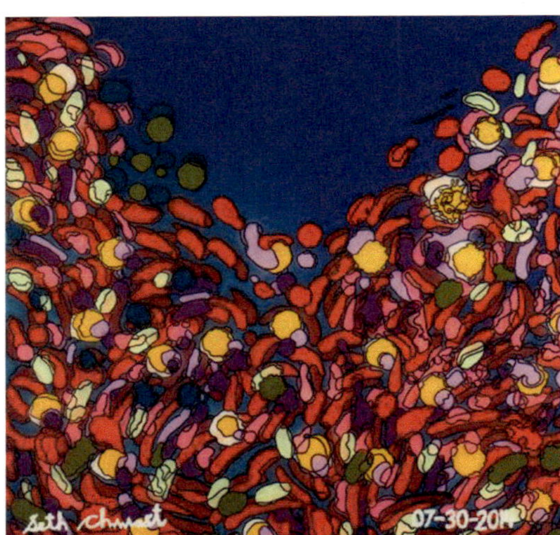

Figure 5.74 Seth Chwast: Purple Cone Flower Abstract. The Big Pink Flower. Acrylic spray on wood panel with polymer, 35" x 36.5", 2014.

Photo courtesy of Seth and Debra Chwast.

Impairments: Autism. He is primarily non-verbal, cannot safely cross the street by himself, rarely speaks and has always lived in his own insular world.

Skills: Artist, painter. Seth has a raw talent for mixing colors and creating works of art that reflect his vision of the world he inhabits. As an artist, he is difficult to classify. He is visionary, intuitive, extremely aware of his surroundings, and free in all things: lines, forms, technique, styles and colors.

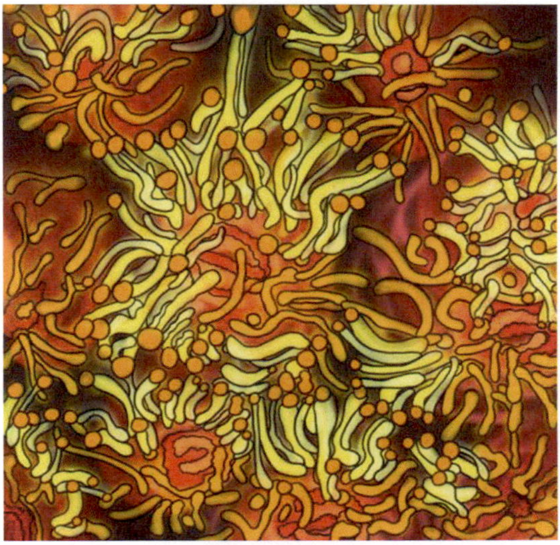

Figure 5.75 Seth Chwast: Sun Coral Abstract. Acrylic spray paint on panel, 36" x 36", 2015.

Photo courtesy of Seth and Debra Chwast.

Below are references, links to some videos, and additional reading about Seth Chwast.

- Seth Chwast's official website: https://www.sethchwastart.com/
- Seth Chwast on Facebook: https://es-la.facebook.com/pg/SethChwastArt/photos/
- Seth Chwast on Instagram: https://www.instagram.com/sethchwast/
- Seth Chwast on Twitter: https://twitter.com/sethchwastart

- Barber-Stetson, C. (2017). A Vibrant Autistic Aesthetic and the Limits of Art Brut. *Journal of Literary & Cultural Disability Studies, 11*(2), 113-131.
- Hunter, K. and Barnbaum, D. (2012). Pragmatic Aesthetics and the Autistic Artist. *The Journal of Aesthetic Education, 46*(4), 48-56.
- Chwast, D. and Chwast, S. (2011). *An Unexpected Life: A Mother and Son's Story of Love, Determination, Autism, and Art.* Sterling Publishing Company.
- Barnbaum, D. (2008). *The ethics of autism: Among them, but not of them.* Indiana University Press.
- Dubuffet, J. (1988). Place à l'incivisme. *Jean Dubuffet,* 103-106.
- *Cardinal, R. (1972). Outsider Art. London: Studio Vista. ISBN 9780289701683.*
- *Treffert, D. Seth Chwast. Agnesian.com* https://www.agnesian.com/page/seth-chwast
- Lappon. K. Seth Chwast – The Critique. International Confederation of Art Critics. https://www.international-confederation-art-critics.org/seth-chwast-critique
- Seth Chwast – A Different Kind of Journey. https://www.youtube.com/watch?v=Vvn4e8wPxZE
- Bai Presents: The Zac Brown Guitar Project | Artist: Seth Chwast. https://www.youtube.com/watch?v=qYQiV2dwZZY
- Natl Gallery presents Seth Chwast. https://www.youtube.com/watch?v=IzSCMtU5d5w
- Seth Chwast – Living With Autism by Dawn Kendrick. https://www.youtube.com/watch?v=ySEgEQupnZQ

5.25 Thristan Mendoza (born 1989)

Thristan "Tum-Tum" Mendoza was born in Quezon City, Philippines in 1989. He is an autistic savant and marimba prodigy. He was able to read and write at the age of two and a half and was later enrolled in a Montessori school. But not everything would turn out as expected. Thristan was solitary by nature, hyperactive, avoided eye contact, did not develop communication skills, and avoided playing with other children. His school suggested a psychological assessment, which was how his parents found out that their son was autistic. They were told they should not expect much of him. His mother has said:

The signs suddenly fell into place. He hated video lights and any form of the shade of red. He could not tolerate the sound of electric drills and food grinders. A loner, he needed a lot of prodding before he would play or interact with others. He did not like looking at the mirror, saying he was too shy to do so. He uttered certain words again and again. (Treffert, 2007).

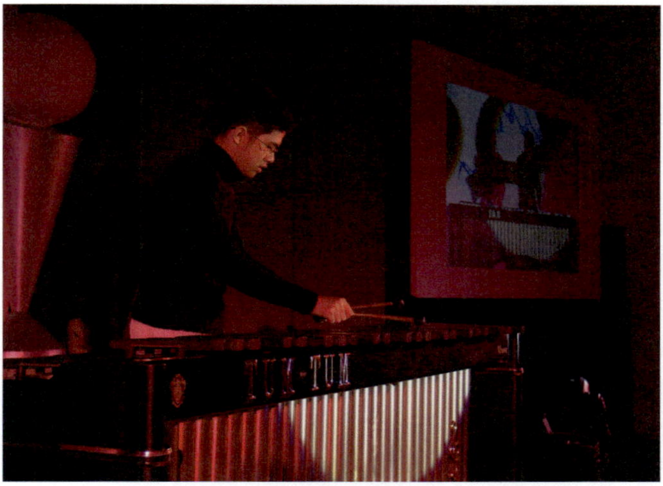

Figure 5.76 Thristan Mendoza.

Photo courtesy of Thristan Tum-Tum Mendoza.

The same year he was diagnosed with autism, Thristan began to play various instruments. He learned to play marimba at age five. Since then, because he has perfect pitch, Thristan excels at practically any instrument he chooses. During his first performance at school, he played the drums, cymbals, and temple block, all at the same time. He also excels at the Japanese Kumon method of mathematics.

Thristan seems to have been born with a pair of drumsticks in his hands. He has received numerous awards around the world. At age ten, "he was almost a veteran with more than 120 performances with the best instrumentalists, composers and percussionists from all over the world" (Treffert, 2007). He is a two-time grand prize winner of the McDonald's Philippines Makabata Awards. The University of the Philippines also named him their gifted child prodigy in 1997. In 2000, he earned the Millennium Dreamer's Award from the Walt Disney Company, McDonald's and UNESCO. In 2012, Thristan graduated from the University of the Philippines College of Music in Diliman with a Bachelor's degree in Music, majoring in Percussion Performance under the tutelage of Professor Leodivino Roque. The international media has also shown great interest in Thristan. He has already given nearly 200 concerts both in his homeland and abroad, especially in countries like the United States and in Brunei, where he performed for the royal family. He has been featured on CNN, Nickelodeon, and NHK Japan.

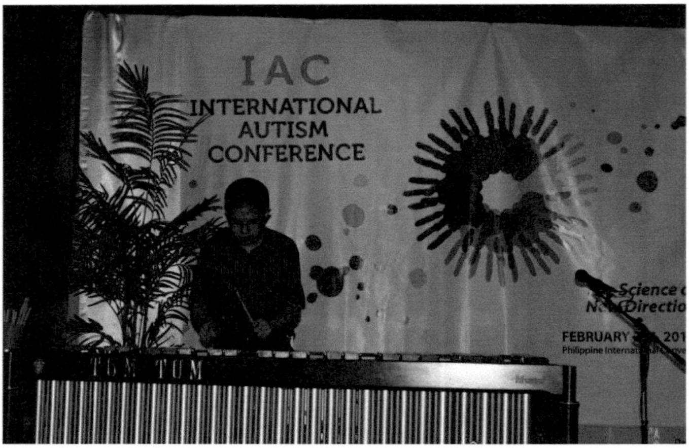

Figure 5.77 Thristan Mendoza: International Autism Conference, 2011.

Photo courtesy of Thristan Tum-Tum Mendoza.

Impairment: Autism. Diagnosed as autistic at the age of two and a half. Social skills are his main deficit. But as he says, "it didn't stop me from being the highly-functioning person I always dreamed to be" (Thristan Mendoza's Facebook page).

Skills: Musician, perfect pitch, marimba virtuoso, mathematics. IQ: 131. Shortly after his diagnosis, he began to play the marimba and, with his perfect pitch, he has become a marimba prodigy, although he excels at practically any instrument he chooses.

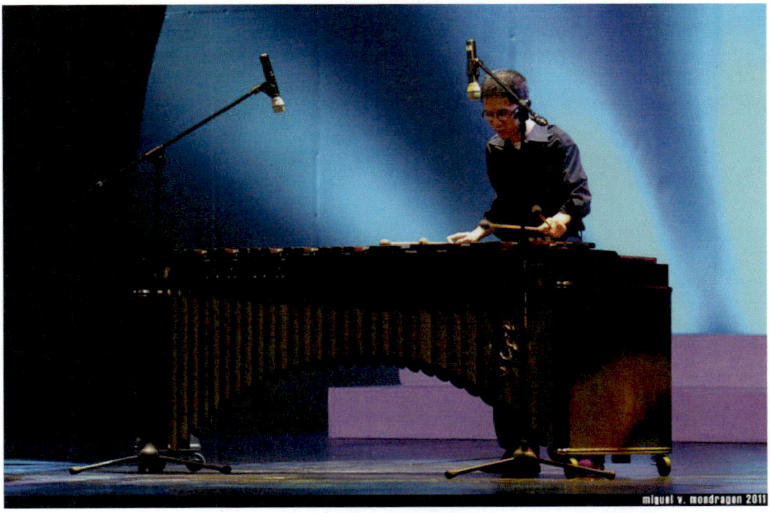

Figure 5.78 Thristan Mendoza, 2011.

Photo courtesy of Thristan Tum-Tum Mendoza.

Below are references, links to some videos, and additional reading about Thristan Mendoza.

- Thristan Mendoza on Facebook: https://www.facebook.com/ToogsToogsToogsToogsWorld
- Treffert, D. (2007). Thristan "Tum-Tum" Mendoza. Agnesian Healthcare. SSM Health. https://www.agnesian.com/page/thristan-tum-tum-mendoza
- Aguila, A. (2004). Music from the inner heart. Philstar. July 11, 2004. https://www.philstar.com/other-sections/starweek-magazine/2004/07/11/257204/music-inner-heart
- WAAD Concert 2008: Tumtum. https://www.youtube.com/watch?v=tWGinEGg7sk
- Filipino child prodigy marimbist with autism. https://www.youtube.com/watch?v=y5WXpmmroFs

- UP Perc Squad: "Samba Battucada feat Billie Jean" – UP Perc Squad feat Thristan Mendoza. https://www.youtube.com/watch?v=INc2NAdqRNs

5.26 Leland Lee (born 1989)

I am deeply indebted to Michele Chang, Leland's language teacher, for her extensive assistance in the final revisions of this profile.

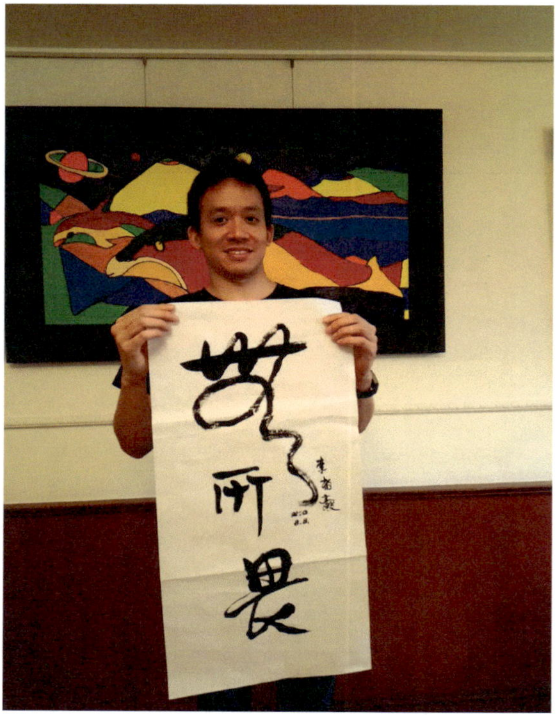

Figure 5.79 Leland Lee. 2019 "Fearless" Chinese calligraphy scroll.

Photo courtesy of Leland Lee and Karen Chien.

Leland Lee was born to a Taiwanese-American family in Los Angeles, California in 1989. He is an artist and an autistic savant. His father worked at NASA while his mother took on the work of caring for Leland. As an infant, Leland began to paint even before speaking, but there was something in his behavior that disturbed his parents despite this oddity. Leland secluded himself, avoided eye contact, did not speak, did not respond to his parents, and threw tantrums for no apparent reason. When Leland was eighteen months old, he was diagnosed with severe autism. The doctor who treated him had devastating news for the child's parents: Leland would have difficulty speaking, walking, and managing in society. This was a common prognosis at the time for children with autism.

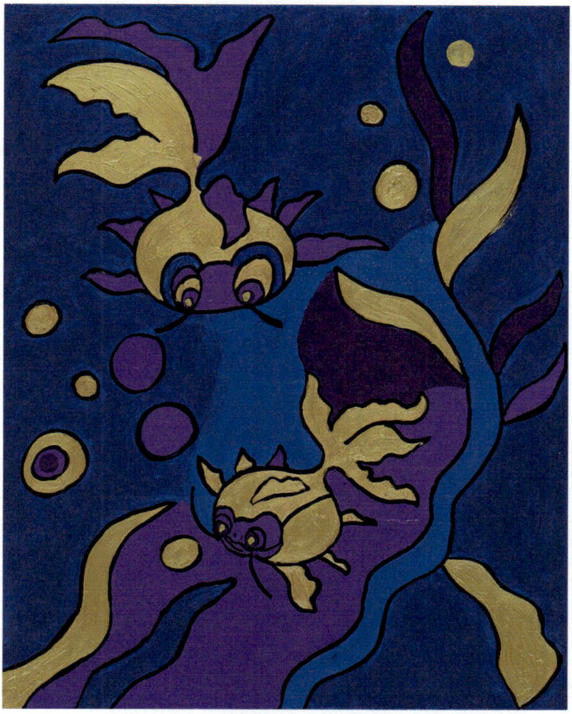

Figure 5.80 Leland Lee. Gold Fish, 2014.

Photo courtesy of Leland Lee and Karen Chien.

Leland began to use his multi-colored artworks as a way to express himself and to communicate with his mother, Karen, and the rest of the world. Leland's parents focused their parenting efforts on Leland's abilities instead of disabilities. Karen believed that Leland should have the same opportunities to learn as his older brother did. Accordingly, Leland has had lessons in Chinese, English, gymnastics, swimming, horseback riding, guitar, Chinese calligraphy, and ping pong, and his mother has even involved him in activities in church, as she is a woman of faith. Karen's dedication and unconditional love, Leland's love for life and zest for learning, and both mother and son's unwavering desire to improve have transformed Leland into a young man who speaks two languages, swims competitively, loves to sing, and plays guitar. Besides being gifted in art, he is a natural athlete. Leland cannot participate in team sports but excels in sports that are repetitive, such as swimming, horseback riding, bowling, and free throw basketball. Leland won Gold and Silver medals at the 2006 Special Olympics swimming competition. Leland is currently under training in the Artistic Swimming Association of Taiwan program run by Coach Julia Startch.

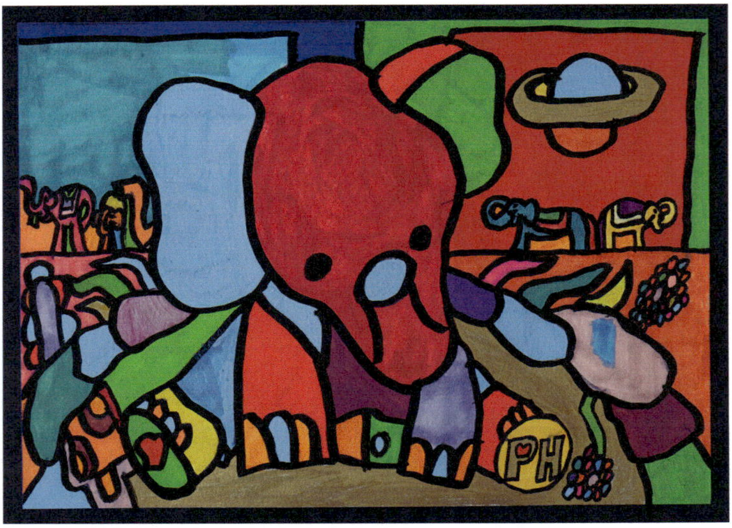

Figure 5.81 Leland Lee. Les Enphants, 2003.

Photo courtesy of Leland Lee and Karen Chien.

The table below shows a typical daily schedule for Leland as a boy.

	Sunday	Monday	Tuesday	Wednesday	Thursday	Friday	Saturday
Daily Routine	Paint Swim Practice Guitar Sing Read bible Write journal	Paint Swim Practice guitar Sing Read bible Write journal	Paint Swim Practice guitar Sing Read bible Write journal	Paint Swim Practice guitar Sing Read bible Write journal	Paint Swim Practice guitar Sing Read bible Write journal	Paint Swim Practice guitar Sing Read bible Write journal	Paint Swim Practice Guitar Sing Read bible Write journal
Lessons			English lesson	Chinese calligraphy lesson	Ping pong league English lesson	Golf lesson	Artistic Swimming lesson

Figure 5.82 Schedule of Leland's daily life.

"Lee attended the Los Angeles Conservatory of Fine Arts between the age of six and seventeen, when his family relocated back to Taiwan" (Bohwongprasert, 2018). Karen never gave up on her son, and relying on her faith in God and the help of Professor Ching-Chih Kuo of the National Taiwan Normal University, who took a genuine interest in Leland's development, she saw Leland begin to progress not only as a painter, but also as a socially outgoing person (Bohwongprasert, 2018).

> Leland likes to use bold colors. Intricate shaped blocks filled with golden yellow, fiery red, bright orange, teal, purple, turquoise, and royal blue, accentuated by gold or silver lines are often found in his compositions. It's remarkable that the strong contrasting colors achieve an incredible harmony, all without the formal training in color theory. This natural talent, untainted by schooling and studying often produces artworks that are joyful and invigorating—a soulful reflection of Leland's person and inner world (Leland's mother, Karen Chien).

Leland often uses modern technology to generate paintings and 3D artworks full of color that express his boundless imagination and the rich life experiences gathered from his travels. Leland creates unique Chinese calligraphy scrolls which he incorporates drawings into to match the theme of the calligraphic writing.

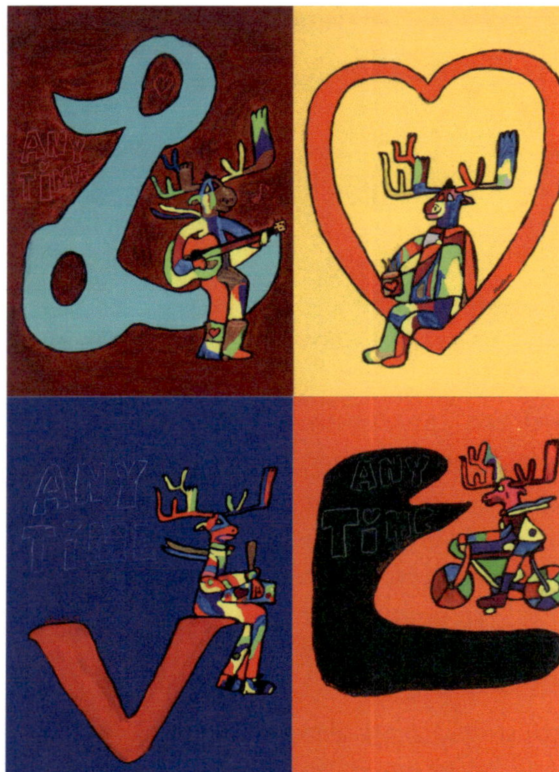

Figure 5.83 Leland Lee. Love, 2009.

Photo courtesy of Leland Lee and Karen Chien.

He has been featured as a savant artist in different countries around the world. His exquisite artwork has brought him critical claim and success. In 2013, Leland was named one of Ten Outstanding Young Persons in Taiwan, and his work was exhibited in Taiwan, China, Europe, the United States, and Canada. In 2014, Leland had a visit with Pope Francis in Rome, where he presented the Pontiff with one of his artworks.

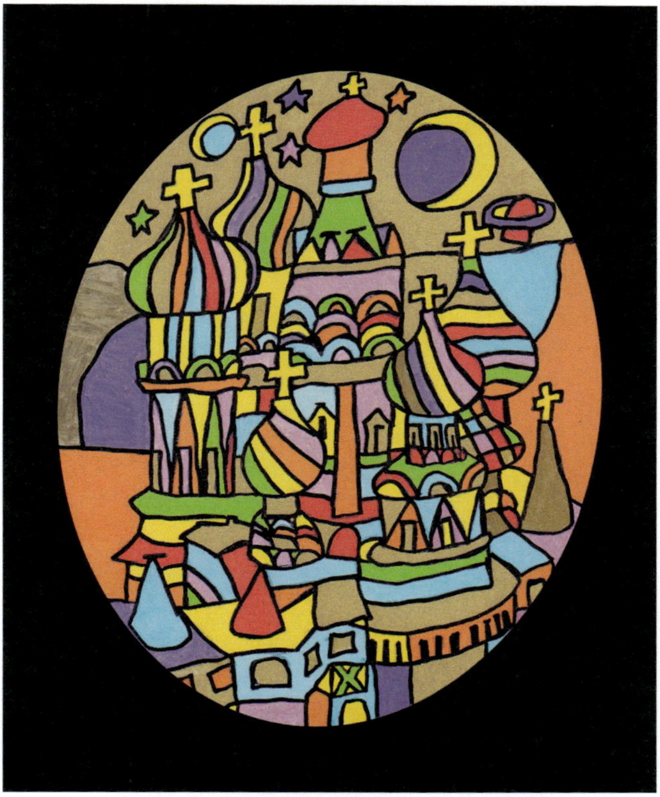

Figure 5.84 Leland Lee. Starry Night in Moscow, 2012.

Photo courtesy of Leland Lee and Karen Chien.

He currently resides in Taipei, Taiwan and works at Café Astoria. Leland and his mother have brought a ray of hope to families with autistic children in Taiwan. They use different platforms and media to promote autism awareness. They are invited to speak at universities and events, and frequently appear on TV programs in Taiwan.

> Leland is like a "friendship ambassador" for autism bringing government, medical science and scholars to work together, all for a common goal for the world to be a friendlier place to autistic children and provide more support for the parents (Karen Chien).

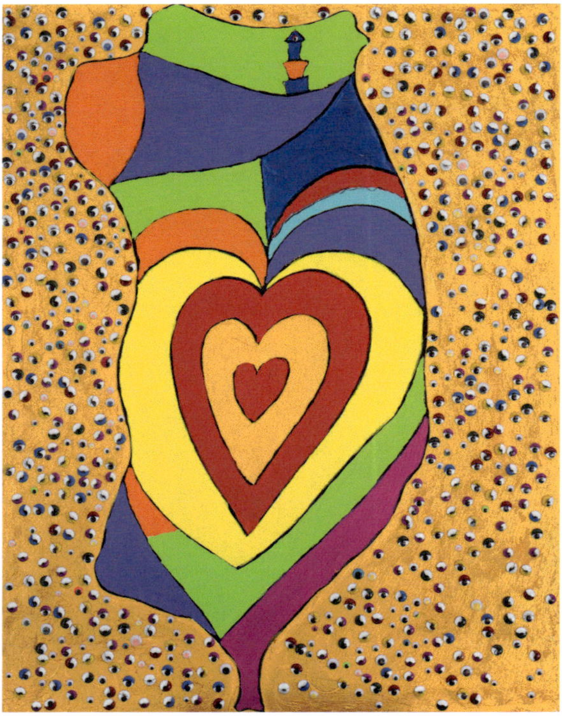

Figure 5.85 Leland Lee. Eye love Taiwan, 2012.

Photo courtesy of Leland Lee and Karen Chien.

Impairments: Autism. During childhood, Leland secluded himself, avoided eye contact, did not speak, did not respond to his parents, and threw tantrums for no apparent reason.

Skills: Artist, painter, competitive swimmer, singer, guitarist. His multi-colored works of art reflect his endless imagination and life experiences, especially from places he has visited.

Below are references, links to some videos, and additional reading about Leland Lee.

- Leland Lee's official website: https://lelandlee.com

- Leland Lee's official website in Chinese: https://lelandlee.wordpress.com
- Chien, K. (2020). Love in the Moment: A Memoir. Amazon. https://www.amazon.com/Love-Moment-Memoir-Karen-Chien/dp/1710270152/ref=sr_1_2?keywords=karen+chien&qid=1583799056&s=digital-text&sr=1-2-catcorr
- Strong, M. (2020). Taiwan artist mixes art and technology at Café Astoria. Taiwan News. Jun 18, 2020. https://www.taiwannews.com.tw/en/news/3950227
- Bohwongprasert, I. (2019). Love is all around. Bangkok Post. September 5, 2019. https://www.bangkokpost.com/life/arts-and-entertainment/1743239/love-is-all-around
- Bohwongprasert, I. (2018). Able artistry. Bangkok Post. September 11, 2018. https://www.bangkokpost.com/life/arts-and-entertainment/1537910/able-artistry
- Babcock, S. (2011). Leland Lee, An International Star from Taiwan Making a Difference. https://lelandlee.wordpress.com/about/leland-lee-an-international-star-from-taiwan/
- Lin, J. (c. 2007). Case Study of an Autistic Young Artist: Leland Lee.
- Leland Lee at the San Francisco Public Library. https://www.youtube.com/watch?v=BrPqj9U0dDY
- Leland Lee: Boundless Creativity. Mount Tabor. February 12, 2018. https://mounttabor.it/boundless-creativity/
- Good Idea Online Art Gallery featuring Leland Lee's ceramic art. https://1121a.101grace.com/en/%E5%B7%A5%E8%97%9D-%E6%9D%8E%E6%9F%8F%E6%AF%85/

5.27 Matt Savage (born 1992)

I greatly appreciate the contributions of Diane Savage, Matt's mother, in reviewing this profile.

Matthew "Matt" Savage was born on May 12, 1992 in Sudbury, Massachusetts. He is an autistic savant and musician. Matt was a child prodigy with what is known as hyperlexia, a syndrome characterized by precocious and unexpected reading skills and abilities beyond a child's chronological age. During his childhood, Matt hated sounds and music. He was also hyperactive and exhibited severe communication problems, particularly in socializing with other children. He was diagnosed with pervasive developmental disorder at age three, which partly explained this behavior.

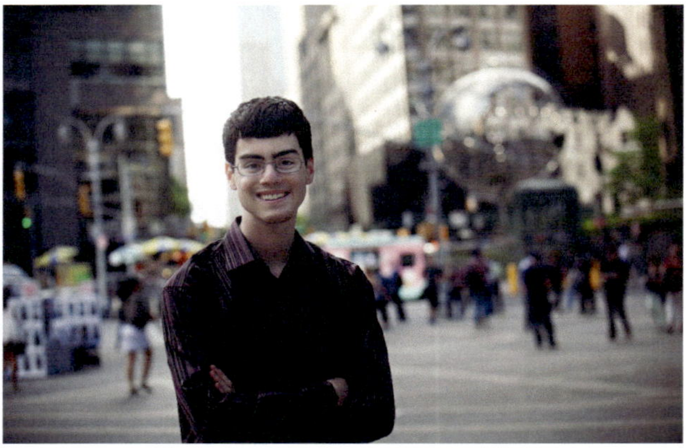

Figure 5.86 Matt Savage, 2015. Photo by Alex Abercrombie.

Photo courtesy of Matt Savage.

Everything changed when Matt reached the age of six. He received auditory integration therapy, and suddenly music returned to his life. Matt taught himself to play piano and read sheet music. He began studying classical music but soon discovered jazz. At the age of seven, he took lessons at the New England Conservatory of Music in Boston, Massachusetts. Since he had perfect pitch, everything regarding music came very easily and naturally to him. "Music just came to me," Matt says.

Matt had the opportunity to perform with Chaka Khan and other popular singers when he was still a child. He also started playing jazz in a club, where he met the musicians who would become his sidemen; bassist John Funkhouser and drummer Steve Silverstein. The three formed the Matt Savage Trio. Since then, Matt has produced thirteen albums (writing almost all the songs), given concerts around the world (including in the United States, Canada, Singapore, Costa Rica, Curacao, Aruba, Spain, India, Japan, and China), and appeared on several TV and radio shows, such as *The Late Show with David Letterman, Late*

Night with Conan O'Brien, The Today Show, and *All Things Considered*, and on channels like the Discovery Channel, BBC, and Telemundo TV.

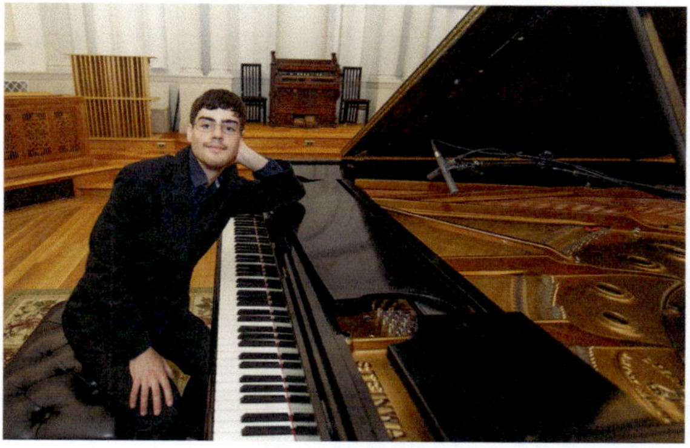

Figure 5.87 Matt Savage. 2016.

Photo courtesy of Matt Savage.

The Wall Street Journal, JazzTimes, JAZZIZ, TIME, WIRED, Der Spiegel, The Jerusalem Report, People Magazine, TIME for Kids, American Way, The Globe and Mail, the Toronto Star, The Boston Globe, the New York Daily News, and others have featured Matt in print (Matt Savage's official website).

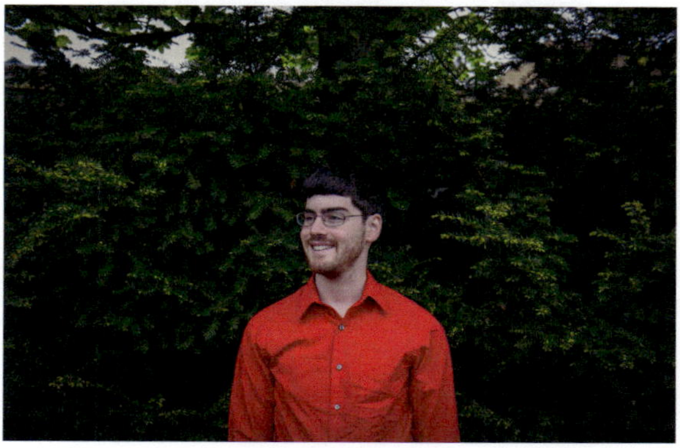

Figure 5.88 Matt Savage, 2019. Photo by Micah Gummel.

Photo courtesy of Matt Savage

Despite his hectic life as a music professional, Matt always made time for studies. He received his B.M. in Performance (Piano) from Berklee College of Music in 2012. A year later, he composed and recorded the score for a full-length documentary film, *Sound of Redemption: The Frank Morgan Story*. In May 2015, Matt received his M.M. in Jazz Performance (Piano) from the Manhattan School of Music.

Matt always says that he is a big fan of numbers, which come to him in dreams and inspire him to compose music. "Forty-Seven," a song from the Matt Savage Trio album *Groovin' on Mount Everest*, is a clear example of the results of this inspiration. Matt, now an acclaimed jazz pianist and composer, currently balances his professional music career with teaching. "Savage has been called 'amazing' by jazz legend Dave Brubeck and been touted as the Mozart of jazz" (Treffert, 2010). He has produced several albums, been offered concerts around the world, and appeared on several TV shows.

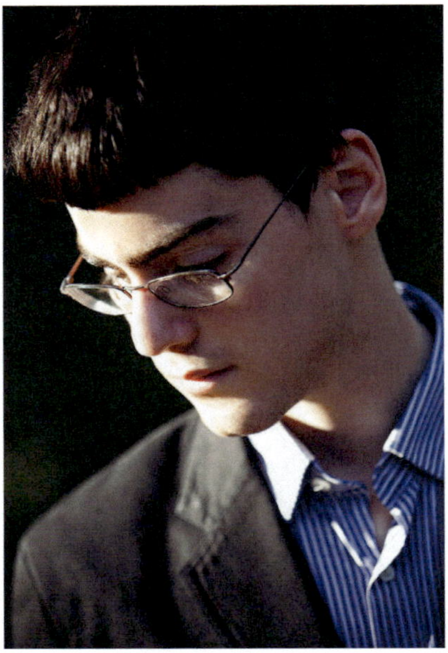

Figure 5.89 Matt Savage, 2015. Photo by Alex Abercrombie.

Photo courtesy of Matt Savage.

Impairments: Autism with hyperlexia. Matt was diagnosed with autism at the age of three.

Skills: Musician, composer perfect tempo, perfect pitch. Highly intelligent.

Below are references, links to some videos, and additional reading about Matt Savage.

- Matt Savage's official website: http://www.savagerecords.com
- Matt Savage on Facebook: https://www.facebook.com/MattSavageOfficial/?tn-str=k*F
- Matt Savage on YouTube: https://www.youtube.com/channel/UCHXQbJ4yzoB5oCQRGaTtk2g
- Varga, K. (2018). From silence to sensation: Prodigy Matt Savage, born with autism, now a music veteran. Democratic & Chronicle. June 17, 2018. https://www.democratandchronicle.com/story/lifestyle/2018/06/17/matt-savage-autistic-savant-and-child-prodigy-plays-jazz-fest-xrijf-rochester-jazz/690534002/
- Solomon, O. (2013). Autism and Affordances of Achievement. *The social life of achievement*, 2, 120.
- Treffert, D. (2010). *Islands of genius: The bountiful mind of the autistic, acquired, and sudden savant*. Jessica Kingsley Publishers.
- Tammet, D. (2009). *Embracing the wide sky: A tour across the horizons of the mind*. Simon and Schuster.
- Biever, C. (2009). The makings of a savant. *New Scientist, 202*(2711), 30-33.
- Matt Savage plays "Blues in 33/8" in New York. https://www.youtube.com/watch?v=RGD1gl0YtfM
- Seven Up – The Matt Savage Trio. https://www.youtube.com/watch?v=l8yrxadl1tE
- Matt Savage- "Spain" by Chick Corea (Live in Spain). https://www.youtube.com/watch?v=gjegFMfvRKQ
- The Matt Savage Trio- "Power Pop" (Live in Japan). https://www.youtube.com/watch?v=Dwv9I7xSPBk
- Matt Savage Trio- "Go On" (Live in Japan 2015). https://www.youtube.com/watch?v=4PQvyfFLIxo

- Matt Savage- "Stella by Starlight." https://www.youtube.com/watch?v=CJV4oSdazW4
- Matt Savage – "Got to Get You Into My Life" (Live at Regattabar). https://www.youtube.com/watch?v=taCBOouZ1Lc

5.28 Ping Lian Yeak (born 1993)

I am deeply indebted to Dr. Rosa Martinez (Strokes of Genius) and Sarah Lee, Ping Lian's mother, for their extensive assistance in the final revisions of this profile.

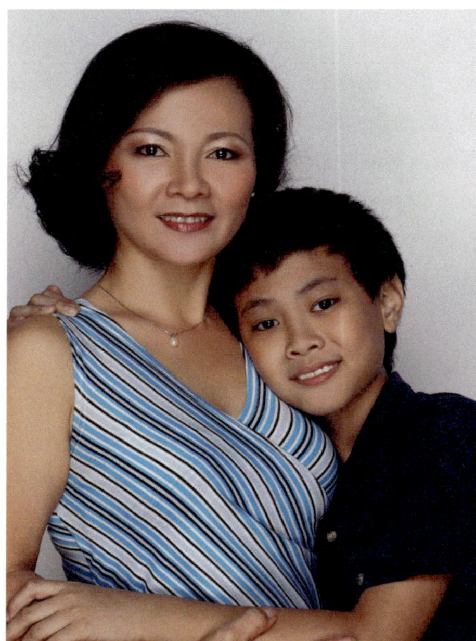

Figure 5.90 Ping Lian and his mother.

Photo courtesy of Sarah SH Lee and Ping Lian Yeak.

Ping Lian Yeak was born in Malaysia on November 18, 1993. He is an autistic savant and artist. He has lived in Sydney, Australia since May 2006. As a child, Ping Lian was hyperactive, lived in his own world, showed no affection nor emotions, and had limited ability to speak, in addition to fine motor control so poor that he could not hold a pencil in his fingers to write. He was four years old when doctors diagnosed him with autism, and things for his family grew worse when his father tragically died of a heart attack when Ping Lian was ten. Yet his mother, Sarah Lee, moved heaven and earth for her son, demonstrating an iron-willed determination to achieve the almost impossible. With her love, Sarah Lee managed to make her son an outstanding artist.

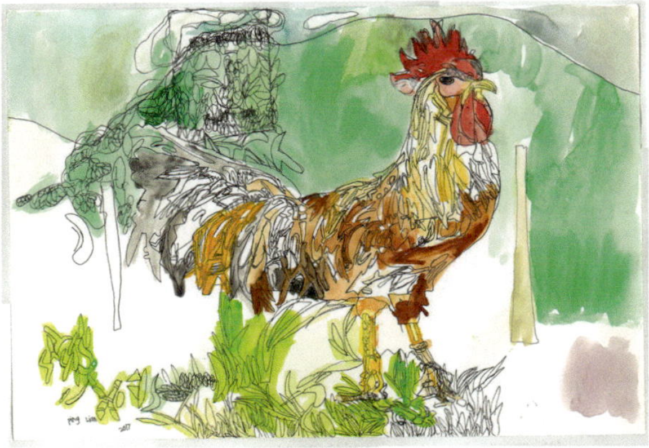

Figure 5.91 Rooster, 17402. Painted in 2017.

Photo courtesy of Sarah SH Lee and Ping Lian Yeak.

After many years of hard work on exercises that focused on developing his fine motor skills (i.e., his home program focused on tracing and coloring activities), Ping Lian began drawing and painting around age eight, and soon it became his favorite activity. He has never stopped since. His talent is immense and apparently limitless. His artworks consist mainly of colorful and intricately detailed depictions of animals and great architectural sites, such as the Sydney Opera house, the Malaysia Twin Towers, and different mosques. He works in acrylic, oil, watercolor, charcoal, and ink, and sometimes combines multiple media. Ping Lian continues to be deficient in the areas of socialization, verbal communication and intellectual ability. However, given the many years of guidance, nurturance and perseverance of Ping Lian's dedicated "Mum," Ping Lian has grown to be an obedient, hardworking, and grateful young man, full of love and affection.

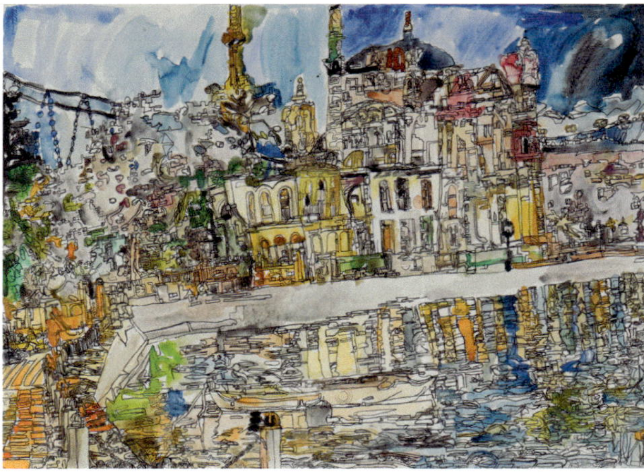

Figure 5.92 Ortaköy Mosque, Istanbul. 14005. Painted in 2014.

Photo courtesy of Sarah SH Lee and Ping Lian Yeak.

Ping Lian's art has been featured in various books, TV programs, and exhibits in New York, Australia, Germany, Japan, UK, South Korea, Singapore, and Malaysia. In 2011 he was featured in a book published in Korea, *Knowledge-e6* by EBS, which also included the Real Rain Man (Kim Peek), Albert Einstein, Abraham Lincoln, Warren Edward Buffett etc. In the same year Ping Lian was featured in *Real Reading: Creating an Authentic Reading Experience.* In 2019, Utah State University acquired six of Ping Lian's original artworks. Dr. Rosa Martínez, the president and founder of Strokes of Genius, says that if Ping Lian did not have autism, "he would be considered a prodigy and a genius based solely on his artistic talents."

Ping Lian is acknowledged as a prodigious savant. The book *I Want To Be Artist: An Autistic Savant's Voice and A Mother's Dream Transformed onto Canvas* written by his mother and published in 2017, "serves as an inspiration not only to the autistic community, but also to the art world at large" (Lee, 2017).

Impairments: Autism. As a child he was hyperactive, lived in his own world, showed no affection or emotions, and could not speak or write. He was four years old when doctors diagnosed him with autism.

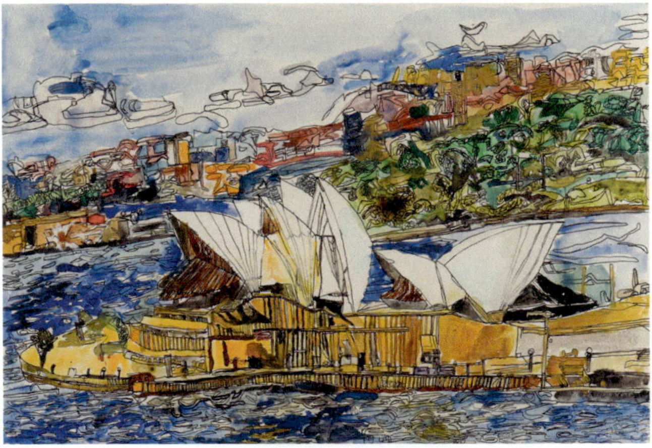

Figure 5.93 Sydney Opera House, Sydney. 15002. Painted in 2015.

Photo courtesy of Sarah SH Lee and Ping Lian Yeak.

Skills: Artist, painter. He began drawing and painting around age eight and has not stopped since. His talent is vast and apparently limitless. His work consists mainly of colorful and intricately detailed depictions of animals and great architectural sites. He works in acrylic, oil, watercolor, charcoal, and ink, and sometimes combines multiple media.

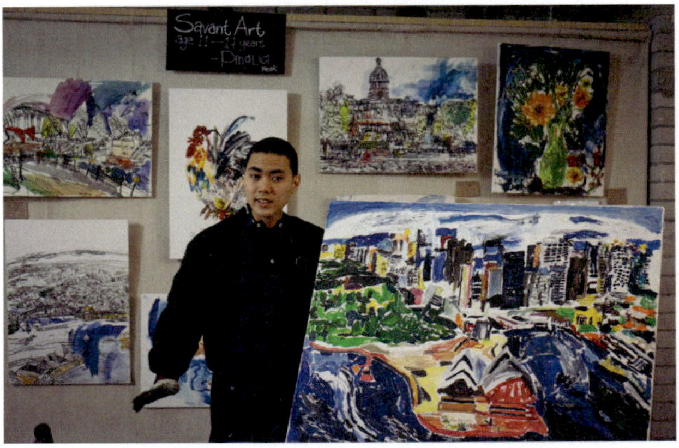

Figure 5.94 Lian at The Rocks. Pop-up project. 2011.

Photo courtesy of Sarah SH Lee and Ping Lian Yeak.

Below are references, links to some videos, and additional reading about Ping Lian Yeak.

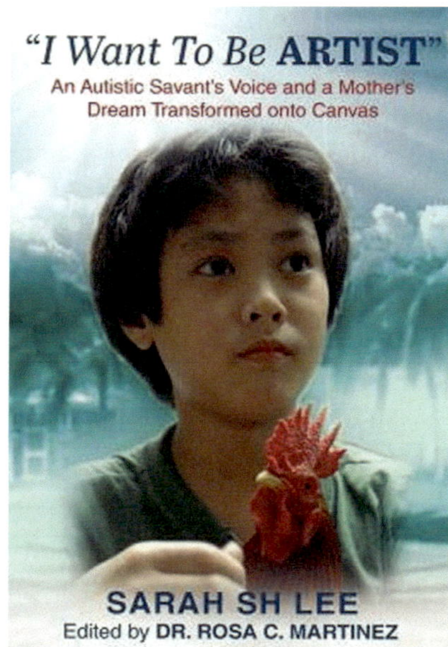

Figure 5.95 Ping Lian Yeak. Cover of the book: "I want to be artist"

Photo courtesy of Sarah SH Lee and Dr. Rosa Martinez

- Ping Lian Yeak website: https://www.pinglian.com/
- Ping Lian Yeak's Facebook page: https://www.facebook.com/pinglianyeak/
- Ping Lian Online Shop: https://pinglian-com.myshopify.com/
- Lee, S. (2017). I Want To Be ARTIST: An Autistic Savant's Voice and A Mother's Dream Transformed onto Canvas. Siew Hong Lee. ISBN: 978-0648035411.
    - "There can be no doubt that Ping Lian owes a debt to his 'tiger mother', Sarah, who recognized his talent at an early age and worked so tirelessly to help him develop his artistic facility. One need not share Sarah's faith in either God or motivational literature to realize she has found a set of techniques that have brought out the best in her son." John McDonald, Art critic for the Sydney Morning Herald.

  - "I Want To Be ARTIST – An Autistic Savant's Voice and a Mother's Dream Transformed onto Canvas is the inspiring story of how a mother nurtured and encouraged her son's ability in art. Find out what your child is good at and then broaden and expand it. My mother always encouraged me to draw many different things. It is important to always "stretch" and expand a child's experiences." Temple Grandin, author.
  - "This book is an owner's manual of sorts, providing a chronicle of what did work—stylized but painfully slowly, for this mother, Sarah Lee, for her son Ping Lian in helping him on the road toward realizing his full potential as an artist. But even more importantly, helping him also to attain the best communication and social skills he could on the road toward eventually being as independent as possible." Darold Treffert, M.D.
  - "I Want To Be ARTIST: An Autistic Savant's Voice and A Mother's Dream Transformed onto Canvas is the story of a mother's desperate struggle to get her autistic son to 'see' her; to 'love' his family and to be a contributing member to society. Readers will be fortunate to capture not just the turmoil but the life lessons and strategies created out of Sarah Lee's desperation that have led to her son's success." Rosa Martínez, Ph.D., BCBA-D. Strokes of Genius, Inc-President and Founder.

- Clark, T. (2016). *Exploring giftedness and autism: A study of a differentiated educational program for autistic savants*. Routledge.
- Ruthsatz, J. and Stephens, K. (2016). *The Prodigy's Cousin: The Family Link Between Autism and Extraordinary Talent*. Current.
- Treffert, D. (2010). *Islands of genius: The bountiful mind of the autistic, acquired, and sudden savant*. Jessica Kingsley Publishers.
- Mullin, J. (2009). *Drawing autism*. Mark Batty Publisher. ISBN 9780981960005
- Bonesteel, L. and Nation, P. (2011). *Real reading: creating an authentic reading experience*. Pearson Longman.
- Autistic Savant Artist, Ping Lian Yeak at age 12. https://www.youtube.com/watch?v=Rq9n6mgWwAI
- Ping Lian Yeak, Autistic Savant Artist at age 12. https://www.youtube.com/watch?v=buktflGp0GE

- Agora Galley, New York. https://www.agoragallery.com/ArtistPage/Ping_Lian_Yeak.aspx

5.29 Buğra Cankir (born 1994)

I am deeply indebted to Kamel Cankir, Buğra's father, for his extensive assistance in the final revisions of this profile.

Buğra Cankir was born in 1994, in Dörtyol, Hatay, Turkey. He is an autistic savant and a gifted musician (a pianist, specifically). Buğra did not speak or understand a word until the age of three. He did not know his name, or even why he was given a name. He also had the socialization and communication problems typical of an autistic person. Buğra was always distant and distracted. His parents struggled to comprehend what was happening with their son, until they received his formal diagnosis with autism disorder at the age of three.

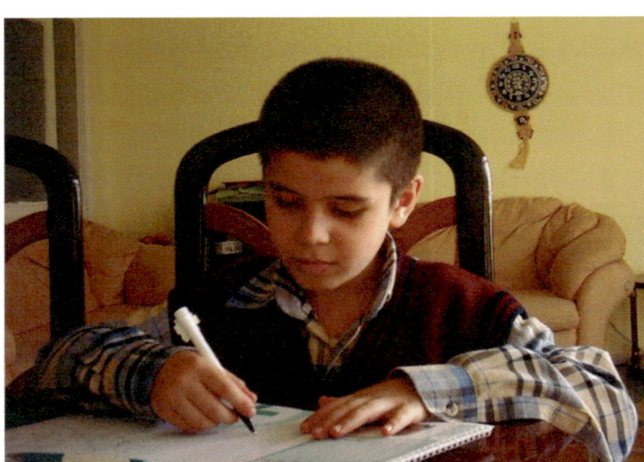

Figure 5.96 Buğra Cankir. Photo courtesy of Buğra and Kamel Cankir.

Buğra's parents went out of their way to give their child the best education possible. They also helped him with different types of therapy. When he was three and a half years old, his parents gave him a puzzle board with letters on it, which Buğra learned to read and write with. This was an important change for him, and it turned out to be a milestone in his education. Buğra has an exceptional memory, is fascinated by music, and is an expert in computer games. He is also a "calendar man," a calendrical savant.

During his entire school life, from primary school to university, Buğra's mother accompanied him like a shadow. It was the only way to be sure he could continue his education. Buğra finished both preschool and elementary school at a Montessori school and then mainstreamed into high school education at the Music Department of the Hatay Bedii Sabuncu High School of Fine Arts.

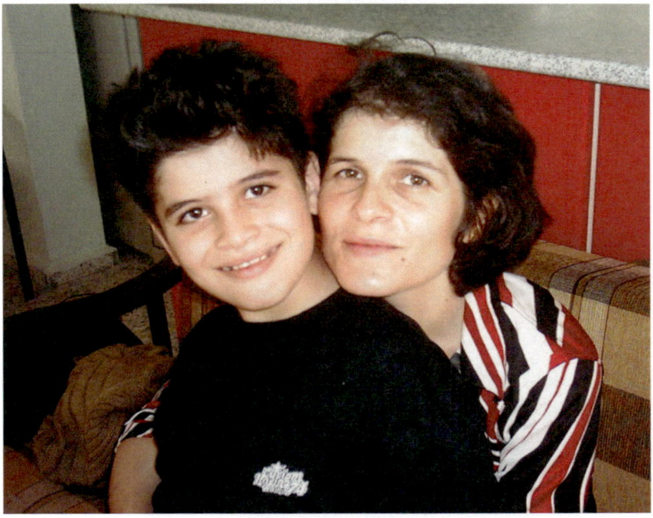

Figure 5.97 Buğra Cankir and his mother.

Photo courtesy of Buğra and Kamel Cankir.

Buğra did not receive any formal piano lessons until he was ten years old. But with perfect pitch and an exceptional talent for music, he soon became a masterful pianist and flutist. From the age of ten, he began practicing between 6 and 10 hours a week with his teacher Victoria Perepelitsa. The speed at which Buğra learned and progressed was a surprise to everyone around him. Perepelitsa reports that Buğra completed her two-year program in just one year.

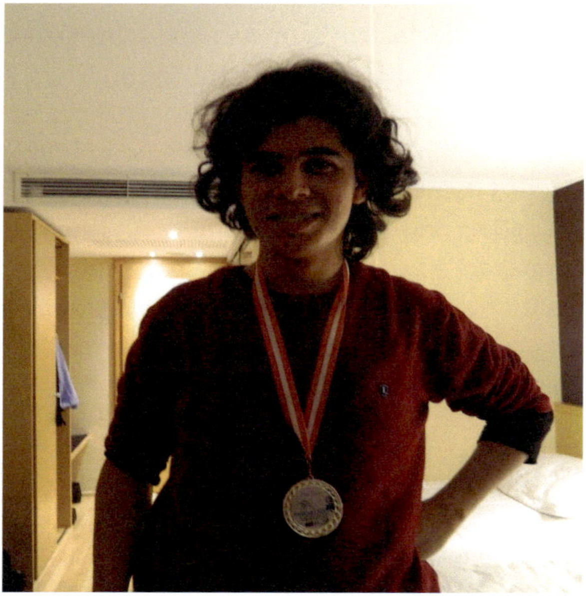

Figure 5.98 Buğra Cankir in Vienna with the bronze medal.

Photo courtesy of Buğra and Kamel Cankir.

In 2006, Buğra was tested by a University of California Genetics of Absolute Pitch study group and was found to have an impressive "perfect score" of 36/36 for both pure tone and piano tone, ranking first among the 664 people who were able to pass the test.

> He was also reported to be the youngest participant who had high absolute pitch score. He also took the Royal Academy exams and received the second top score in the history of the exam, then was invited to Cambridge University in England (Erden & Reyhanoglu, 2019).

Buğra's many accomplishments did not come easily, and required hard work. He wanted to receive a formal music education at a conservatory but was not accepted, despite his superior grades. The argument was always the same: we don't have teachers trained to work with autistic youth. Buğra, however, had one major advantage: his parents, who had been closely involved in his education from the beginning, would not give up until their son had a chance to reach his goals.

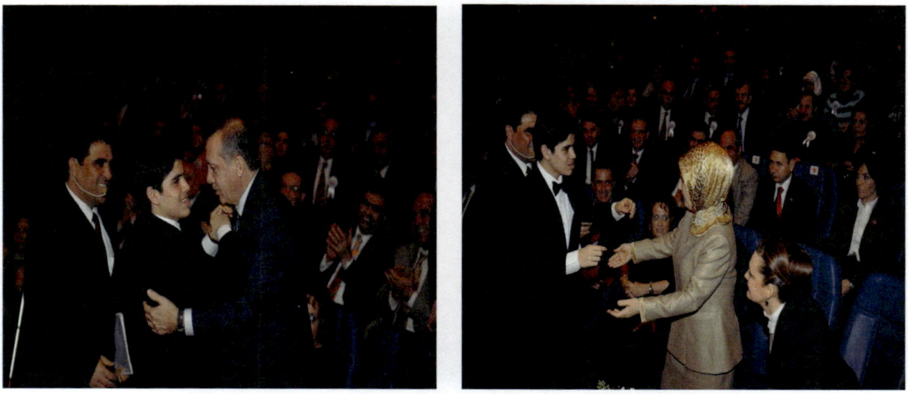

Figure 5.99 Recital for the President Recep Tayyip Erdoğan and First Lady of Turkey, Emin Erdoğan.

Photo courtesy of Buğra and Kamel Cankir.

Finally, in 2006, Buğra was accepted into the Associated Board of the Royal School of Music education system. His instructors also had to overcome various obstacles, since they did not have sufficient knowledge of or experience with his special condition (Erden & Reyhanoglu, 2019). Buğra, like other autistic people, did not follow rules for long. His tolerance was very limited. In class, he would sometimes get up without warning, scratch his body, burp if he felt like it, lose concentration, or laugh for no apparent reason. Despite these obstacles, Buğra's performance from the first year was consistently outstanding.

It is increasingly evident that individuals within the ASD think and behave differently from other individuals. They often attend schools that do not recognize their special needs, which affects not only these children, whose needs are not met and who feel completely misunderstood, but also their teachers, who lack the experience and information to support them in their education. This creates an opportunity to develop new careers around the world that specialize in the care and treatment of children on the autism spectrum.

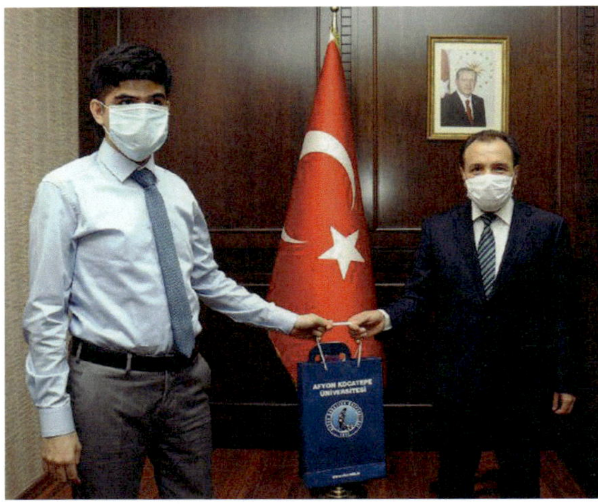

Figure 5.100 Buğra Cankir and the Rector of Afyon Kocatepe University. June 2020. Photo courtesy of Buğra and Kamel Cankir.

In 2006, Buğra performed at an art and music conference hosted by the Autism Research Centre of the University of Cambridge in London, with eleven other exceptional musicians who were diagnosed with autism or Asperger Syndrome. These included Derek Paravicini, Stephen Wiltshire, Gilles Trehin, and Ping Liang Yeak, who also displayed their artwork at the event. In 2013, Buğra was awarded with the "Best Value-Added Artist of the Year" award in the field of art. Buğra has given piano recitals at national and international events and has enraptured audiences with his performance of Rachmaninoff's "Elegie." The same year, he represented Turkey as a finalist at the International Piano Competition in Vienna. He won the Bronze Medal in his category.

Buğra received his Bachelor's degree from the Iskenderun Technical University's Mustafa Yazıcı State Conservatory in 2012. In June 2020, Buğra earned his Master's degree at the Afyon Kocatepe University (AKU)

Conservatory. He currently lives in Iskenderun (historically known as Alexandretta), Hatay, on the Mediterranean coast of Turkey.

Impairments: Autism. Buğra did not speak or understand a word until the age of three. He did not know his name or why he was given a name. He had also the behavioral, socialization, and communication problems typical of an autistic person.

Skills: Musician. Pianist and flutist. Perfect pitch. Exceptional memory. Expert in computer games.

Below are references, links to some videos, and additional reading about Buğra Cankir.

- Erden, S., & Reyhanoglu, G. (2019). Conservatory education of a musical savant with autism: a case study in Turkey. *Advances in Autism*.
- Treffert, D. Bugra Cankir. Agnesian. SSMHealth. https://www.agnesian.com/page/bugra-cankir
- İSTİKLAL MARŞI Piyano Buğra Çankır. https://www.youtube.com/watch?v=qy9qYB9VnB8
- Chopin Fantaisie-Impromptu (BUGRA CANKIR). https://www.youtube.com/watch?v=OuJ-BoRcs1Q
- Bugra CANKIR plays Flute piece Bach, Badinerie with Orchestra. https://www.dailymotion.com/video/xpq76c
- Shostakovich, Waltz no 2, Flute and Piano. https://www.youtube.com/watch?v=Es4iSUE3lXc
- Buğra Çankır – Musical Supervisor. https://www.youtube.com/watch?v=1mGiWqa8ARw
- Bugra CANKIR Show TV haberde. https://www.youtube.com/watch?v=kSr2mz4f1eY
- Bugra CANKIR plays Pathetique Rondo with Antalya SYMPHONY ORCHESTRA. https://www.youtube.com/watch?v=yYDjUqlxndk
- Yeteneksizsiniz Bugra CANKIR Engelleri Kaldiralim piyano performansı https://www.youtube.com/watch?v=3suIVdDO1WM

5.30 Rex Lewis-Clack (born 1995)

I am deeply indebted to Cathleen Lewis, Rex's mother, for her extensive assistance in the final revisions of this profile.

Rex Lewis-Clack was born in California, United States, on June 24, 1995. He is autistic, blind, and a prodigious musical savant. He is one of the few people in history to combine this rare triad of blindness, autism, and musical genius. Rex was born with a cerebral arachnoid cyst and with a form of blindness called septo-optic dysplasia. Rex's disabilities made educational specialists fear he might never walk, talk, eat solid food by himself, or do much of anything.

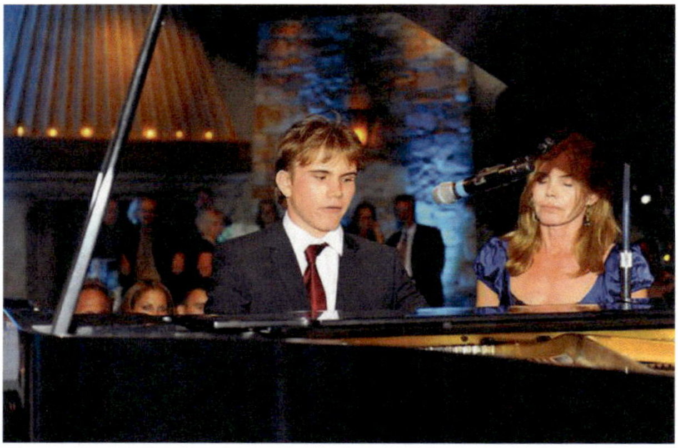

Figure 5.101 Rex playing Chopin for Best Buddies International at the Tehama Country Club in Carmel, California to help celebrate the mission of "Friendship for everyone."

Photo courtesy of Rex Lewis-Clack and Cathleen Lewis.

Arachnoid cysts are cerebrospinal fluid sacs that are located on the arachnoid membrane that covers the brain and the spinal cord. In most cases, arachnoid cysts are present at birth, stable (not requiring treatment), and are usually asymptomatic throughout an individual's life. Septo-optic dysplasia, on the other hand, is a disorder of early brain and eye development. Although its symptoms generally vary, the condition is traditionally defined by three main features: underdevelopment of the optic nerves (which carry visual information from the eyes to the brain), abnormal formation of structures along the midline of the brain, and a small pituitary gland (hypoplasia). Two of these features must be present for a clinical diagnosis. As a result, people with optic nerve hypoplasia have impaired vision (or complete blindness) in one or both eyes.

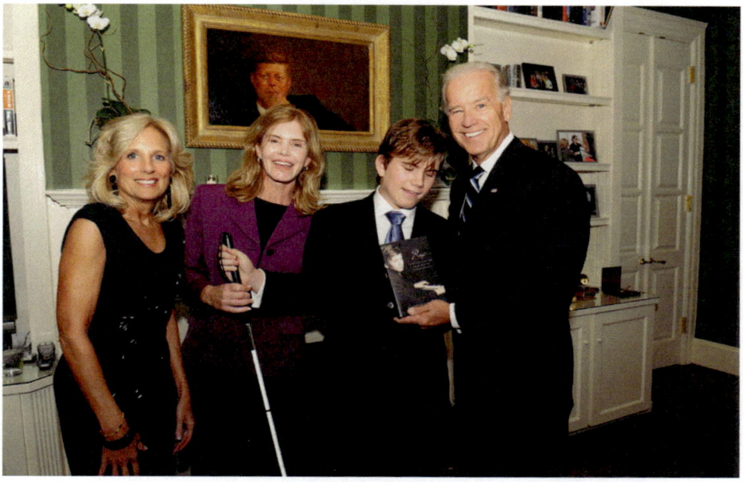

Figure 5.102 Rex performing at the President's (Joe Biden) residence at a VIP reception to celebrate the life and work of Eunice Kennedy Shriver (Anthony Shriver founded Best Buddies International).

Photo courtesy of Rex Lewis-Clack and Cathleen Lewis.

Rex cannot tie his shoes, needs some assistance to dress himself, and at times struggles to orient himself, which causes him to get turned around when moving about his own home. Rex also has difficulty carrying on a basic conversation, although he can express himself with regard to his daily wants and needs. He requires special assistance on a constant basis. Rex began walking around the age of two, talking at three, and has been educated in the public school system since the age of 5, but his path has not been an easy one, and his education was fraught with difficulty.

Rex began to perform on a piano keyboard, a gift from his father, at the age of two, and it instantly became his favorite activity. He began piano lessons at the age of five, and his talent exploded. The piano seems to have awakened him in the most wonderful and unimaginable way. Within months of starting his lessons, he could instantly identify any note that was played for him. One day, one of his teachers showed him a scale, and he then ran the other 11 scales back. At the age of 11, Rex could play Mozart or Schubert, note by note, perfectly (without reading music or seeing the piano keys) after hearing it only once. He can also improvise from other themes with little effort. Undoubtedly, there is an element of magic (the evident ability to produce results that are contrary to natural laws) in his condition. His mother Cathleen wonders, "... how can an 11-year old boy hear a Mozart fantasy for the first time and play it back note-for-note perfectly—but struggle to navigate the familiar surroundings of his own home?" (Lewis, 2008).

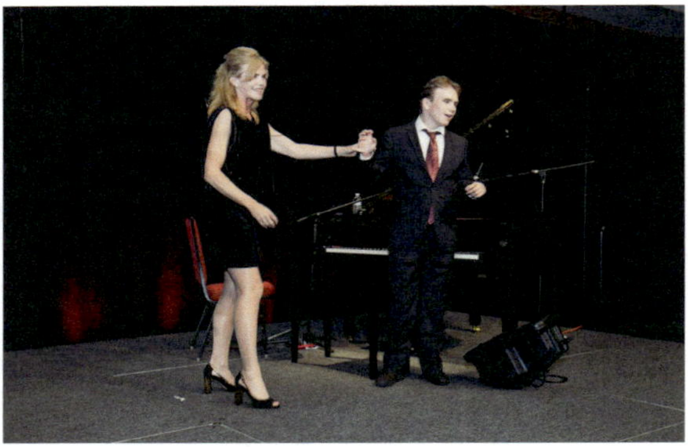

Figure 5.103 Rex taking a bow after a fundraiser in Maryland, at an "I Have a Voice" Gala--giving a voice to individuals with disabilities.

Photo courtesy of Rex Lewis-Clack and Cathleen Lewis.

Rex Lewis-Clack came to national attention in 2003 at age eight, when he appeared on CBS's *60 Minutes*, which began following his life and development. In 2006, he was the recipient of the "Winspiration Award" in Germany. In 2011, The Science Channel presented "The Boy with the Musical Mind," an episode of the documentary series *Ingenious Minds*, which focused on Rex. He has had the opportunity to travel and perform nationwide and abroad, always in the company of his mother (a graduate of Stanford University and a former foreign-exchange trader), sharing his life and his gifts on the piano. In 2013, Rex and Cathleen launched the Rex & Friends foundation, which supports musical education for individuals who are blind or autistic.

Impairments: Autism, blindness. He was born with a cerebral arachnoid cyst and septo-optic dysplasia. Rex is unable to tie his own shoes or dress himself independently and struggles with basic conversations and spatial orientation, even in familiar environments. He requires special assistance at all times.

Skills: Musical genius, pianist. Rex can hear a Mozart or Schubert work just once, and then play it back impeccably without missing a note. He can also improvise from other themes with little effort.

Below are references, links to some videos, and additional reading about Rex Lewis-Clack.

- Rex Lewis-Clack's official website: https://en.wikipedia.org/wiki/Rex_Lewis-Clack
- Rex Lewis-Clack on Facebook: https://www.facebook.com/Rex-Lewis-Clack-184911764774/
- Margulis, E. (2017). Neuroscience: How music meets mind. *Nature*, 546(7658), 351-351.
- Marsa, L. (2016). Extraordinary Minds: The link between savantism and autism. Spectrum. January 13, 2016. https://www.spectrumnews.org/features/deep-dive/extraordinary-minds-the-link-between-savantism-and-autism/
- Lewis, C. (2008). *Rex: A mother, her autistic child, and the music that transformed their lives*. Thomas Nelson.
- Ockelford, A., Pring, L., Welch, G. and Treffert, D. (2006). Focus on music.
- Pring, L. and Ockelford, A. (2005). Children with septo-optic dysplasia-musical interests, abilities and provision: the results of a parental survey. *British Journal of Visual Impairment*, 23(2), 58-66.
- Tormented by Genius original version of Rex, Full (21–minute), can be found on Vimeo, but not on YouTube. This was posted on Vimeo by the Editor, before some final changes were made, and it was retitled "Ingenious Minds." https://vimeo.com/18989003
- Musically Speaking. Original 60 Minutes profile on Rex (2003) called Musically Speaking, can only be found on Rex's Facebook Page (posted in

2013). You can find Derek Paravicini at the end of the profile, as an example of where 8-year-old Rex's savant gift might go by age 24 (as Derek was when this was filmed). https://www.facebook.com/watch/?v=10151750987604775

- Catching Up With Rex. https://www.youtube.com/watch?v=cCF1xSgyKXg
- Rex Lewis-Clack Tormented by Genius AKA Ingenious Minds. https://www.youtube.com/watch?v=sKcJjWwSa8U
- Rex Lewis-Clack plays Beethoven's Moonlight Sonata III Movement-presto. https://www.youtube.com/watch?v=WTqVanXWylM
- Rex Lewis-Clack plays Chopin Revolutionary Etude. https://www.youtube.com/watch?v=xYGVYMMmLts
- Rex Lewis Clack plays Rachmaninoff Prelude in G Minor. https://www.youtube.com/watch?v=auEoawNQmfE
- Gabriela Montero and Rex Lewis Clack Improvising on We Wish you a Merry Christmas. https://www.youtube.com/watch?v=cFK4QazQFxQ
- Piano Savant | Rex Lewis-Clack // 60 Second Docs+. https://www.youtube.com/watch?v=PoYQHR0aANQ
- TV Südbaden: Genialer Autist am Klavier. https://www.youtube.com/watch?v=NaHlPrKXNil
- Rex Lewis-Clack – Beethoven's Moonlight Sonata, the 3rd Movement, Presto – Breath of Love Benefit. https://www.youtube.com/watch?v=8M9t6MSko6Q
- Catching Up With Rex. https://www.youtube.com/watch?v=cCF1xSgyKXg&t=181s
- A Musical Savant Shows Talent. https://www.youtube.com/watch?v=3oZaCrkCxu8

5.31 Grant Maniér (born 1995)

I am deeply indebted to Julie Coy, Grant's mother, for her extensive assistance in the final revision of this profile.

Grant Maniér was born in Florida, United States. He is autistic and a very special artistic savant who has made a name for himself by combining his autism with a tremendous talent in the genre of "eco art," which "uses recycled resources to help improve our relationship with the earth." From a very early age, he exhibited the behavior uniquely associated with autistic children: he had difficulties in socializing, combined with anxiety and repetitive behavior. When Grant was five years old, his mother was able to confirm her son's diagnosis: Asperger syndrome. From then on, she was better able to understand what was going on with her son.

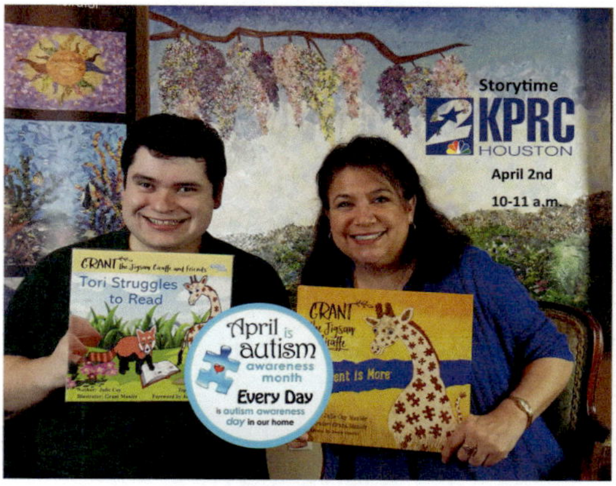

Figure 5.104 Grant Maniér and Julie Coy. Photo courtesy of Grant Maniér.

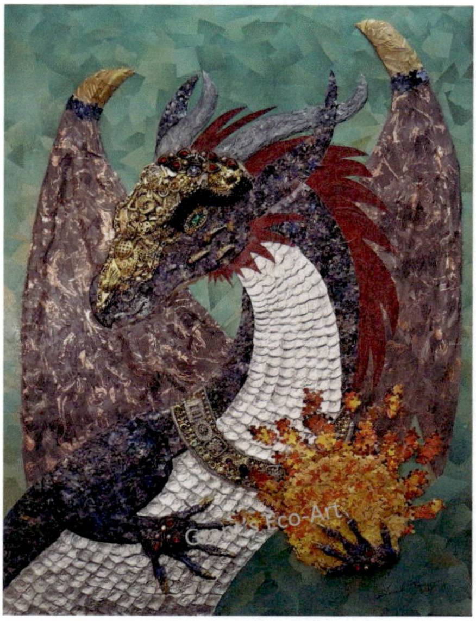

Figure 5.105 Grant Maniér. Eco-Art, 2020.

Photo courtesy of Grant Maniér and Julie Coy.

When Grant was only a young child, he began to collect and recycle paper materials, including puzzles, magazines, calendars, and posters, among others. This not only served as a kind of art therapy but soon made Grant an expert in the technique of collage, the practice of creating art by combining fragments of different media, colors, shapes, and textures on a surface. He is now recognized as a promising figure in the art world. As Grant puts it, "It's not what I can't do, it's what I can do that makes a difference ... (add) because I am doing it!" Practically since he was a child, Grant was very clear on the idea that we must focus on our strengths, our abilities, our talent, rather than on our impairments and on what we cannot do. "It feels incredible to be an artist. I am honored to call myself an artist – and I'm only 17" (Luks, 2013). Grant is also mentored in art and business by Dr. Temple Grandin, who he met in 2008 at age 13.

Grant attended a private school for children with autism until the age of eight. He then began school at a public school that did not recognize his special needs. Life as a student was hard, and he was teased and bullied constantly. Realizing that mainstream schooling was not working for Grant (Grant Maniér's official website), his mother enrolled him at the Focus Academy, a center that serves children and young people on the autism spectrum. He went to school twice a week and completed the rest of the curriculum online from home (Lucks, 2013).

Grant has been featured on TV shows and radio and in newspapers, magazines, and documentaries. He has also received many awards and recognition for his striking artwork, including the 2011 Disabilities Youth Advocate of the Year and the Houston's Mayor Award 2012. Some of Grant's art pieces have sold for more than $6,000.

> He has been recognized by the United States Congress, the Texas State Senate, the Texas Governor, the Mayor of Houston, the Austin Rodeo as Grand Champion, and other prestigious notable awards (Maniér's website).

Grant works part-time at a local supply office in Houston. Job skills outside the art business are important to him and his mother. Grant spends around 20 hours a week doing his collage works and the rest of his time speaking and raising money for student scholarships, therapies, and camps. Grant says:

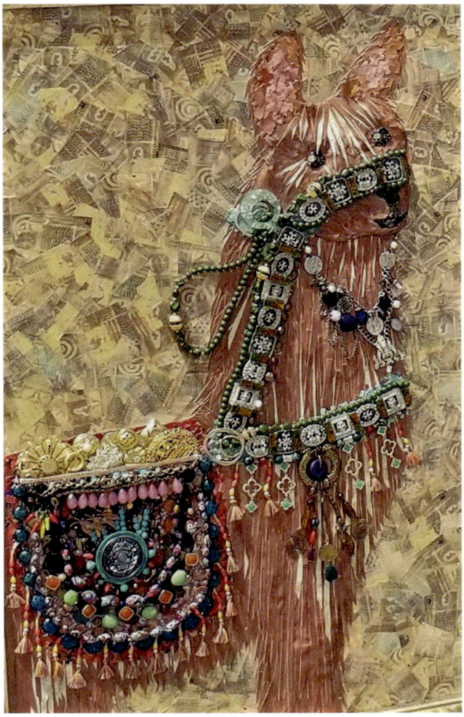

Figure 5.106 Grant Maniér. Eco-Art.

Photo courtesy of Grant Maniér and Julie Coy.

> My goal for this art exhibit is to help teach others the importance of protecting our planet and the beautiful animals that are fighting for survival every day. Living with autism, I understand challenges and struggles, but it's not about what I can't do, it's about what I *can* do to make a difference (Pearl Fincher, Museum of Fine Arts).

Impairments: Asperger syndrome. As a child he suffered from difficulties in socializing combined with anxiety and repetitive behavior.

Skills: Artist. Eco art. Grant is an expert in the technique of collage, the practice of creating art by combining fragments of different media, colors, shapes, and textures on a surface.

Below are references, links to some videos, and additional reading about Grant Maniér.

- Grant Maniér's official website: https://jigsawgrant.com/
- Grant Maniér's Facebook Page: https://www.facebook.com/jigsawgrant
- Grant Maniér's Instagram account: https://www.instagram.com/jigsawgrant/?hl=es-la
- Jigsaw Grant on YouTube: https://www.youtube.com/channel/UC9IGgwJf1nvZ38idMeUknLg?view_as=subscriber
- Eco-Artist Grant Maniér on YouTube: https://www.youtube.com/results?search_query=eco-artist+grant+manier
- Maniér, J. (2017). Grant the Jigsaw Giraffe. Long Tale Publishing.
- Luks, J. (2013). Autistic artist Grant Manier is a rising star: "Coolages" king racks up awards and changes thinking. Culturemap. March 8, 2013. https://houston.culturemap.com/news/city-life/03-08-13-austic-artist-grant-manier-is-a-rising-star-teen-of-coolages-racks-up-awards-challenges-false-notions/#slide=0
- Feldman, C. (2013). Young eco-artist views his disability as a gift. Houston Chronicle. March 8, 2013. https://www.houstonchronicle.com/life/article/Young-eco-artist-views-his-disability-as-a-gift-4339850.php
- Pearl Fincher. Museum of Fine Arts. https://www.pearlmfa.org/manier.html
- Grant Manier wins Houston's Mayor Award 2012. https://www.youtube.com/watch?v=7JLBi1FVoMw
- The Autistic Eco-Artist (Grant Manier). Autism Live. https://www.youtube.com/watch?v=UvCmvODjtS4

5.32 Amanda LaMunyon (born 1995)

I am deeply indebted to Sherry LaMunyon, Amanda's mother, for her extensive assistance in the final revisions of this profile.

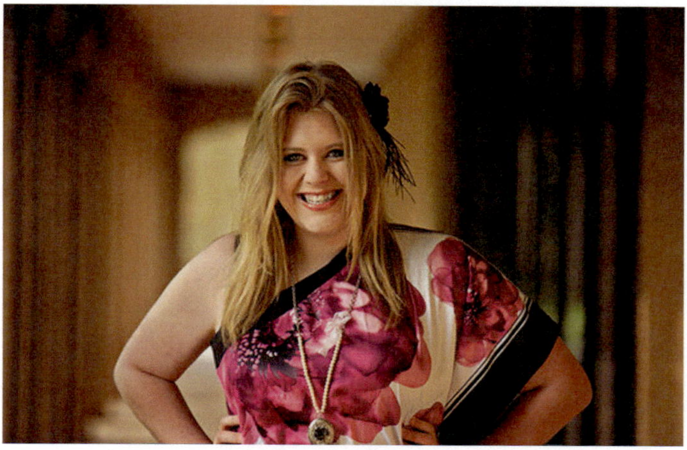

Figure 5.107 Amanda LaMunyon.

Photo courtesy of Erin Haney Designs.

Amanda LaMunyon was born in Oklahoma, United States, on April 14, 1995. She is an impressionist painter artistic savant who has Asperger syndrome. Amanda was clearly different from a young age. She was diagnosed with Asperger syndrome when she was eight years old (Amanda LaMunyon's official website). Her youth was not easy, as she had trouble understanding the world around her. When she became nervous or felt out of place, she would throw herself on the floor and begin to scream, and no one could stop her or understand why. This was her habitual reaction, especially when encountering a large number of strangers. As she grew older, she began understand what caused this behavior, which helped her to control the situation. She had also a hard time at school, mainly because she was always distracted and simply couldn't sit still, so when she became too restless, she would simply get up and go for a walk.

Amanda's story is fascinating. She loves to express herself through singing and painting. Her contact with art began when she was seven years old. Soon, Amanda began to paint and draw the songs she loved. This was her way of expressing herself and gaining self-confidence when she could not find the right words. At that moment, her spirit blossomed. She identifies with Impressionism and likes painters like Monet, Van Gogh, and the French Impressionists. Amanda paints landscapes and flowers with relatively thin yet visible brush strokes, open composition, emphasis on the capture of variations of light and color in nature, and a remarkable ability to evoke movement in a still image.

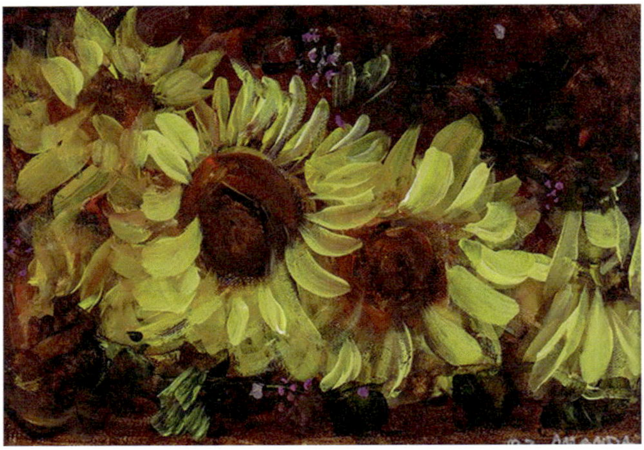

Figure 5.108 Amanda LaMunyon. Sunflowers. Painted in 2002.

Photo courtesy of Amanda and Jerry LaMunyon.

Amanda has become a prolific speaker about the "World of Autism" that she lives in (Amanda LaMunyon's official website). Because of this, and for many other reasons, she has received many awards in her life, including the Temple Grandin Award and the Prudential Spirit of Community Award for community service in fundraising efforts for autism research and children's health. She has had the honor of presenting President George W. Bush with her painting "Our Flag Still There" and former First Lady Nancy Reagan, with her portrait of President Ronald Reagan (Amanda LaMunyon's official website). She has also been featured in several books on autism, including *Genius Island*, by Dr. Darold Treffert, *Drawing of Autism*, by Jill Mullin, *Artism: The Art of Autism* by Debbie Hosseini, *Girls Under the Umbrella of the Autism Spectrum* by Lori Ernsperger and Danielle Wendell, and *A Girl's Guide to Achieving the Arts* by Dr. Kristen Stephens and Dr. Frances Karnes. Amanda LaMunyon's art has been displayed in galleries like Carnegie Hall in New York City. She has also been featured on several national TV programs such as *Megyn Kelly Today*.

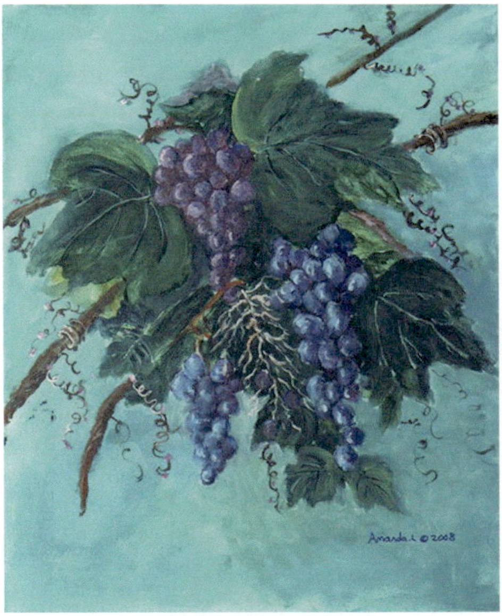

Figure 5.109 Amanda LaMunyon. Grapes for children. Painted in 2008.

Photo courtesy of Amanda and Jerry LaMunyon.

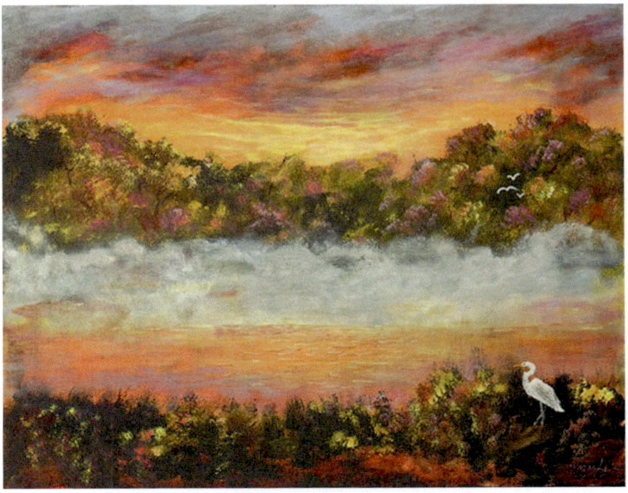

Figure 5.110 Amanda LaMunyon. Shenandoah. Painted in 2008.

Photo courtesy of Amanda and Jerry LaMunyon.

Amanda has overcome many challenges, and she has learned to live with others. She has travelled the world to raise awareness about ASD and to help others with learning differences or problems of any kind, encouraging them to not give up, to be patient, and to dream big. She also works with a number of organizations helping to raise money for children's health and autism research. Amanda is currently attending college, where she is majoring in art and psychology. She hopes to obtain a degree in Psychology with a specialization in autism and AS, and to work with people in the autism spectrum.

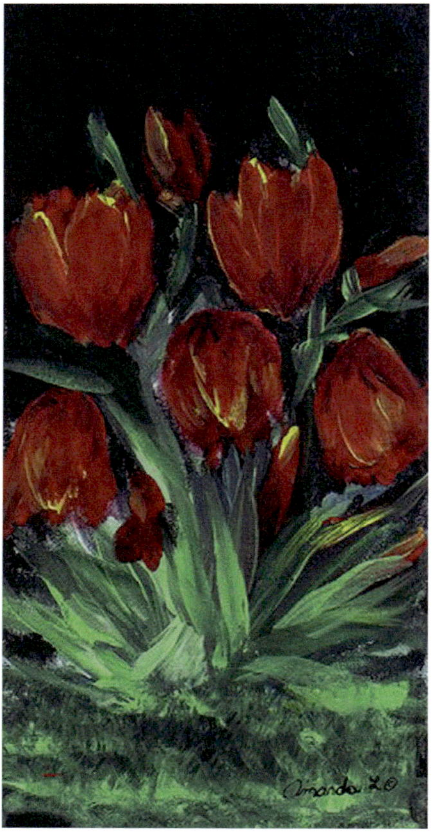

Figure 5.111 Amanda LaMunyon. Red tulips. Painted in 2002.

Photo courtesy of Amanda and Jerry LaMunyon

"I do not look at myself as a person with a disability. I see myself as someone with something to give," Amanda said when she received the Prudential Spirit of Community Award.

Impairments: Asperger syndrome. Distracted, terribly restless.

Skills: Artist, impressionist painter, singer. She has travelled the world to raise awareness about ASD and to help others with learning differences not to give up, be patient and to have big dreams. She is also committed with many organizations to help raise money for children's health and for finding the cause of autism.

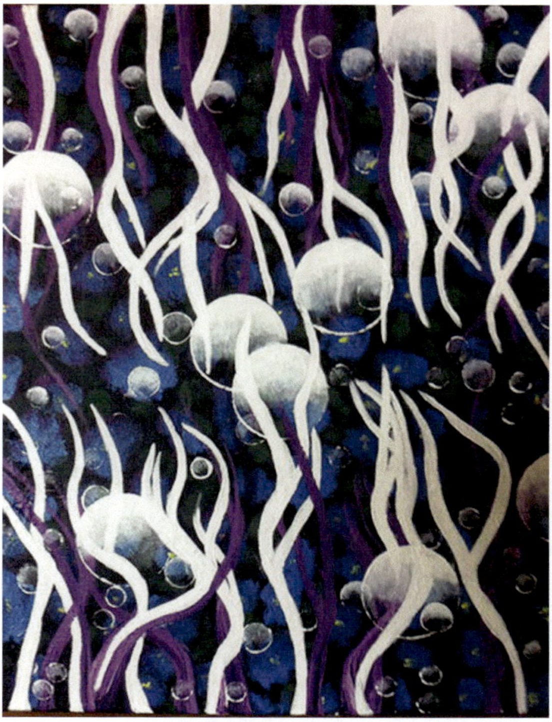

Figure 5.112 Amanda LaMunyon. Bubbles, ribbons and flowers. Painted in 2013.

Photo courtesy of Amanda and Jerry LaMunyon.

Below are references, links to some videos, and additional reading about Amanda LaMunyon.

- Amanda LaMunyon's official website: https://amandalamunyon.com/
- Amanda LaMunyon on Twitter: https://twitter.com/amandalamunyon
- Mullin, J. (2014). *Drawings of Autism*. Akashic Books.
- Hosseini, D., Hosseini, D. and Martinez, R. (2011). *Artism: The Art of Autism*. Autism Today.
- Treffert, D. (2010). *Islands of genius: The bountiful mind of the autistic, acquired, and sudden savant*. Jessica Kingsley Publishers.
- Ernsperger, L. and Wendel, D. (2007). *Girls under the umbrella of autism spectrum disorders: Practical solutions for addressing everyday challenges*. AAPC Publishing.

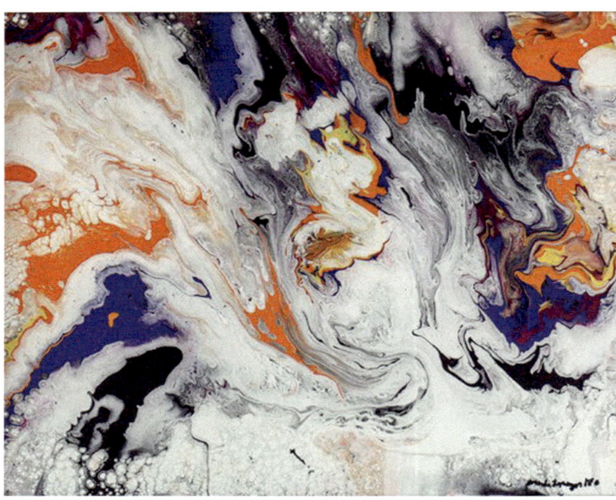

Figure 5.113 Amanda LaMunyon. Abstract. Lost in the Moment. Painted in 2018.

Photo courtesy of Amanda and Jerry LaMunyon.

- Karnes, F. and Stephens, K. (2007). A Girl's Guide to Achieving in the Arts. Royal Fireworks Publishing
- Treffert, D. Amanda LaMunyon: https://www.agnesian.com/page/amanda-lamunyon

- Amanda LaMunyon – "A Little Secret" at the United Nations. https://www.youtube.com/watch?v=ydkjrqV8Ztk
- Amanda LaMunyon – Impressions of Grace (1080).mov https://www.youtube.com/watch?v=a2e_MaylmXM
- How Painting Unlocked 1 Woman's Abilities As A Savant | Megyn Kelly TODAY. https://www.youtube.com/watch?v=uY6-raLF8nU
- Creative outlet opens doors for Enid girl with Asperger's syndrome – Article Photos. The Oklahoman. https://oklahoman.com/gallery/articleid/3535375

5.33 Kodi Taehyun Lee (born 1996)

I am deeply indebted to Tina Lee, Kodi's mother, for her extensive assistance in the final revisions of this profile.

Kodi Lee was born at the Mission Viejo Hospital in California, on July 7, 1996. He is an American singer, composer, and pianist, and is autistic savant. Kodi was born with optic nerve hypoplasia (ONH), causing him to become legally blind. Kodi also survived a life-saving surgery at 5 days old. He was diagnosed with autism at an early age and suffers from Addison's disease, and also grew up with serious communication and socialization problems. Kodi cannot dress by himself or have a simple conversation. Despite all the impairments in his brain, however, Kodi is a musical genius.

ONH is a congenital anomaly produced from the underdevelopment or absence of the optic nerves. It can present unilaterally or bilaterally. It is often associated with endocrinopathies (hormone deficiencies), developmental delay, pituitary problem and brain malformations. The optic nerves are responsible for transmitting impulses (visual signals) from the retina of the eye to the brain. A normal person has more than a million nerve fibers. People diagnosed with ONH, however, have fewer optic nerve axons. Most people with ONH have abnormal eye movements (nystagmus), problems with light perception and/or mild to severe visual impairment of one or both eyes. ONH is the leading ocular cause of blindness and visual impairment in young children.

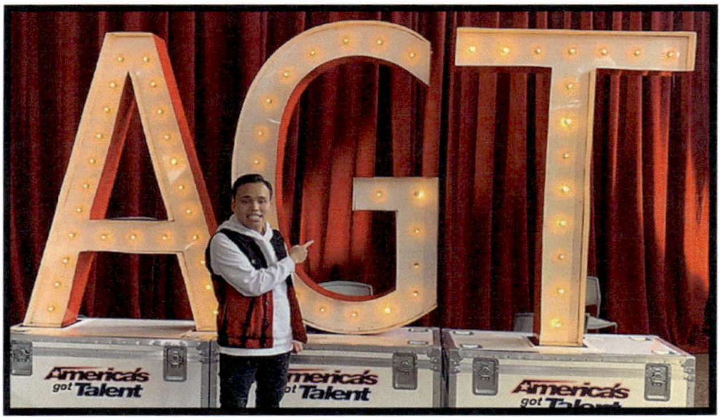

Figure 5.114 Kodi Lee at AGT.

Photo courtesy of Kodi and Tina Lee.

Addison's disease, on the other hand, also called adrenal insufficiency or hypoadrenalism, is a long-term endocrine disorder in which the body does not produce enough steroid hormones for normal functioning. In Addison's disease, the adrenal glands, located just above the kidneys, produce too little cortisol and, often, too little aldosterone. Symptoms generally develop slowly and may include extreme fatigue, abdominal pain, low mood, weakness, darkening skin, and weight loss.

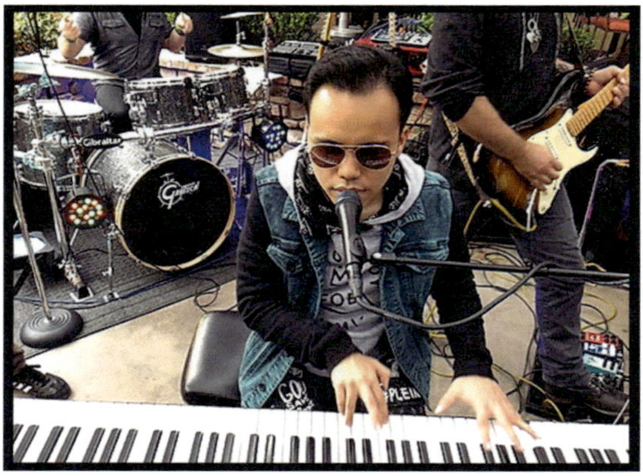

Figure 5.115 Kodi and Midnight Satellites. Miramonte Winery. May 26, 2018.

Photo courtesy of Kodi and Tina Lee.

Kodi's life has not been easy for him and his family. At times simply going out was a conflict too complex for all family members. Suddenly, however, music appeared in Kodi's life and completely changed it forever. Kodi has perfect pitch and passion for all forms of music. He can store a song in his memory after listening to it just once. His brain is like a record store with thousands of songs available. In addition to his musical talent, he is also a skilled tap dancer. As Kodi's father says:

> Music to him is like air. I mean it's not like he's an autistic, blind boy who likes music. I mean it's really a part of him and he's driving himself to do better (Yeates, 2008).

Kodi rose to fame after entering and winning season 14 of the reality competition *America's Got Talent* in 2019. Kodi's audition for the show had over 50 million views on the internet within two weeks. In May of the same year, Lee sang Donny Hathaway's version of "A Song for You," and with the approval of the competition's judges, quickly went on to the next round. The performance was viewed more than 300 million times online across social media platforms, including Facebook and YouTube. In August, Kodi sang Simon and Garfunkel's "Bridge over Troubled Water," easily entering the semi-finals. In this stage, he moved the audience and judges singing Calum Scott's "You Are the Reason," and gained a seat in the finals. In the final stage of the competition, Kodi performed "Lost Without You" by Freya Ridings and, as he had throughout the entire contest, moved all the judges and received a standing ovation from the entire theater. The prize was one million dollars. "One of the most beautiful things I've ever, ever heard," judge Simon Cowell said at the song's finish. After that resounding success, Kodi has traveled the world performing his songs. He was recently invited to perform at the prestigious Carnegie Hall in New York City. He has been featured on a number of national TV programs and documentaries.

> Kodi's amazing gift lies within his musical expression, perfect pitch, and passion for all forms of music. Kodi has an audio photographic memory, in which he can recall music he hears after just one listen. An

unbelievable gift in itself, but his musical expression and prowess top even that (Kodi Lee's official website).

Kodi continues to pursue his musical career and his dream is to be a rock star, performing for thousands of fans.

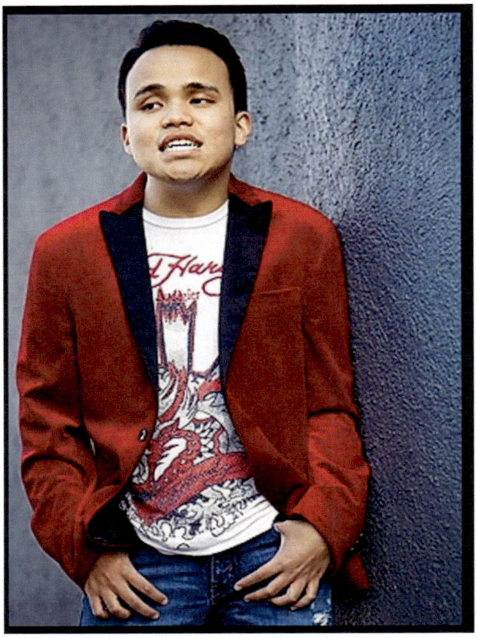

Figure 5.116 Kodi Lee.

Photo courtesy of Kodi and Tina Lee.

Impairments: Autism. Born with optic nerve hypoplasia, which caused legal blindness. Kodi survived a life-saving surgery at five days old. He was diagnosed with autism at an early age and suffers from Addison's disease. Kodi cannot dress himself or have a simple conversation.

Skills: Singer, composer, pianist, tap dancing. Kodi has perfect pitch and passion for all forms of music. He can store a song in his memory after listening to it just once. His brain is like a record store with thousands of songs available.

Below are references, links to some videos, and additional reading about Kodi Lee.

- Kodi Lee's official website: https://www.kodileerocks.com/
- Kodi Lee on Twitter: https://twitter.com/kodileerocks?lang=es
- Kodi Lee on Instagram: https://www.instagram.com/kodileerocks/?hl=es-la
- Billboard (2020). Kodi Lee Breaks Hearts With 'AGT' Performance as Five Advance to Semis: Watch. Billboard Staff. August 13, 2020. https://www.billboard.com/articles/news/9433594/kodi-lee-agt-performance-five-advance-semis
- Lankston, C. and Stern, C. (2019). 'He has no disabilities on stage': Mother of blind autistic singer who left America's Got Talent judges in TEARS calls him an 'innocent soul' who transforms when he performs music. Daily Mail. May 30, 2019. https://www.dailymail.co.uk/femail/article-7087405/Mom-blind-autistic-singer-Kodi-Lee-Americas-Got-Talent-says-no-disabilities-stage.html
- Brinsford, J. The inspiring story of America's Got Talent winner Kodi Lee as he wows a nation. Mirror. September 20, 2919. https://www.mirror.co.uk/3am/celebrity-news/inspiring-story-americas-talent-winner-20095187
- Gonzalez, M. (2019). Spotlight on the incredible musical prodigy Kodi Lee. The Independent. https://theindependent.sg/spotlight-on-the-incredible-musical-prodigy-kodi-lee/
- Keveney, B. (2019). Kodi Lee celebrates his 'AGT' victory: 'Heck, yeah! I'm the winner'. USA Today. September 19, 2019. https://www.usatoday.com/story/entertainment/tv/2019/09/19/agt-champ-kodi-lee-and-his-mom-tina-talk-season-14-victory/2371754001/
- Martin, R. (2019). Who is America's Got Talent 2019 winner Kodi Lee? Metro. September 19, 2019. https://metro.co.uk/2019/09/19/americas-got-talent-2019-winner-kodi-lee-10771648/
- Mizoguchi, K. (2019). Kodi Lee, Singing Phenom Who Is Blind and Has Autism, 22, Wins *America's Got Talent* Season 14. People. September 18, 2019. https://people.com/tv/kodi-lee-wins-americas-got-talent-season-14/

- Kabbany, J. (2012). LAKE ELSINORE: Musical savant eyes stardom. The San Diego Union Tribune. October 1, 2012. https://www.sandiegouniontribune.com/sdut-lake-elsinore-musical-savant-eyes-stardom-2012oct01-story.html
- Yeates, E. (2008). Disabled boy a musical genius. KSL. https://www.ksl.com/article/2664997/disabled-boy-a-musical-genius
- Kodi Lee Performs "Sign of the Times" by Harry Styles – America's Got Talent: The Champions. https://www.youtube.com/watch?v=zv67C01rSPg
- Kodi Lee: Blind Autistic Singer SHOCKS The World Again In The Live Show! | America's Got Talent 2019. https://www.youtube.com/watch?v=AIXgLR4wFuU
- Kodi Lee: America Loves Kodi Gets STANDING Ovation in Semifinals! | America's Got Talent 2019. https://www.youtube.com/watch?v=2ww0ylpiM2c
- Kodi Lee With Leona Lewis Grand Finale. https://www.youtube.com/watch?v=bKzfAs11uCY
- Performance! | America's Got Talent 2019. https://www.youtube.com/watch?v=g7yqx8p0zJI
- Kodi Lee: Finals Performance Will Have You Say "Heck Yeh!" | America's Got Talent 2019. https://www.youtube.com/watch?v=aki-_-vLwQ4&pbjreload=10
- KODI LEE WINS AMERICA'S GOT TALENT SEASON 14! – America's Got Talent 2019. https://www.youtube.com/watch?v=Y3Mf53LeKfA
- Golden Buzzer: Kodi Lee Wows You With A Historical Music Moment! – America's Got Talent 2019. https://www.youtube.com/watch?v=pDPdRYF7hTQ
- Kodi Lee: Blind Autistic Singer WOWS And Gets GOLDEN BUZZER! | America's Got Talent 2019. https://www.youtube.com/watch?v=pDPdRYF7hTQ

5.34 Jodi DiPiazza (born 2001)

I greatly appreciate the contributions of Thomas DiPiazza, Jodi's father, in reviewing this profile.

Jodi was born in the United States on October 3, 2001. She is an American singer, composer, musician, and an autistic savant. She was diagnosed with autism before her second birthday, so her parents were aware of the reasons for Jodi's behavior early on. Tom DiPiazza, her father has said "What they told us was there's no cure for it. It's a life-long disability and don't expect too much" (Murphy, 2012). Instead of panicking, however, the DiPiazzas began to plan a complete education and stimulation program, full of learning experiences for Jodi. She started Applied Behavior Analysis (ABA) therapy at home as a toddler for a full school day, "with an additional two hours of tutoring in the evening" (Wallis and Goehner, 2006). Despite the impairment in her brain, Jodi is a musical genius. Once again, we are able to see the power of music for individuals on the autism spectrum disorder.

Jodi has perfect pitch and an extraordinary talent for music. She began playing the piano at the age of three, when she was barely able to form sentences. Jodi could listen to a song and reproduce it perfectly by listening to it only once. She is hyperlexic and taught herself to read at the age of two, long before she could speak. From that moment on, and with her parents' help in ensuring she had everything she needed to do so, Jodi has grown steadily.

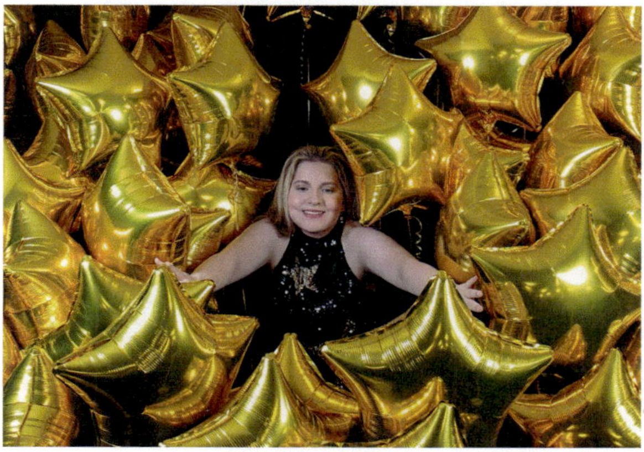

Figure 5.117 Jodi DiPiazza.

Photo courtesy of Jodi and Thomas DiPiazza

Jodi likes to perform many different genres and is skilled at several instruments: piano, guitar, ukulele, voice, drums, and clarinet. In 2012, she had the opportunity to perform "Firework" with Katy Perry at an annual Comedy Central fundraiser for autism programs at the Beacon Theater in New York. Perry tweeted, "I will never forget last night. It was the most important moment thus far of what I do" (@katyperry). The concert raised more than four million dollars for autism education. Since then, Jodi has been featured on various TV shows and documentaries, including *Good Morning America* (2012), Fox News (2013), and *El Tiempo* (Colombian broadcast TV, 2013). In April 2016, she sang the American national anthem on autism awareness night at a New York Red Bulls soccer game. She has performed with Matt Savage, Laura Benanti, Jon Batiste, Stephanie Block, Cynthia Erivo, and "Weird Al" Yankovic at several events. Jodi has worked tirelessly to present another face for autistic children and youth and prove to them if that if the conditions are right, they too can achieve something important. Jodi has performed at over 200 fundraisers and community events to benefit individuals who are on the autism spectrum disorder and various disabilities.

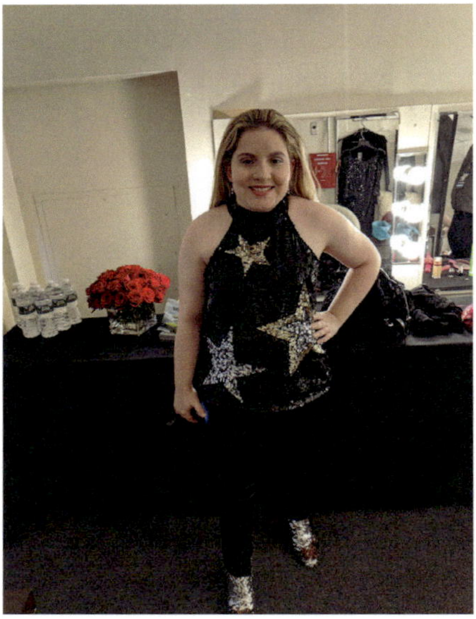

Figure 5.118 Jodi DiPiazza.

Photo courtesy of Jodi and Thomas DiPiazza.

According to her official website, Jodi is currently a student at the Mannes College of Music Preparatory Division, where she studies voice, piano, conducting, music theory, and composition.

Impairments: Autism. As a child, she displayed typically autistic behaviors.

Skills: Musician, singer, conductor, composer. Jodi has perfect pitch and an extraordinary talent for music.

Below are references, links to some videos, and additional reading about Jodi DiPiazza.

- Jodi DiPiazza's official website: https://www.jodigirl.com/
- Jodi DiPiazza Facebook page: https://www.facebook.com/jodigirl2001/
- Jodi DiPiazza on Twitter: https://twitter.com/jodidipiazza
- Lewis, R. (2015). Weird Al Yankovic, young people with autism sing 'Yoda' on telethon. Los Angeles Times. March 9, 2015. https://www.latimes.com/entertainment/music/posts/la-et-ms-weird-al-yankovic-yoda-autism-telethon-jodi-dipiazza-20150309-story.html#
- Murphy, E. (2012). Autistic Girl, Jodi DiPiazza, Performs with Katy Perry. ABC News. October 19, 2012. https://abcnews.go.com/blogs/entertainment/2012/10/autistic-girl-jodi-dipiazza-performs-with-katy-perry/
- McQueeney, K. (2012). The heart-warming moment autistic girl performs Firework with her idol Katy Perry. Daily Mail. October 19, 2012. https://www.dailymail.co.uk/tvshowbiz/article-2220146/Night-Of-Too-Many-Stars-Katy-Perry-performs-Firework-autistic-girl-Jodi-DiPiazza-benefit.html
- Kaplan, R. (2012). Music Therapy for Individuals with Autism. *The Huffington Post.*
- Wallis, C. and Goehner, A. (2006). A tale of two schools. *Time, 20,* 48-51.
- Jodi DiPiazza singing the Star Spangled Banner at the Red Bulls 2016. https://www.youtube.com/watch?v=56_KdNzWvv4
- Jodi DiPiazza performing live at Disney World. https://www.youtube.com/watch?v=-Mj6DYgTI9I

- Weird Al Yankovic and Jodi DiPiazza sing "Yoda". https://www.youtube.com/watch?v=J2Ql74_42Ro
- Queen Bohemian Rhapsody 2015 performed by Jodi DiPiazza. https://www.youtube.com/watch?v=EKSU5heCKKo
- Katy Perry & Jodi DiPiazza – Firework 2012. https://www.youtube.com/watch?v=Ke_JrWF7vE4
- Jodi playing Levon on her new Piano Elton John. https://www.youtube.com/watch?v=bFreE-MDtqY

5.35 Iris Grace Halmshaw (born 2009)

I am deeply indebted to Arabella Carter-Johnson, Iris's mother, for her extensive assistance in the final revisions of this profile.

Iris was born in Leicestershire, England in 2009. She is an artist and severely autistic savant. Her autism was evident very early in her life: she rarely spoke or smiled, did not establish visual contact even with those closest to her, had serious socialization problems, did not want to play with other children, had irregular sleep patterns, and was extremely obsessive. She was highly sensitive to noise and other stimuli. Her mother recalls that "Iris seemed to be trapped in her own world, unreachable" (Carter-Johnson, 2016).

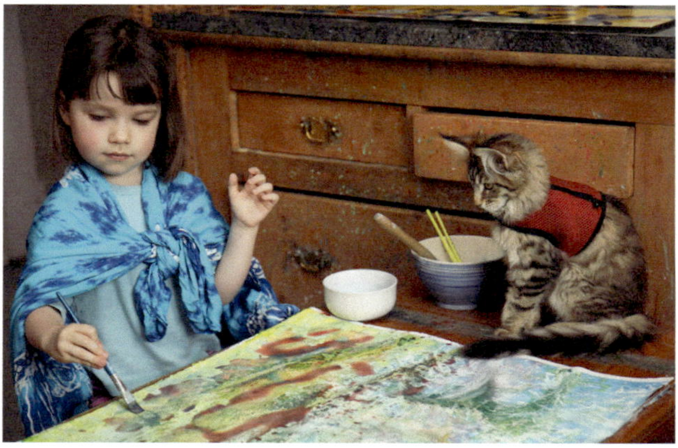

Figure 5.119 Iris Grace Halmshaw with her cat Thula.

Photo courtesy of Iris Grace Halmshaw and Arabella Carter-Johnson.

Iris was diagnosed as severely autistic when she was two years old. Since then, her parents have been working hard to help their daughter connect with the world. After her parents tried equine therapy, which did not yield results, some friends suggested that they try a cat. This was how Thula, a Maine Coon cat, came into Iris Grace's life. Thula and Iris formed an inseparable bond: wherever Iris goes, Thula is sure to follow. There are no secrets between the two of them, they understand each other, almost as equals. If Thula perceives that Iris is upset about something, she comes over and sits on her lap until the girl calms down. If Iris wakes up frightened during the night, Thula keeps her company until Iris falls asleep again.

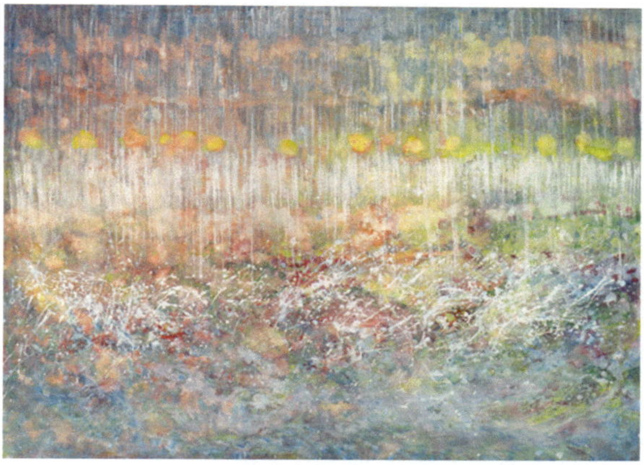

Figure 5.120 Iris Grace Halmshaw. Anima. 9.05 inches x 12.20 inches.

Photo courtesy of Iris Grace Halmshaw and Arabella Carter-Johnson.

With Thula's soothing presence, Iris soon found her way of communicating with the world through painting. "She created colorful abstract pieces that appeared to express deep emotion" (Mohney, 2014). Her talent at capturing this emotion in her paintings is astonishing—so much so that she has earned the nickname "little Monet", comparing her colors and lines with those of the great French painter, one of the creators of impressionism.

Iris is inspired mainly by nature and English landscapes. All of her paintings are titled. At first it was Iris's parents who gave each work a title based either on what they looked like, Iris's mood while painting, or the music she was listening to. Now Iris titles her paintings herself.

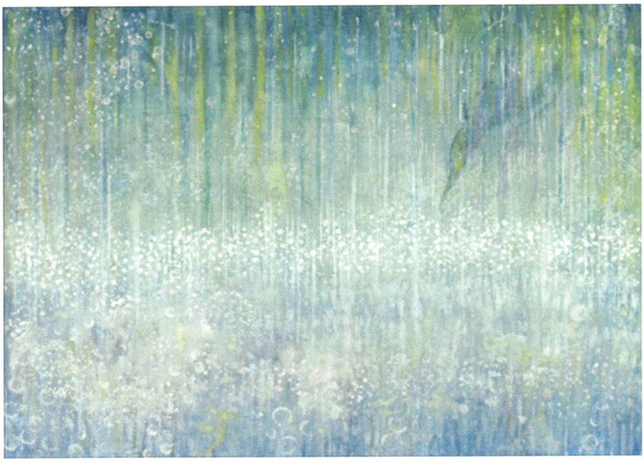

Figure 5.121 Iris Grace Halmshaw. Water Dance. 9.05 inches x 12.20 inches. Photo courtesy of Iris Grace Halmshaw and Arabella Carter-Johnson.

Iris' mother, Arabella Carter-Johnson, a professional photographer, has written a book called *Iris Grace* that became a *Sunday Times* bestseller. The book documents her daughter's journey and the remarkable progress Iris has made over the years. Today, Iris's paintings have been sold around the world and are owned by private art collectors in the UK and elsewhere, some selling for as much as £1,500. Even Angelina Jolie has bought one of Iris's paintings.

For Iris, painting is a way of gaining calm and peace. It illuminates her world and lets her express herself: it lets her fly. In her spare time, Iris likes to swim, play with toys, and ride bikes with her parents. When she falls asleep, as always, Thula is by her side. Arabella writes in her book that "different is brilliant." When speaking of Iris, that seems unquestionable.

Impairments: Severe autism. She rarely spoke or smiled, did not establish visual contact even with those closest to her, had serious socialization problems, did not want to play with other children, had irregular sleep patterns, and was extremely obsessive.

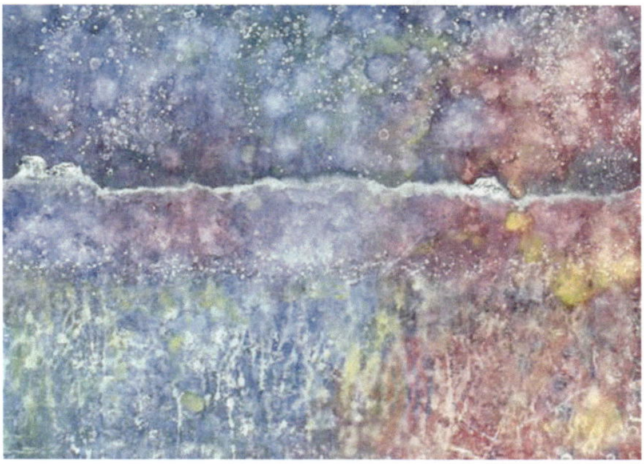

Figure 5.122 Iris Grace Halmshaw. Tumpty Tum. 9.05 inches x 12.20 inches.

Photo courtesy of Iris Grace Halmshaw and Arabella Carter-Johnson.

Skills: Artist, painter. Her extraordinary talent has earned her the nickname "little Monet."

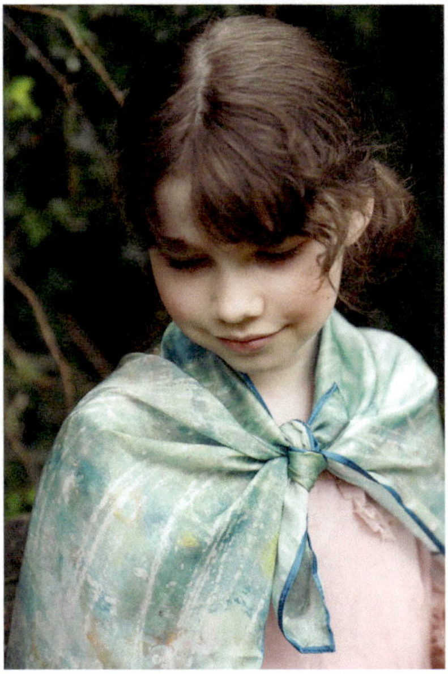

Figure 5.123 Iris Grace Halmshaw.

Photo courtesy of Iris Grace Halmshaw and Arabella Carter-Johnson.

Below are references, links to some videos, and additional reading about Iris Grace Halmshaw.

- Iris Grace's official website: https://irisgracepainting.com/
- Iris Grace on Facebook: https://www.facebook.com/IrisGracePainting/
- Carter-Johnson, A. (2016). *Iris Grace*. Penguin UK.
- Grant, K. (2016). Iris Grace Halmshaw, profile: Six-year-old painter with a reputation as an internationally renowned artist. Independent. March 3, 2016. https://www.independent.co.uk/news/people/profiles/iris-grace-halmshaw-profile-six-year-old-painter-reputation-internationally-renowned-artist-a6908281.html
- Strickland, A. (2016). Portrait of a 6-year-old artist with autism and her therapy cat. CNN. March 11, 2016. https://edition.cnn.com/2016/03/11/health/turning-points-iris-grace-autism/index.html
- Brannen, A. (2016). Unbreakable bond between an autistic little girl and her cat: Six-year-old who didn't talk paints, cycles and SWIMS with the feline who helped her find her voice. Daily Mail. March 15, 2016. https://www.dailymail.co.uk/femail/article-3491674/Autistic-six-year-old-paints-cycles-SWIMS-tabby-feline-helped-voice.html
- Mohney, G. (2014). After Autistic Girl Finds Success in Art World, Parents Shield Her From Spotlight. ABC News. September 30, 2014. https://abcnews.go.com/Health/autistic-girl-finds-success-art-world-parents-shield/story?id=25865752
- Iris Grace: Autism Speech Breakthroughs with Gemiini | Gemiini Testimonial – Speech Support. https://www.youtube.com/watch?v=uyBMZbuxMZ4
- Maine Coon Cat Helps Autistic Girl Overcome Her Fear of Water – ITV 15-06-2016. https://www.youtube.com/watch?v=nZNB2tRcha0
- 6 year old autistic girl Iris and her cat Thula…wonderful story – 23rd Match 2016. https://www.youtube.com/watch?v=d1UcTZwP0v0
- Iris Grace Painting. https://www.youtube.com/watch?v=Ftv0FUuoBK0
- The Miracle Of Little Miss Masterpiece – AMAZING!! Iris Grace Painting. https://www.youtube.com/watch?v=N4wwCK_jeRA
- Iris and Thula at home. https://www.youtube.com/watch?v=lBBZqRZRMuM
- Different is Brilliant. https://www.youtube.com/watch?v=Rx4h1XsghsY

6

DISCUSSION

For many years, it was believed that exceptional talents could only be found in extraordinarily intelligent individuals. It is now evident, however, that talent can be found in individuals who differ enormously in general levels of intelligence. Savant syndrome, in which this paradox is most dramatically embodied, is a concrete reality, and the existence of such individuals poses a serious challenge to theories that posit general intelligence factors as the primary source of individual differences in skill (Miller, 1989). The hallmark of savantism is remarkable intelligence in a particular domain or isolated area of knowledge, supporting the idea that intelligence is modular in nature (Pring, 2005; Andersson, 1998). The study of such individuals is not only valuable in that it can allow savants themselves to gain a better self-understanding, but in that also gives hope that comprehension of the atypical can shed light on the typical (Winner, 2000).

Individuals with savant syndrome often have a prodigious memory and spatial visualization abilities, are attracted to numbers and calendars, and are generally fascinated by music and art. Their skills emerge spontaneously; they are literal, not symbolic; and their skills are not generally the result of practice. They exercise these skills out of intrinsic enjoyment, not to improve their performance (Pring, 2005). Savants' motivation to perform their skill is exclusively internal. Miller (1989) described several musical savants who seemed to have an inextinguishable appetite for musical interactions of various kinds.

Although there are several hypotheses that offer inroads to understanding savant syndrome, no one cognitive theory has been found to be completely sufficient on its own. There is a lack of unifying definitions and a wide spectrum of prodigiousness, all of which refute the idea of savant syndrome as a monolithic condition (Ammari, 2011). One of the more plausible explanations for savant syndrome is that it is related to a dysfunction of the left hemisphere of the brain, but this theory does not explain all cases. The most promising line of research is doubtless that which relates to Autism Spectrum Disorder, or ASD. Most autistic individuals and those with savant syndrome share similar brains. Our knowledge of the anatomical and functional characteristics of the autistic brain can therefore enhance our understanding of savant syndrome (Mottron et al., 2013). For example, future research may explore the role of enhanced perception in the development of expertise (Mottron et al., 2009) as well as sensory hypersensitivity (Baron-Cohen et al., 2009). Clearly the combination of heightened perception, sensory hypersensitivity, and obsessive behavior contribute to and explain much of a savant's expertise.

Throughout this text, we have seen the ways in which a seemingly elusive concept such as talent manifests in reality, revealing how far we are from possessing a functional understanding of the brain. This complex organ has shown itself to be an intriguing, highly distributed, self-organizing system (Singer, 2009) with a tremendous compensatory capacity in which the complexity of cellular and molecular organization of neural connections determines the brain's own capacity (Cairó, 2017), the attributes of the person it belongs to, and, indeed, the self (Singer, 2009).

At present, there is another point we must consider in coming years when making distinctions between different types of savants. This is the multiple combinations (n x n) that arise between the degree of mental disabilities (1-mild, 2-moderate, 3-severe) and the degree of ability (1-average, 2-high average, 3-superior). These combination gives rise to six different results, i.e.: 1 (1x1), 2 (1x2, 2x1), 3 (3x1, 1x3), 4 (2x2), 6 (2x3, 3x2), and 9 (3x3). While the first three results of the combinations (1, 2, 3) raise serious doubts as to whether individuals with these combinations should be considered savants, there is no doubt with regard to the remaining three (4, 6, 9). If we do not make a clear distinction in the combination of these factors, we run the serious risk of generating confusion.

Likewise, until only a few years ago the United States and the United Kingdom were home to 95% of the savants that had been detected. We know, however, that neither talent nor impairment distinguish between geographic regions. In the years ahead, with advances in medicine, the generation of new knowledge, and massive distribution of information through the internet and social networks, dozens of savants are sure to emerge all over the world.

There are other daunting questions that must be answered, which open the door to fascinating new lines of research: Does the human brain have latent savant-like abilities? Do our higher cognitive functions somehow block these abilities? Can these abilities be temporarily induced by artificial means? Might neuropsychological research give us a better understanding of the neuroscience of giftedness? We do not yet have the answers to these questions.

> The more we learn about the brain the more abstract will the descriptions become because we shall be dealing with increasingly complex assemblies (Singer, 2009).

Over the coming years, researchers will continue to search for insights into what happens within and between the regions and hemispheres of the brain, especially in autistic individuals or those with the savant syndrome. Upon reviewing the relevant literature, it is evident that many questions about the existence and nature of savant syndrome remain unanswered, and that numerous issues exist which obviously require much further research.

REFERENCES

Aguila, A. (2004). Music from the inner heart. Philstar. July 11, 2004. https://www.philstar.com/other-sections/starweek magazine/2004/07/11/257204/music-inner-heart

Allen, V. (2010). Family wins right to control future of piano prodigy known as 'Human iPod'. Daily Mail. May 14, 2010. https://www.dailymail.co.uk/news/article-1278253/Human-iPod-Derek-Paravicini-Family-win-right-control-piano-prodigys-future.html

Allen, N. (2009). Kim Peek: The 'RealRainMan' dies. The Telegraph. December 22, 2009. https://www.telegraph.co.uk/news/obituaries/medicine-obituaries/6867567/Kim-Peek.html

Allen, J. (2005). Perfect. Diremakers. News Review. https://www.newsreview.com/sacramento/diremakers/content?oid=35264

Ally, B., Hussey, E. and Donahue, M. (2013). A case of hyperthymesia: Rethinking the role of the amygdala in autobiographical memory. *Neurocase, 19*(2), 166-181.

Amato. D. (2013). My Beautiful Disaster: My Brain Injury, My Gift, My Life. CreateSpace Independent Publishing Platform (January 1, 2014). Amazon.

Amato, D. (2012). Experience: a head injury made me a musical prodigy. The Guardian. October 12, 2012. https://www.theguardian.com/lifeandstyle/2012/oct/12/experience-head-injury-musical-prodigy

Ammari, E. (2011). Prodigious Polyglot Savants: The Enigmatic Adjoining of Language Acquisition and Emaciated Potentials. *International Journal of Business and Social Science*, 2(7).

Anderson, M. (1998). Mental retardation general intelligence and modularity. *Learning and individual differences, 10*(3), 159-178.

Andrade, P. and Bhattacharya, J. (2003). Brain tuned to music. *Journal of the Royal Society of Medicine, 96*(6), 284-287.

Ankan, J. (2011). Derek Paravicini: Musician or a Superhuman? EFI News. December 21, 2011. https://web.archive.org/web/20120509054943/http://www.efi-news.com/2011/12/derek-paravicini-musician-or-superhuman.html

Arnott, S. and Alain, C. (2014). A brain guide to Sound Galleries. *The Multisensory Museum, Cross-Disciplinary Perspectives on Touch, Sound, Smell, Memory, and Space*, 85-108.

Arnott, S., Thaler, L., Milne, J., Kish, D. and Goodale, M. (2013). Shape-specific activation of occipital cortex in an early blind echolocation expert. *Neuropsychologia, 51*(5), 938-949.

Arsalidou, M. and Taylor, M. (2011). Is 2+ 2= 4? Meta-analyses of brain areas needed for numbers and calculations. *Neuroimage, 54*(3), 2382-2393.

Ash, L. (2015). Drawing what our mouths cannot say. BBC News. June 12, 2015.

Asperger, H. (1944). Die „Autistischen Psychopathen" im Kindesalter. *Archiv für psychiatrie und nervenkrankheiten, 117*(1), 76-136.

Attwood, T. (1997). *Asperger's syndrome: A guide for parents and professionals.* Jessica Kingsley Publishers.

Azoulai, S., Hubbard, E. and Ramachandran, V. (2005). Does synesthesia contribute to mathematical savant skills. *Journal of cognitive neuroscience, 69*(1).

Babcock, S. (2011). Leland Lee, An International Star from Taiwan MakingaDifference.https://lelandlee.wordpress.com/about/leland-lee-an-international-star-from-taiwan/

Bailey, A., Luthert, P., Dean, A., Harding, B., Janota, I., Montgomery, M., ... and Lantos, P. (1998). A clinicopathological study of autism. *Brain: a journal of neurology, 121*(5), 889-905.

Bailey, A., Palferman, S., Heavey, L. and Le Couteur, A. (1998a). Autism: The phenotype in relatives. *Journal of autism and developmental disorders,* 28(5), 369-392.

Barber-Stetson, C. (2017). A Vibrant Autistic Aesthetic and the Limits of Art Brut. *Journal of Literary & Cultural Disability Studies, 11*(2), 113-131.

Barker, A., Jalinous, R. and Freeston, I. (1985). Non-invasive magnetic stimulation of human motor cortex. *The Lancet,* 325(8437), 1106-1107.

Barnbaum, D. (2008). *The ethics of autism: Among them, but not of them.* Indiana University Press.

Baron-Cohen, S. (2012). Autism and the technical mind. *Scientific American, 307*(5), 72-75.

Baron-Cohen, S., Ashwin, E., Ashwin, C., Tavassoli, T. and Chakrabarti, B. (2009). Talent in autism: hyper-systemizing, hyper-attention to detail and sensory hypersensitivity. *Philosophical Transactions of the Royal Society of London B: Biological Sciences, 364*(1522), 1377-1383.

Baron-Cohen, S. (2009a). Autism: the empathizing–systemizing (E-S) theory *Annals of the New York Academy of Sciences, 1156*(1), 68-80.

Baron-Cohen, S., Bor, D., Billington, J., Asher, J., Wheelwright, S. and Ashwin, C. (2007). Savant memory in a man with colour form-number synaesthesia and asperger. *Journal of consciousness studies, 14*(9-10), 237-251.

Baron-Cohen, S. (2006). The hyper-systemizing, assortative mating theory of autism. *Progress in Neuro-Psychopharmacology and Biological Psychiatry, 30*(5), 865-872.

Baron-Cohen, S. and Wheelwright, S. (2004). The empathy quotient: an investigation of adults with Asperger syndrome or high functioning autism, and normal sex differences. *Journal of autism and developmental disorders, 34*(2), 163-175.

Baron-Cohen, S., Richler, J., Bisarya, D., Gurunathan, N. and Wheelwright, S. (2003). The systemizing quotient: an investigation of adults with Asperger syndrome or high–functioning autism, and normal sex differences. *Philosophical Transactions of the Royal Society of London B: Biological Sciences, 358*(1430), 361-374.

Baron-Cohen, S. and Hammer, J. (1997). Parents of children with Asperger syndrome: what is the cognitive phenotype?. *Journal of cognitive neuroscience, 9*(4), 548-554.

Baron-Cohen, S. and Harrison, J. (1997). *Synaesthesia: Classic and contemporary readings*. Blackwell Publishing.

Barr, M. (1910). *Mental defectives, their history, treatment and training*. P. Blakiston's Son & Company.

Barry, A. (1997). *Visual intelligence: Perception, image, and manipulation in visual communication*. SUNY Press.

Bäzner, H. and Hennerici, M. (2006). Stroke in painters. *International review of neurobiology, 74*, 165-191.

Bashir, S., Mizrahi, I., Weaver, K., Fregni, F. and Pascual-Leone, A. (2010). Assessment and modulation of neural plasticity in rehabilitation with transcranial magnetic stimulation. *PM&R*, 2(12), S253-S268.

Baskin, J., Sperber, M. and Price, B. (2006). Asperger syndrome revisited. *Rev Neurol Dis*, 3(1), 1-7.

Bates, E. (1997). On language savants and the structure of the mind. *International Journal of Bilingualism*, 1, 163-179.

Bauman, M. and Kemper, T. (2005). Neuroanatomic observations of the brain in autism: a review and future directions. *International journal of developmental neuroscience*, 23(2-3), 183-187.

Bäzner, H. and Hennerici, M. (2006). Stroke in painters. *International review of neurobiology*, 74, 165-191.

Becker, E. and Stoodley, C. (2013). Autism spectrum disorder and the cerebellum. In *International review of neurobiology* (Vol. 113, pp. 1-34). Academic Press.

Beeferman, L. (2006). Artists on Artists: Leah Beeferman on Gregory Blackstock. *Bomb*, (97), 32-33.

Beeman, M. (1998). Coarse semantic coding and discourse comprehension. *Right hemisphere language comprehension: Perspectives from cognitive neuroscience*, 255-284.

Bellos, A. (2013). George Widener: the incredible life of the man who makes art for robots. https://www.theguardian.com/science/alexs-adventures-in-numberland/2013/jun/17/mathematics

Biever, C. (2009). The makings of a savant. *New Scientist*, 202(2711), 30-33.

Billobard (2020). Kodi Lee Breaks Hearts With 'AGT' Performance as Five Advance to Semis: Watch. Billboard Staff. August 13, 2020. https://www.billboard.com/articles/news/9433594/kodi-lee-agt-performance-five-advance-semis

Billington, J., Baron-Cohen, S. and Wheelwright, S. (2007). Cognitive style predicts entry into physical sciences and humanities: Questionnaire and performance tests of empathy and systemizing. *Learning and Individual Differences*, 17(3), 260-268.

Blackstock, G. (2006). *Blackstock's Collections: The Drawings of an Artistic Savant*. Princeton Architectural Press.

Bohwongprasert, I. (2019). Love is all around. Bangkok Post. September 5, 2019.

https://www.bangkokpost.com/life/arts-and-entertainment/1743239/love-is-all-around

Bohwongprasert, I. (2018). Able artistry. Bangkok Post. September 11, 2018. https://www.bangkokpost.com/life/arts-and-entertainment/1537910/able-artistry

Bókkon, I., Salari, V., Scholkmann, F., Dai, J. and Grass, F. (2013). Interdisciplinary implications on autism, savantism, Asperger syndrome and the biophysical picture representation: Thinking in pictures. *Cognitive Systems Research*, 22, 67-77.

Bohning, D., Shastri, A., McConnell, K., Nahas, Z., Lorberbaum, J., Roberts, D., and George, M. (1999). A combined TMS/fMRI study of intensity-dependent TMS over motor cortex. *Biological psychiatry*, 45(4), 385-394.

Bonatti, L. (1998). Neil Smith and Ianthi-Maria Tsimpli, The mind of a savant: language learning and modularity. Oxford: Basil Blackwell, 1995. Pp. xviii+ 243. *Journal of Linguistics*, *34*(1), 227-297.

Bonesteel, L. and Nation, P. (2011). *Real reading: creating an authentic reading experience*. Pearson Longman.

Bookheimer, S. (2002). Functional MRI of language: new approaches to understanding the cortical organization of semantic processing. *Annual review of neuroscience*, 25(1), 151-188.

Booth, R. and Happé, F. (2018). Evidence of reduced global processing in autism spectrum disorder. *Journal of autism and developmental disorders*, *48*(4), 1397-1408.

Bor, D., Billington, J. and Baron-Cohen, S. (2008). Savant memory for digits in a case of synaesthesia and Asperger syndrome is related to hyperactivity in the lateral prefrontal cortex. *Neurocase*, *13*(5-6), 311-319.

Boroojerdi, B., Phipps, M., Kopylev, L., Wharton, C., Cohen, L. and Grafman, J. (2001). Enhancing analogic reasoning with rTMS over the left prefrontal cortex. *Neurology*, 56(4), 526-528.

Bottini, G., Corcoran, R., Sterzi, R., Paulesu, E., Schenone, P., Scarpa, P., ... and Frith, D. (1994). The role of the right hemisphere in the interpretation of figurative aspects of language A positron emission tomography activation study. *Brain*, *117*(6), 1241-1253.

Boucher, J. (2017). *Autism spectrum disorder: Characteristics, causes and practical issues*. SAGE.

Bouvet, L., Donnadieu, S., Valdois, S., Caron, C., Dawson, M. and Mottron, L. (2014). Veridical mapping in savant abilities, absolute pitch, and synesthesia: an autism case study. *Frontiers in psychology*, 5, 106.

Bower, G. (1970). Analysis of a mnemonic device: Modern psychology uncovers the powerful components of an ancient system for improving memory. *American Scientist*, 58(5), 496-510.

Bölte, S. and Poustka, F. (2004). Comparing the intelligence profiles of savant and nonsavant individuals with autistic disorder. *Intelligence*, 32(2), 121-131.

Bradford, T. (2020). Renowned North Shore artist to show work at Princeton. The Salem News. January 2, 2020. https://www.salemnews.com/news/north_of_boston/renowned-north-shore-artist-to-show-work-at-princeton/article_67bdb742-4286-5d6b-8fb0-6a7035f3ec73.html

Brannen, A. (2016). Unbreakable bond between an autistic little girl and her cat: Six-year-old who didn't talk paints, cycles and SWIMS with the feline who helped her find her voice. Daily Mail. March 15, 2016. https://www.dailymail.co.uk/femail/article-3491674/Autistic-six-year-old-paints-cycles-SWIMS-tabby-feline-helped-voice.html

Breathnach, C. & Ward, C. (2005). The Victorian genius of Earlswood–a review of the case of James Henry Pullen. *Irish journal of psychological medicine*, 22(4), 151-155.

Brink, T. (1980). Idiot savant with unusual mechanical ability: an organic explanation. *The American journal of psychiatry*.

Brinsford, J. The inspiring story of America's Got Talent winner Kodi Lee as he wows a nation. Mirror. September 20, 2919. https://www.mirror.co.uk/3am/celebrity-news/inspiring-story-americas-talent-winner-20095187

Broadus, V. (2011). For woman with Williams Syndrome, music was the key. Lexington Herald Leader. May 11, 2011. https://www.kentucky.com/news/local/community/article44095050.html

Brogaard, B. and Marlow, K. (2015). *The superhuman mind: Free the genius in your brain*. Penguin.

Brogaard, B., Vanni, S. and Silvanto, J. (2013). Seeing mathematics: perceptual experience and brain activity in acquired synesthesia. *Neurocase*, 19(6), 566-575.

Brogaard, B. and Marlow, K. (2013). Hearing colours. *The Philosophers' Magazine*, (63), 28-35.

Brogaard, B: (2013). Hidden Talent Unleashed. Psychology Today. September 9, 2013. https://www.psychologytoday.com/intl/blog/the-superhuman-mind/201309/hidden-talent-unleashed

Buchen, L. (2011). Scientists and autism: When geeks meet. *Nature News*, *479*(7371), 25-27.

Burke, B. (2003). 'Rain Man' reigns in Casper. Casper Star Tribune. March 13, 2003. https://trib.com/news/local/rain-man-reigns-in-casper/article_0c374fd8-9737-51b8-87e8-f896ad30d317.html

Bushak, L. (2015). Watch How A Traumatic Brain Injury Turned This Lawyer Into A Talented Artist. Medical Daily. February 20, 2015. https://www.medicaldaily.com/watch-how-traumatic-brain-injury-turned-lawyer-talented-artist-322972

Butterworth, B. (2005). The development of arithmetical abilities. *Journal of Child Psychology and Psychiatry*, *46*(1), 3-18.

BBC News, 2004. 21 June 2004. Creative side unlocked by stroke. http://news.bbc.co.uk/2/hi/health/3826857.stm

Cairo, O. (2017). Assessing Relevance of External Cognitive Measures. *Frontiers in integrative neuroscience, 11.*

Cairo Battistutti, O. (2011). *El hombre artificial: el futuro de la tecnología* (No. 004.8 006.3). Alfaomega Grupo Editor. ISBN 978-607-707-260-7.

Calautti, C., Naccarato, M., Jones, P., Sharma, N., Day, D., Carpenter, A., ... and Baron, J. (2007). The relationship between motor deficit and hemisphere activation balance after stroke: a 3T fMRI study. *Neuroimage*, *34*(1), 322-331.

Cardinal, R. (2009). Outsider Art and the autistic creator. *Philosophical Transactions of the Royal Society B: Biological Sciences*, *364*(1522), 1459-1466.

Cardinal, R. and Rhodes, C. (2009). The art of George Widener. Oculeum. Henry Boxer Gallery. https://www.blurb.co.uk/b/570362-the-art-of-george-widener

Cardinal, R. (2005). The calendars of George Widener. *Raw Vision, 51*, 42-47.

Cardinal, R. (1972). *Outsider Art. London: Studio Vista. ISBN 9780289701683.*

Carter-Johnson, A. (2016). *Iris Grace*. Penguin UK.

Cassidy, S., Bradley, P., Robinson, J., Allison, C., McHugh, M. and Baron-Cohen, S. (2014). Suicidal ideation and suicide plans or attempts in adults with

Asperger's syndrome attending a specialist diagnostic clinic: a clinical cohort study. *The Lancet Psychiatry, 1*(2), 142-147.

Cavallera, G., Giudici, S. and Tommasi, L. (2012). Shadows and darkness in the brain of a genius: Aspects of the neuropsychological literature about the final illness of Maurice Ravel (1875–1937). *Medical science monitor: international medical journal of experimental and clinical research, 18*(10), MH1.

Charan, S. (2012). Childhood disintegrative disorder. *Journal of pediatric neurosciences, 7*(1), 55.

Charuchandra, S. (2020). Savant in the Limelight, 1988-2009. The Scientist. May 1, 2020. https://www.the-scientist.com/foundations/savant-in-the-limelight-19882009-67446

Chatterjee, A. (2015). The neuropsychology of visual art. *Art, Aesthetics, and the Brain, 341.*

Chatterjee, A. (2006). The neuropsychology of visual art: Conferring capacity. *International Review of Neurobiology, 74*, 39-49.

Chien, K. (2020). Love in the Moment: A Memoir. Amazon. https://www.amazon.com/Love-Moment-Memoir-Karen-Chien/dp/1710270152/ref=sr_1_2?keywords=karen+chien&qid=1583799056&s=digital-text&sr=1-2-catcorr

Christian, S. (1990). Perfect Pitch: Gloria Lenhoff Is a 'Musical Savant' Who Sings and Plays Beautifully but Can't Understand Mathematics. https://www.latimes.com/archives/la-xpm-1990-12-23-vw-9838-story.html

Chwast, D. and Chwast, S. (2011). *An Unexpected Life: A Mother and Son's Story of Love, Determination, Autism, and Art.* Sterling Publishing Company.

Cicoria, T. (2014). The electrifying story of the accidental pianist & composer. *Missouri medicine, 111*(4), 308-308.

Clark, T. (2016). *Exploring giftedness and autism: A study of a differentiated educational program for autistic savants.* Routledge.

Clarke, T., Lupton, M., Fernandez-Pujals, A., Starr, J., Davies, G., Cox, S., ... and Smith, B. (2016). Common polygenic risk for autism spectrum disorder (ASD) is associated with cognitive ability in the general population. *Molecular psychiatry, 21*(3), 419-425.

Cohen, L., Lehéricy, S., Henry, C., Bourgeois, M., Larroque, C., Sainte-Rose, C., ... and Hertz-Pannier, L. (2004). Learning to read without a left occipital lobe:

Right-hemispheric shift of visual word form area. *Annals of Neurology: Official Journal of the American Neurological Association and the Child Neurology Society*, 56(6), 890-894.

Cooperrider, J. (2011). Dr. Temple Grandin: a neuroimaging case study. In *Poster Presented at the International Meeting for Autism Research (IMFAR), San Diego, CA, USA*.

Corrigan, N., Richards, T., Treffert, D. and Dager, S. (2012). Toward a better understanding of the savant brain. *Comprehensive psychiatry*, 53(6), 706-717.

Cosslett, R. (2017). This was my form of language: the artist who draws cities from memory. https://www.theguardian.com/cities/2017/may/04/artist-draws-cities-memory-stephen-wiltshire

Cowan, R. and Frith, C. (2009). Do calendrical savants use calculation to answer date questions? A functional magnetic resonance imaging study. *Philosophical Transactions of the Royal Society B: Biological Sciences*, 364(1522), 1417-1424.

Cowan, R., O'Connor, N. and Samella, K. (2003). The skills and methods of calendrical savants. *Intelligence*, 31(1), 51-65.

Dabell, J. (2019). Nadia's Drawings. January 5, 2019.

Daily Mail Reporter (2010). Ex-street fighter, 60, turned into a fanatical artist by a brain haemorrhage that physically altered his mind. March 15, 2010. https://www.dailymail.co.uk/news/article-1256967/Man-survived-brain-haemorrhage-transformed-fanatical-artist-paints-18-hours-day.html

Darius, H. (2007). Savant syndrome-theories and empirical findings. http://www.diva-portal.org/smash/get/diva2:2901/FULLTEXT01.pdf

DeBlois, J. and Felix, A. (2005). *Some kind of genius: The extraordinary journey of musical savant Tony DeBlois*. Rodale.

Dehaene, S. (2011). *The number sense: How the mind creates mathematics*. OUP USA.

Dehaene, S., Molko, N., Cohen, L. and Wilson, A. (2004). Arithmetic and the brain. *Current opinion in neurobiology, 14*(2), 218-224.

Dehaene, S. (2001). Is number sense a patchwork?. *Mind and Language, 16*(1), 89-100.

Démonet, J., Thierry, G. and Cardebat, D. (2005). Renewal of the neurophysiology of language: functional neuroimaging. *Physiological reviews*, 85(1), 49-95.

De Bruijn, J. (2011). *Managing professionals.* Routledge de Bruin, E., Ferdinand, R., Meester, S., de Nijs, P. and Verheij, F. (2007). High rates of psychiatric co-morbidity in PDD-NOS. *Journal of autism and developmental disorders, 37*(5), 877-886.

Dileone, M., Carrasco-López, M., Segundo-Rodriguez, J., Mordillo-Mateos, L., López-Ariztegui, N., Alonso-Frech, F., ... and Foffani, G. (2017). Dopamine-dependent changes of cortical excitability induced by transcranial static magnetic field stimulation in Parkinson's disease. *Scientific Reports, 7*(1), 4329.

Dorman, C. (1991). Exceptional calendar calculation ability after early left hemispherectomy. *Brain and cognition*, 15(1), 26-36.

Down, J. (1887). Lettsomian Lectures on some of the Mental Affections of Childhood and Youth. *British medical journal, 1*(1362), 256.

Drues, M. (2014). Secrets Of The De Novo Pathway, Part 1: Why Aren't More Device Makers Using It? Med Device Online. https://www.meddeviceonline.com/doc/secrets-of-the-de-novo-pathway-part-why-aren-t-more-device-makers-using-it-0001

Dubischar-Krivec, A., Neumann, N., Poustka, F., Braun, C., Birbaumer, N. and Bölte, S. (2009). Calendar calculating in savants with autism and healthy calendar calculators. *Psychological medicine*, 39(08), 1355-1363.

Dubuffet, J. (1988). Place à l'incivisme. *Jean Dubuffet*, 103-106.

Duguid, S. (2007). First Person: Tony Cicoria. September 21, 2007. *Financial Times.* https://www.ft.com/content/c69f7968-6655-11dc-9fbb-0000779fd2ac

Dwyer, J. (2009). Like a skyline is etched in his head. The New York Times. October 27, 2009. https://www.nytimes.com/2009/10/28/nyregion/28about.html

Dykens, E., Sutcliffe, J. and Levitt, P. (2004). Autism and 15q11-q13 disorders: Behavioral, genetic, and pathophysiological issues. *Mental retardation and developmental disabilities research reviews*, 10(4), 284-291.

D'Souza, D., Booth, R., Connolly, M., Happé, F. and Karmiloff-Smith, A. (2016). Rethinking the concepts of 'local or global processors': evidence from Williams syndrome, Down syndrome, and Autism Spectrum Disorders. *Developmental science, 19*(3), 452-468.

Edelson, S., Edelson, M., Kerr, D. and Grandin, T. (1999). Behavioral and physiological effects of deep pressure on children with autism: A pilot study evaluating the efficacy of Grandin's Hug Machine. *American Journal of Occupational Therapy*, 53(2), 145-152.

Edelstyn, N. (2006). Creativity and the brain. *The Psychologist*, *19*(10), 616.

Edgers, G. A changed man. The Boston Globe. June 11, 2006. http://archive.boston.com/ae/theater_arts/articles/2006/06/11/a_changed_man/

Eisenberg, N. (2002). Empathy-related emotional responses, altruism, and their socialization. *Visions of compassion: Western scientists and Tibetan Buddhists examine human nature*, *135*, 131-164.

Emmerton, J., Lohmann, A., & Niemann, J. (1997). Pigeons' serial ordering of numerosity with visual arrays. *Animal Learning & Behavior*, 25(2), 234-244.

English, L. (2018). A Book Review on Musicophilia by Oliver Sacks. *Trent Notes on Linguistics*, *1*, 89-92.

Erden, S., & Reyhanoglu, G. (2019). Conservatory education of a musical savant with autism: a case study in Turkey. *Advances in Autism*.

Erickson, K., Voss, M., Prakash, R., Basak, C., Szabo, A., Chaddock, L., Kim, J., Heo, S., Alves, H., White, S., Wojcicki, T., Mailey, E., Vieira, V., Martin, S., Pence, B., Woods, J., McAuley, E., Kramer, A. and Gage, F. (2011). Exercise training increases size of hippocampus and improves memory. *Proceedings of the National Academy of Sciences*, 108(7), 3017-3022.

Ernsperger, L. and Wendel, D. (2007). *Girls under the umbrella of autism spectrum disorders: Practical solutions for addressing everyday challenges*. AAPC Publishing.

Ewen, J., Marvin, A., Law, K. and Lipkin, P. (2019). Epilepsy and autism severity: a study of 6,975 children. *Autism Research*, *12*(8), 1251-1259.

Fatemi, S., Reutiman, T., Folsom, T. and Sidwell, R. (2008). The role of cerebellar genes in pathology of autism and schizophrenia. *The Cerebellum*, *7*(3), 279-294.

Feldman, D. and Morelock, M. (2011). Prodigies and savants. *The Cambridge handbook of intelligence*, 210-234.

Feldman, C. (2013). Young eco-artist views his disability as a gift. Houston Chronicle. March 8, 2013. https://www.houstonchronicle.com/life/article/Young-eco-artist-views-his-disability-as-a-gift-4339850.php

Fernández, M., Sierra-Arregui, T. and Peñagarikano, O. (2019). The Cerebellum and Autism: More than Motor Control. In *Behavioral Neuroscience*. IntechOpen.

Ferstl, E., Rinck, M. and Cramon, D. (2005). Emotional and temporal aspects of situation model processing during text comprehension: An event-related fMRI study. *Journal of cognitive Neuroscience, 17*(5), 724-739.

Fine, C. (2010). *Delusions of gender: How our minds, society, and neurosexism create difference*. WW Norton & Company.

Fitzgerald, P. and Daskalakis, Z. (2013). *Repetitive Transcranial Magnetic Stimulation for Depressive Disorders*. Berlin Heidelberg: Springer-Verlag. pp. 81–90. doi:10.1007/978-3-642-36467-9.

Fombonne, E. (2009). Epidemiology of pervasive developmental disorders. *Pediatric research, 65*(6), 591-598.

Fombonne, E. and Tidmarsh, L. (2003). Epidemiologic data on Asperger disorder. *Child and Adolescent Psychiatric Clinics, 12*(1), 15-21.

Fombonne, E. (2002). Prevalence of childhood disintegrative disorder. *Autism, 6*(2), 149-157.

Fox, D. (2002). The inner savant. *Discover*, 23(2), 44-9.

Frisch, D. (2017). Wynn Newhouse Awards: Gregory Blackstock. https://www.wnewhouseawards.com/gregoryblackstock.html

Frith, U. (2008). *Autism: A very short introduction* (Vol. 195). Oxford University Press.

Frith, U. (1989). *Autism: Explaining the enigma* (Vol. 1989). Blackwell Scientific Publications: Oxford.

Garavan, H., Ross, T. and Stein, E. (1999). Right hemispheric dominance of inhibitory control: an event-related functional MRI study. *Proceedings of the National Academy of Sciences, 96*(14), 8301-8306.

Gazzaniga, M. (1983). Right hemisphere language following brain bisection: A 20-year perspective. *American Psychologist, 38*(5), 525.

Gersner, R., Oberman, L., Sanchez, M., Chiriboga, N., Kaye, H., Pascual-Leone, A., ... and Rotenberg, A. (2016). H-coil repetitive transcranial magnetic stimulation for treatment of temporal lobe epilepsy: A case report. *Epilepsy & behavior case reports*, 5, 52-56.

Geschwind, N. and Galaburda, A. (1985). Cerebral lateralization: Biological mechanisms, associations, and pathology: I. A hypothesis and a program for research. *Archives of neurology*, 42(5), 428-459.

Giles, J. (2004). Change of mind. https://www.nature.com/articles/430014a

Gillberg, I., Helles, A., Billstedt, E. and Gillberg, C. (2016). Boys with Asperger syndrome grow up: psychiatric and neurodevelopmental disorders 20 years after initial diagnosis. *Journal of Autism and Developmental Disorders, 46*(1), 74-82.

Gillberg, I. and Gillberg, C. (1989). Asperger syndrome—some epidemiological considerations: a research note. *Journal of child psychology and psychiatry, 30*(4), 631-638.

Goel, V. and Dolan, R. (2001). The functional anatomy of humor: segregating cognitive and affective components. *Nature neuroscience, 4*(3), 237-238.

Gómez, E. (2009). On the Border. *Art & Antiques Magazine*, February Issue.

Gonzalez, M. (2019). Spotlight on the incredible musical prodigy Kodi Lee. The Independent. https://theindependent.sg/spotlight-on-the-incredible-musical-prodigy-kodi-lee/

Gorvett, Z. (2018). The mystery of why some people become sudden geniuses. January 6, 2018. *BBC Future.* https://www.bbc.com/future/article/20180116-the-mystery-of-why-some-people-become-sudden-geniuses

Gottlieb, A. (2007). Take Five, and Call Me. October 28, 2007 . *The New York Times.* https://www.nytimes.com/2007/10/28/books/review/Gottlieb-t.html

Gottfredson, L. S. (1997). Mainstream science on intelligence: An editorial with 52 signatories, history, and bibliography: 13-23.

Grandin, T. (Ed.). (2019). *Livestock handling and transport.* Cabi.

Grandin, T. (Ed.). (2015). *Improving animal welfare: a practical approach.* Cabi.

Grandin, T. and Panek, R. (2013). *The autistic brain: Thinking across the spectrum.* Houghton Mifflin Harcourt.

Grandin, T. (2012). Temple Grandin Inducted into Colorado Women's Hall of Fame. March 8, 2012. https://web.archive.org/web/20131228000859if_/http://www.wherefoodcomesfrom.com/article/2281/Temple-Grandin-Inducted-into-Colorado-Womens-Hall-of-Fame#.Ur4Wmyj7TIU

Grandin, T. (2011). *The way I see it: A personal look at autism & Asperger's.* Future Horizons.

Grandin, T. (2009). How does visual thinking work in the mind of a person with autism? A personal account. *Philosophical Transactions of the Royal Society B: Biological Sciences, 364*(1522), 1437-1442.

Grandin, T. and Johnson, C. (2009). *Animals in translation: Using the mysteries of autism to decode animal behavior*. SUNY Press.

Grandin, T. (2008). *Thinking in pictures, expanded edition: My life with autism*. Vintage.

Grandin, T. (2006). *Thinking in pictures: And other reports from my life with autism*. Vintage.

Grandin, T. (1992). Calming effects of deep touch pressure in patients with autistic disorder, college students, and animals. *Journal of child and adolescent psychopharmacology*, 2(1), 63-72.

Grandin, T. (1992b). An inside view of autism. In *High-functioning individuals with autism* (pp. 105-126). Springer, Boston, MA.

Grant, K. (2016). Iris Grace Halmshaw, profile: Six-year-old painter with a reputation as an internationally renowned artist. Independent. March 3, 2016. https://www.independent.co.uk/news/people/profiles/iris-grace-halmshaw-profile-six-year-old-painter-reputation-internationally-renowned-artist-a6908281.html

Green, C. (2013). The blind pianist who led our reporter to a closed courtroom. Independent. May 2, 2013. https://www.independent.co.uk/news/uk/home-news/the-blind-pianist-who-led-our-reporter-to-a-closed-courtroom-8601774.html

Green, C. (2009). The human iPod: Meet the musical savant. Independent. May 28, 2009. https://www.independent.co.uk/arts-entertainment/music/news/the-human-ipod-meet-the-musical-savant-1691818.html

Griffin, D. (1958). Listening in the dark: the acoustic orientation of bats and men.

Griffin, D. (1944). Echolocation by blind men, bats and radar. *Science, 100*(2609), 589-590.

Grosbras, M. and Paus, T. (2002). Transcranial magnetic stimulation of the human frontal eye field: effects on visual perception and attention. *Journal of cognitive neuroscience*, 14(7), 1109-1120.

Grover, V. (2015). Autistic Savants: Making Child Really Special. *International Journal of Science and Research*, *4*(1), 1824-1827.

Guerin, P., Lyon, G., Barthelemy, C., Sostak, E., Chevrollier, V., Garreait, B., and Lelord, G. (1996). Neuropathological study of a case of autistic syndrome with severe mental retardation. *Developmental Medicine & Child Neurology*, *38*(3), 203-211.

Haensly, P. and Reynolds, C. (1989). Creativity and intelligence. In *Handbook of creativity* (pp. 111-132). Springer, Boston, MA.

Hamblin, D. (1966). They are idiot savants: wizards of the calendar. *Life*, *60*, 106-8.

Hanson, F. (2018). Tony DeBlois is on the move. The Patriot Ledger. https://www.patriotledger.com/news/20180517/tony-deblois-is-on-move

Happé, F. (2018). Why are savant skills and special talents associated with autism?. *World Psychiatry*, *17*(3), 280.

Happé, F. and Vital, P. (2009). What aspects of autism predispose to talent?. *Philosophical Transactions of the Royal Society of London B: Biological Sciences*, *364*(1522), 1369-1375.

Happé, F. and Frith, U. (2006). The weak coherence account: detail-focused cognitive style in autism spectrum disorders. *Journal of autism and developmental disorders*, *36*(1), 5-25.

Happé, F., Ronald, A. and Plomin, R. (2006). Time to give up on a single explanation for autism. *Nature neuroscience*, 9(10), 1218-1220.

Happé, F., Frith, U. and Briskman, J. (2001). Exploring the cognitive phenotype of autism: weak "central coherence" in parents and siblings of children with autism: I. Experimental tests. *The Journal of Child Psychology and Psychiatry and Allied Disciplines*, 42(3), 299-307.

Happé, F. (1996). Studying weak central coherence at low levels: children with autism do not succumb to visual illusions. A research note. *Journal of child psychology and psychiatry*, *37*(7), 873-877.

Heaton, P. (2009). Assessing musical skills in autistic children who are not savants. *Philosophical Transactions of the Royal Society B: Biological Sciences*, *364*(1522), 1443-1447.

Heaton, P. and Wallace, G. (2004). Annotation: The savant syndrome. *Journal of child psychology and psychiatry*, *45*(5), 899-911.

Heavey, L., Hermelin, B., Crane, L. and Pring, L. (2012). The structure of savant calendrical knowledge. *Developmental Medicine & Child Neurology*, 54(6), 507-513.

Henley, D. (1989). Nadia revisited: A study into the nature of regression in the autistic savant syndrome. *Art Therapy*, 6(2), 43-56.

Henshaw, J. (2012). *A tour of the senses: how your brain interprets the world.* JHU Press.

Hermelin, B., Pring, L., Buhler, M., Wolff, S. and Heaton, P. (1999). A visually impaired savant artist: Interacting perceptual and memory representations. *Journal of Child Psychology and Psychiatry, 40*(7), 1129-1139.

Hermelin, B. and O'Connor, N. (1986). Idiot savant calendrical calculators: Rules and regularities. *Psychological medicine,* 16(04), 885-893.

Hernando, S. (2017). Daniel Tammet: un talento incalculable. El País. May 30, 2017. https://elpais.com/elpais/2017/05/31/eps/1496181949_149618.html

Hersh, R. (1998). The Number Sense: How the Mind Creates Mathematics. *The American Mathematical Monthly,* 105(10), 975.

Herrnstein, R. & Murray, C. (2010). *The bell curve: Intelligence and class structure in American life.* Simon and Schuster.

Herwig, U., Padberg, F., Unger, J., Spitzer, M. and Schönfeldt-Lecuona, C. (2001). Transcranial magnetic stimulation in therapy studies: examination of the reliability of "standard" coil positioning by neuronavigation. *Biological psychiatry,* 50(1), 58-61.

Hill, E. (2011). Altered mind: creation of an artist. *The Lancet Neurology, 10*(11), 957-958.

Hill, A. (1978). Savants: Mentally retarded individuals with special skills. *International review of research in mental retardation,* 9, 277-298.

Ho, E., Tsang, A. and Ho, D. (1991). An investigation of the calendar calculation ability of a Chinese calendar savant. *Journal of autism and developmental disorders, 21*(3), 315-327.

Hoffman, R. and Cavus, I. (2002). Slow transcranial magnetic stimulation, long-term depotentiation, and brain hyperexcitability disorders. *American Journal of Psychiatry,* 159(7), 1093-1102.

Hogart, A., Wu, D., LaSalle, J. and Schanen, N. (2010). The comorbidity of autism with the genomic disorders of chromosome 15q11. 2-q13. *Neurobiology of disease,* 38(2), 181-191.

Hollis, F., Kanellopoulos, A. and Bagni, C. (2017). Mitochondrial dysfunction in Autism Spectrum Disorder: clinical features and perspectives. *Current opinion in neurobiology, 45,* 178-187.

Horstkötter, D. and Snoek, A. (2013). The importance of the self for autonomous behavior. *AJOB Neuroscience*, *4*(4), 62-63.

Horvath, J., Perez, J., Forrow, L., Fregni, F. and Pascual-Leone, A. (2011). Transcranial magnetic stimulation: a historical evaluation and future prognosis of therapeutically relevant ethical concerns. *Journal of medical ethics*, 37(3), 137-143.

Horwitz, W., Deming, W. and Winter, R. (1969). A further account of the idiots savants, experts with the calendar. *American Journal of Psychiatry*, 126(3), 412-415.

Horwitz, W., Kestenbaum, C., Person, E. and Jarvik, L. (1965). Identical Twin—"idiot savants"—calendar calculators. *American Journal of Psychiatry*, *121*(11), 1075-1079.

Hosseini, D., Hosseini, D. and Martinez, R. (2011). *Artism: The Art of Autism*. Autism Today.

Howe, M. and Smith, J. (1988). Calendar calculating in 'idiots savants': How do they do it? *British Journal of Psychology*, 79(3), 371-386.

Howlin, P. and Magiati, I. (2017). Autism spectrum disorder: Outcomes in adulthood. *Current Opinion in Psychiatry*, *30*(2), 69-76.

Howlin, P., Goode, S., Hutton, J. and Rutter, M. (2009). Savant skills in autism: psychometric approaches and parental reports. *Philosophical Transactions of the Royal Society B: Biological Sciences*, *364*(1522), 1359-1367.

Hu, S., Lai, J., Xu, D., Qi, H., Peterson, B., Bao, A., ... and Hu, J. (2016). Efficacy of repetitive transcranial magnetic stimulation with quetiapine in treating bipolar II depression: a randomized, double-blinded, control study. *Scientific reports*, *6*, 30537.

Hudmon, A. (2009). *Learning and memory*. Infobase Publishing.

Hughes, J. (2010). A review of Savant Syndrome and its possible relationship to epilepsy. *Epilepsy & behavior*, *17*(2), 147-152.

Humphries, C., Willard, K., Buchsbaum, B. and Hickok, G. (2001). Role of anterior temporal cortex in auditory sentence comprehension: an fMRI study. *Neuroreport*, *12*(8), 1749-1752.

Hunter, K. and Barnbaum, D. (2012). Pragmatic Aesthetics and the Autistic Artist. *The Journal of Aesthetic Education*, *46*(4), 48-56.

Hyltenstam, K. (Ed.). (2016). *Advanced proficiency and exceptional ability in second languages* (Vol. 51). Walter de Gruyter GmbH & Co KG.

Hyltenstam, K. (2016b). The exceptional ability of polyglots to achieve high-level proficiency in numerous languages. *Advanced Proficiency and Exceptional Ability in Second Languages. Boston, MA: De Gruyter Mouton,* 241-272.

Inspiration Matters (2017). Alonzo Clemons Interview. https://www.inspirationmatters.org/interviewshow.aspx?name=alonzo%20clemons&id=58&totalrec=8&alpha=a

Johnson, R. (2005). A genius explains. The Guardian, February 12, 2005. https://www.theguardian.com/theguardian/2005/feb/12/weekend7.weekend2

Jung-Beeman, M. (2005). Bilateral brain processes for comprehending natural language. *Trends in cognitive sciences*, 9(11), 512-518.

Jury, L. (2006). Austistic man with prodigious eye for art opens own gallery. Independent. October 28, 2006. https://www.independent.co.uk/news/uk/this-britain/autistic-man-with-prodigious-eye-for-art-opens-own-gallery-421992.html

Kabbany, J. (2012). LAKE ELSINORE: Musical savant eyes stardom. The San Diego Union Tribune. October 1, 2012. https://www.sandiegouniontribune.com/sdut-lake-elsinore-musical-savant-eyes-stardom-2012oct01-story.html

Kanner, L. (1943). Autistic disturbances of affective contact. *Nervous child*, 2(3), 217-250.

Kaplan, R. (2012). Music Therapy for Individuals with Autism. *The Huffington Post.*

Karnes, F. and Stephens, K. (2007). A Girl's Guide to Achieving in the Arts. Royal Fireworks Publishing

Karpinski, R., Kolb, A., Tetreault, N. and Borowski, T. (2018). High intelligence: A risk factor for psychological and physiological overexcitabilities. *Intelligence, 66,* 8-23.

Kaufman, S. (2014). Where do savant skills come from. *Scientific American Beautiful Minds Blog, 1.*

Keating, S. (2019). The violent attack that turned a man into a maths genius. https://www.bbc.com/future/article/20190411-the-violent-attack-that-turned-a-man-into-a-maths-genius

Kellman, J. (1996). Making sense of seeing: Autism and David Marr. *Visual Arts Research*, 76-89.

Keveney, B. (2019). Kodi Lee celebrates his 'AGT' victory: 'Heck, yeah! I'm the winner'. USA Today. September 19, 2019. https://www.usatoday.com/story/entertainment/tv/2019/09/19/agt-champ-kodi-lee-and-his-mom-tina-talk-season-14-victory/2371754001/

Kilian, A., Yaman, S., von Fersen, L., & Güntürkün, O. (2003). A bottlenose dolphin discriminates visual stimuli differing in numerosity. *Animal Learning & Behavior*, *31*(2), 133-142.

Kirby, T. (2006). Honour for autistic man who speaks through art. https://www.independent.co.uk/news/uk/this-britain/honour-for-autistic-man-who-speaks-through-art-6112727.html

Kish, D. (2009). Human echolocation: How to "see" like a bat. *New Scientist*, *202*(2703), 31-33.

Klappholz, A. (2008). Jon Sarkin: A Medical mystery and artist savant. Vanity Fair. December 18, 2008. https://www.vanityfair.com/news/2008/12/jon-sarkin-artist-savant

Klin, A. (2006). Autismo e síndrome de Asperger: uma visão geral. *Brazilian Journal of Psychiatry*, *28*, s3-s11.

Knipper, M., Van Dijk, P., Nunes, I., Rüttiger, L. and Zimmermann, U. (2013). Advances in the neurobiology of hearing disorders: recent developments regarding the basis of tinnitus and hyperacusis. *Progress in neurobiology*, *111*, 17-33.

Koldewyn, K., Jiang, Y., Weigelt, S. and Kanwisher, N. (2013). Global/local processing in autism: Not a disability, but a disinclination. *Journal of autism and developmental disorders*, *43*(10), 2329-2340.

Landa, R., Folstein, S. and Isaacs, C. (1991). Spontaneous narrative-discourse performance of parents of autistic individuals. *Journal of Speech, Language, and Hearing Research*, 34(6), 1339-1345.

Lankston, C. and Stern, C. (2019). 'He has no disabilities on stage': Mother of blind autistic singer who left America's Got Talent judges in TEARS calls him an 'innocent soul' who transforms when he performs music. Daily Mail. May 30, 2019. https://www.dailymail.co.uk/femail/article-7087405/Mom-blind-autistic-singer-Kodi-Lee-Americas-Got-Talent-says-no-disabilities-stage.html

Lauerman, C. (1988). *Extraordinary People*. Chicago Tribune. https://www.chicagotribune.com/news/ct-xpm-1988-08-28-8801250943-story.html

Lenhoff, H., Perales, O. and Hickok, G. (2001). Absolute pitch in Williams syndrome. *Music Perception: An Interdisciplinary Journal, 18*(4), 491-503.

Lenhoff, H., Wang, P., Greenberg, F. and Bellugi, U. (1997). Williams syndrome and the brain. *Scientific American, 277*(6), 68-73.

Lehrer, J. (2009). Learn to Think Better: Tips from a Savant. Scientific American. April 2009. https://www.scientificamerican.com/article/think-better-tips-from-a-savant/

Leung, R. (2004). A very special brain. 60 Minutes. CBS News. https://www.cbsnews.com/news/a-very-special-brain-06-01-2004/

Levine, R. and Oron, Y. (2015). Tinnitus. In *Handbook of clinical neurology* (Vol. 129, pp. 409-431). Elsevier.

Lewald, J., Foltys, H. and Töpper, R. (2002). Role of the posterior parietal cortex in spatial hearing. *The Journal of neuroscience: the official journal of the Society for Neuroscience*, 22(3), RC207-RC207.

Lewis, R. (2015). Weird Al Yankovic, young people with autism sing 'Yoda' on telethon. Los Angeles Times. March 9, 2015. https://www.latimes.com/entertainment/music/posts/la-et-ms-weird-al-yankovic-yoda-autism-telethon-jodi-dipiazza-20150309-story.html#

Lewis, C. (2008). *Rex: A mother, her autistic child, and the music that transformed their lives*. Thomas Nelson.

Li, H., Wang, J., Li, C. and Xiao, Z. (2014). Repetitive transcranial magnetic stimulation (rTMS) for panic disorder in adults. *The Cochrane Library*.

Lin, J. (c. 2007). Case Study of an Autistic Young Artist: Leland Lee.

Lindell, A. (2006). In your right mind: Right hemisphere contributions to language processing and production. *Neuropsychology review, 16*(3), 131-148.

Lion, V. (2020). Disrupting Temple Grandin. *Disability and Animality: Crip Perspectives in Critical Animal Studies.*

Lopez, B. and Leekam, S. R. (2003). Do children with autism fail to process information in context? *Journal of child psychology and psychiatry, 44*(2), 285-300.

Luber, B. and Lisanby, S. (2014). Enhancement of human cognitive performance using transcranial magnetic stimulation (TMS). *Neuroimage, 85*, 961-970.

Luks, J. (2013). Autistic artist Grant Manier is a rising star: "Coolages" king racks up awards and changes thinking. Culturemap. March 8, 2013. https://houston.culturemap.com/news/city-life/03-08-13-austic-artist-grant-manier-is-a-rising-star-teen-of-coolages-racks-up-awards-challenges-false-notions/#slide=0

Lythgoe, M., Pollak, T., Kalmus, M., De Haan, M. and Chong, W. (2005). Obsessive, prolific artistic output following subarachnoid hemorrhage. *Neurology*, 64(2), 397-398.

Ma, D., Jaworski, J., Menold, M., Donnelly, S., Abramson, R., Wright, H.,... and Cuccaro, M. (2005). Ordered-subset analysis of savant skills in autism for 15q11-q13. *American Journal of Medical Genetics Part B: Neuropsychiatric Genetics*, 135(1), 38-41.

McFarland, H. and Fortin, D. (1982). Amusia due to right temporoparietal infarct. *Archives of Neurology*, 39(11), 725-727.

Maeda, F., Keenan, J., Tormos, J., Topka, H. and Pascual-Leone, A. (2000). Modulation of corticospinal excitability by repetitive transcranial magnetic stimulation. *Clinical Neurophysiology*, 111(5), 800-805.

Maguire, E., Valentine, E., Wilding, J. and Kapur, N. (2003). Routes to remembering: the brains behind superior memory. *Nature neuroscience*, 6(1), 90-95.

Maher, B. (2001). Music, the brain, and Williams syndrome: rare disorder offers insight into the genetic basis of cognition.(focus on Genes and Genomics). *The Scientist*, 15(23), 20-22.

Manier, J. (2017). Grant the Jigsaw Giraffe. Long Tale Publishing.

Margulis, E. H. (2017). Neuroscience: How music meets mind. *Nature*, 546(7658), 351-351.

Martin, R. (2019). Who is America's Got Talent 2019 winner Kodi Lee? Metro. September 19, 2019. https://metro.co.uk/2019/09/19/americas-got-talent-2019-winner-kodi-lee-10771648/

Marqués, M. and González, P. (2016). Savants músicos y oído absoluto. http://revistadigital2.csmvalencia.es/wp-content/uploads/2016/05/Savants-m%C3%BAsicos-y-o%C3%ADdo-absoluto.pdf

Marsa, L. (2016). Extraordinary Minds: The link between savantism and autism. Spectrum. January 13, 2016. https://www.spectrumnews.org/features/deep-dive/extraordinary-minds-the-link-between-savantism-and-autism/

Mashal, N., Faust, M., Hendler, T. and Jung-Beeman, M. (2007). An fMRI investigation of the neural correlates underlying the processing of novel metaphoric expressions. *Brain and language, 100*(2), 115-126.

Mattila, M. L., Kielinen, M., Jussila, K., Linna, S. L., Bloigu, R., Ebeling, H. and Moilanen, I. (2007). An epidemiological and diagnostic study of Asperger syndrome according to four sets of diagnostic criteria. *Journal of the American Academy of Child & Adolescent Psychiatry, 46*(5), 636-646.

McCarthy, G. (2019). Around Cape Ann: Celebrating art on the working waterfront. Gloucester Daily Tomes. January 10, 2019. https://www.gloucestertimes.com/news/the_catch/around-cape-ann-celebrating-art-on-the-working-waterfront/article_30b85cdb-be96-5f95-908e-a8cff4ba55e5.html

McConnell, K., Nahas, Z., Shastri, A., Lorberbaum, J., Kozel, F., Bohning, D. and George, M. (2001). The transcranial magnetic stimulation motor threshold depends on the distance from coil to underlying cortex: a replication in healthy adults comparing two methods of assessing the distance to cortex. *Biological psychiatry*, 49(5), 454-459.

McKenzie, R. (2012). A different way to think about creativity: The case of autism and outsider art. In *Creative Engagements with Children: International Perspectives and Contexts* (pp. 107-119). Brill.

McQueeney, K. (2012). The heart-warming moment autistic girl performs Firework with her idol Katy Perry. Daily Mail. October 19, 2012. https://www.dailymail.co.uk/tvshowbiz/article-2220146/Night-Of-Too-Many-Stars-Katy-Perry-performs-Firework-autistic-girl-Jodi-DiPiazza-benefit.html

Mehra, C., Sil, A., Hedderly, T., Kyriakopoulos, M., Lim, M., Turnbull, J., ... and Absoud, M. (2019). Childhood disintegrative disorder and autism spectrum disorder: a systematic review. *Developmental Medicine & Child Neurology, 61*(5), 523-534.

Meilleur, A., Jelenic, P. and Mottron, L. (2015). Prevalence of clinically and empirically defined talents and strengths in autism. *Journal of autism and developmental disorders, 45*(5), 1354-1367.

Mell, J., Howard, S. and Miller, B. (2003). Art and the brain: The influence of frontotemporal dementia on an accomplished artist. *Neurology*, 60(10), 1707-1710.

Mendez, M. (2004). Dementia as a window to the neurology of art. *Medical hypotheses, 63*(1), 1-7.

Meyer, M., Friederici, A. and von Cramon, D. (2000). Neurocognition of auditory sentence comprehension: event related fMRI reveals sensitivity to syntactic violations and task demands. *Cognitive Brain Research, 9*(1), 19-33.

Michaud, J. (2010). Back Issues: Franco Magnani. The New Yorker. August 24, 2010. https://www.newyorker.com/books/double-take/back-issues-franco-magnani

Miller, B., Boone, K., Cummings, J., Read, S. and Mishkin, F. (2000). Functional correlates of musical and visual ability in frontotemporal dementia. *The British Journal of Psychiatry*, 176(5), 458-463.

Miller, L. (1998). Defining the savant syndrome. *Journal of Developmental and Physical Disabilities, 10*(1), 73-85.

Miller, B., Ponton, M., Benson, D., Cummings, J. and Mena, I. (1996). Enhanced artistic creativity with temporal lobe degeneration. *The Lancet, 348*(9043), 1744-1745.

Miller, L. (1989). *Musical savants: Exceptional skill in the mentally retarded.* Hillsdale, NJ: Lawrence Erlbaum Associates.

Minda, J. (2019). Treffert autism center hosts author Temple Grandin. December 15, 2019. https://www.chausa.org/publications/catholic-health-world/archives/issues/december-15-2019/treffert-autism-center-hosts-author-temple-grandin

Mitchell, R. and Crow, T. (2005). Right hemisphere language functions and schizophrenia: the forgotten hemisphere?. *Brain, 128*(5), 963-978.

Mizoguchi, K. (2019). Kodi Lee, Singing Phenom Who Is Blind and Has Autism, 22, Wins *America's Got Talent* Season 14. People. September 18, 2019. https://people.com/tv/kodi-lee-wins-americas-got-talent-season-14/

Mohney, G. (2014). After Autistic Girl Finds Success in Art World, Parents Shield Her From Spotlight. ABC News. September 30, 2014. https://abcnews.go.com/Health/autistic-girl-finds-success-art-world-parents-shield/story?id=25865752

Montgomery, S. and Grandin, T. (2012). *Temple Grandin: How the girl who loved cows embraced autism and changed the world.* Houghton Mifflin Harcourt.

Monty, S. (2013). *May's boy: The rest of the history*. CreateSpace Independent Publishing Platform (February 13, 2013). Amazon.

Monty, S. (1981). *May's boy: an incredible story of love*. Thomas Nelson Publishers.

Morgan, G., Smith, N., Tsimpli, I. and Woll, B. (2007). Classifier learning and modality in a polyglot savant. *Lingua, 117*(7), 1339-1353.

Morgan, G., Smith, N., Tsimpli, I. and Woll, B. (2002). Language against the odds: The learning of British Sign Language by a polyglot savant. *Journal of Linguistics*, 1-41.

Morris, C., Lenhoff, H. and Wang, P. (Eds.). (2006). *Williams-Beuren syndrome: Research, evaluation, and treatment*. JHU Press.

Moss, S. (2007). He attacked the keyboard. The Guardian. April 30, 2007. https://www.theguardian.com/music/2007/apr/30/classicalmusicandopera.jazz

Mottron, L., Bouvet, L., Bonnel, A., Samson, F., Burack, J.., Dawson, M. and Heaton, P. (2013). Veridical mapping in the development of exceptional autistic abilities. *Neuroscience & Biobehavioral Reviews, 37*(2), 209-228.

Mottron, L. (2011). The power of autism. *Nature, 479*(7371), 33-35.

Mottron, L., Dawson, M. and Soulières, I. (2009). Enhanced perception in savant syndrome: patterns, structure and creativity. *Philosophical Transactions of the Royal Society B: Biological Sciences, 364*(1522), 1385-1391.

Mottron, L., Dawson, M., Soulieres, I., Hubert, B. and Burack, J. (2006). Enhanced perceptual functioning in autism: an update, and eight principles of autistic perception. *Journal of autism and developmental disorders, 36*(1), 27-43.

Mottron, L., Burack, J., Stauder, J. and Robaey, P. (1999). Perceptual processing among high-functioning persons with autism. *Journal of Child Psychology and Psychiatry, 40*(2), 203-211.

Mukerji C., Mottron L. and McPartland J. (2013) Enhanced Perceptual Functioning. In: Volkmar F.R. (eds) Encyclopedia of Autism Spectrum Disorders. Springer, New York, NY.

Mullin, J. (2014). *Drawings of Autism*. Akashic Books.

Mullin, J. (2009). *Drawing autism*. Mark Batty Publisher. ISBN 9780981960005

Murphy, E. (2012). Autistic Girl, Jodi DiPiazza, Performs with Katy Perry. ABC News. October 19, 2012. https://abcnews.go.com/blogs/entertainment/2012/10/autistic-girl-jodi-dipiazza-performs-with-katy-perry/

Murray, S. (2008). *Representing autism: Culture, narrative, fascination*. Oxford University Press.

Nash, A. and Grossi, G. (2007). Picking Barbie™'s brain: Inherent sex differences in scientific ability? *Journal of Interdisciplinary Feminist Thought*, 2(1), 5.

Neal, M. (2012). 'Acquired savant' Derek Amato becomes musical prodigy after hitting his head hard diving into shallow end of pool. New York Daily News. June 7, 2012. https://www.nydailynews.com/news/national/acquired-savant-derek-amato-musical-prodigy-hitting-head-hard-diving-shallow-pool-article-1.1091812

Neisser, U., Boodoo, G., Bouchard Jr, T., Boykin, A., Brody, N., Ceci, S., ... & Urbina, S. (1996). Intelligence: knowns and unknowns. *American psychologist*, *51*(2), 77.

Nevins, T. (2017). Brain Injury Transforms Prominent Attorney into Impassioned Artist—Patrick Fagerberg. Medium. April 11, 2017. https://medium.com/@toddnevins/brain-injury-transforms-prominent-attorney-into-impassioned-artist-patrick-fagerberg-e243219493f4

Neumann, N., Dubischar-Krivec, A., Braun, C., Löw, A., Poustka, F., Bölte, S. and Birbaumer, N. (2010). The mind of the mnemonists: an MEG and neuropsychological study of autistic memory savants. *Behavioural brain research*, *215*(1), 114-121.

Normann, C. and Berger, M. (2008). Neuroenhancement: status quo and perspectives. *European archives of psychiatry and clinical neuroscience*, 258(5), 110-114.

Nurmi, E., Dowd, M., Tadevosyan-Leyfer, O., Haines, J., Folstein, S. and Sutcliffe, J. (2003). Exploratory subsetting of autism families based on savant skills improves evidence of genetic linkage to 15q11-q13. *Journal of the American Academy of Child & Adolescent Psychiatry*, 42(7), 856-863.

Nutt, A. (2011). *Shadows bright as glass: The remarkable story of one man's journey from brain trauma to artistic triumph*. Simon and Schuster.

Nutt, A. (2011b). The man who couldn´t stop drawing. The Guardian. July 29, 2011. https://www.theguardian.com/artanddesign/2011/jul/29/jon-sarkin-couldnt-stop-drawing

Oberman, L., Enticott, P., Casanova, M., Rotenberg, A., Pascual-Leone, A. and McCracken, J. (2016). Transcranial magnetic stimulation in autism spectrum disorder: challenges, promise, and roadmap for future research. *Autism Research*, 9(2), 184-203.

Ockelford, A. (2013). *Music, language and autism: Exceptional strategies for exceptional minds*. Jessica Kingsley Publishers.

Ockelford, A. (2009). *In the key of genius: The extraordinary life of Derek Paravicini*. Random House.

Ockelford, A. (2008). *In the Key of Genius: The Extraordinary Life of Derek Paravicini*. Arrow, 2008

Ockelford, A. (2007). A music module in working memory? Evidence from the performance of a prodigious musical savant. *Musicae Scientiae, 11*(2_suppl), 5-36.

Ockelford, A., Pring, L., Welch, G. and Treffert, D. (2006). Focus on music.

Ockelford, A. and Pring, L. (2005). Learning and creativity in a prodigious musical savant. In *International Congress Series* (Vol. 1282, pp. 903-907). Elsevier.

O'Connell, D. (2009). *The Ballad of Blind Tom, Slave Pianist: America's Lost Musical Genius*. ABRAMS.

O'Connor, N., Cowan, R. and Samella, K. (2000). Calendrical calculation and intelligence. *Intelligence*, 28(1), 31-48.

O'Connor, N., Smith, N., Frith, C. and Tsimpli, I. M. (1994). Neuropsychology and linguistic talent. *Journal of Neurolinguistics*, 8(2), 95-107.

O'Connor, N. and Hermelin, B. (1989). The memory structure of autistic idiot☒savant mnemonists. *British Journal of Psychology*, 80(1), 97-111.

O'Dwyer, L. (2016). A Tale of Two Hemispheres. TheScientist. https://www.the-scientist.com/opinion/opinion-a-tale-of-two-hemispheres-32333

Opitz, J., Smith, J. and Santoro, L. (2008). The FG syndromes (online mendelian inheritance in man 305450): Perspective in 2008. *Advances in pediatrics*, 55(1), 123-170.

Ozonoff, S., Strayer, D., McMahon, W. and Filloux, F. (1994). Executive function abilities in autism and Tourette syndrome: An information processing approach. *Journal of child Psychology and Psychiatry*, 35(6), 1015-1032.

Paine, S. (1981). *Six children draw*. Academic Press.

Pariser, D. and Zimmerman, E. (2004). Learning in the visual arts: Characteristics of gifted and talented individuals. *Handbook of research and policy in art education*, 379-405.

Pariser, D. (1981). Nadia's drawings: Theorizing about an autistic child's phenomenal ability. *Studies in Art Education*, 22(2), 20-31.

Park, D. and Reuter-Lorenz, P. (2009). The adaptive brain: aging and neurocognitive scaffolding. *Annual review of psychology*, *60*, 173-196.

Park, C. (1978). Review of Nadia: a case of extraordinary drawing ability in an autistic child. *Journal of Autism and Childhood Schizophrenia*, *8*(4), 457-472.

Parker, E., Cahill, L. and McGaugh, J. (2006). A Case of Unusual Autobiographical Remembering. *Psychology Press*, 12, 35–49.

Pascual-Leone, A., Valls-Solé, J., Wassermann, E. and Hallett, M. (1994). Responses to rapid-rate transcranial magnetic stimulation of the human motor cortex. *Brain*, 117(4), 847-858.

Peek, F. and Hanson, L. (2008). *The life and message of the real Rain Man: The journey of a mega-savant*. Port Chester, N.Y: Dude Pub.

Peek, F. (1996). *The real rain man, Kim Peek*. Salt Lake City, Utah: Harkness Pub. Consultants.

Peek, F. (1996). *The real rain man, Kim Peek*. Harkness Pub. Consultants.

Pellicano, E., Maybery, M., Durkin, K. and Maley, A. (2006). Multiple cognitive capabilities/deficits in children with an autism spectrum disorder:" Weak" central coherence and its relationship to theory of mind and executive control. *Development and psychopathology*, 18(1), 77.

Philby, C. (2009). My secret life: Stephen Wiltshire, artist, 34. https://www.independent.co.uk/arts-entertainment/art/features/my-secret-life-stephen-wiltshire-artist-34-1488487.html

Piazza, M., Izard, V., Pinel, P., Le Bihan, D. and Dehaene, S. (2004). Tuning curves for approximate numerosity in the human intraparietal sulcus. *Neuron*, *44*(3), 547-555.

Piechowski-Jozwiak, B. and Bogousslavsky, J. (2020). Painting in Neurology. In *Brain and Art* (pp. 41-52). Springer, Cham.

Piedmont-Palladino, S. (2007). *Tools of the imagination: Drawing tools and technologies from the eighteenth century to the present*. Princeton Architectural Press.

Pilkington, E. (2009). The real Rain Man dies of heart attack in home town of Salt Lake City, aged 58. The Guardian. December 22, 2009. https://www.theguardian.com/world/2009/dec/22/kim-peek-rain-man-dies

Plaisted, K. (2015). Reduced generalization in autism: An alternative to weak central coherence.

Plank, A. (2006). Interview with Temple Grandin. WrongPlanet.net. January 2, 2006. https://wrongplanet.net/interview-with-temple-grandin/

Pring, L., Ryder, N., Crane, L. and Hermelin, B. (2012). Creativity in savant artists with autism. *Autism, 16*(1), 45-57.

Pring, L. (2008). Memory characteristics in individuals with savant skills. In: J. Boucher and D. Bowler, eds. *Memory in Autism.* Cambridge: Cambridge University Press, pp. 210-230.

Pring, L. (2005). Savant talent. *Developmental Medicine & Child Neurology,* 47(7), 500-503. doi:10.1017/S0012162205000976

Pring, L. and Ockelford, A. (2005). Children with septo-optic dysplasia-musical interests, abilities and provision: the results of a parental survey. *British Journal of Visual Impairment,* 23(2), 58-66.

Pring, L., & Hermelin, B. (2002). Numbers and letters: exploring an autistic savant's unpractised ability. *Neurocase, 8*(4), 330-337.

Pring, L., Hermelin, B., Buhler, M. and Walker, I. (1997). Native savant talent and acquired skill. *Autism, 1*(2), 199-214.

Pring, L. and Hermelin, B. (1993). Bottle, tulip and wineglass: semantic and structural picture processing by savant artists. *Journal of Child Psychology and Psychiatry, 34*(8), 1365-1385.

Pulsifer, M., Brandt, J., Salorio, C., Vining, E., Carson, B. and Freeman, J. (2004). The cognitive outcome of hemispherectomy in 71 children. *Epilepsia,* 45(3), 243-254.

Ramachandran, V. and Hubbard, E. (2001). Synaesthesia--a window into perception, thought and language. *Journal of consciousness studies,* 8(12), 3-34.

Ratey, J., Grandin, T. and Miller, A. (1992). Defense behavior and coping in an autistic savant: the story of Temple Grandin, PhD. *Psychiatry,* 55(4), 382-391.

Rayala, M. (1981). On "Nadia's Drawings: Theorizing about an Autistic Child's Phenomenal Ability". *Studies in Art Education,* 22(2), 70-72.

Rehagen, T. (2016). Uncharted Waters. Southwest, pp56-59. October 2016. https://issuu.com/southwestmag/docs/oct2016/60?e=18825507%2F39247819

Reznikova, Z. and Ryabko, B. (2011). Numerical competence in animals, with an insight from ants. *Behaviour, 148*(4), 405-434.

Rimland, B. and Fein, D. (1988). Special talents of autistic savants. In Obler, L. and Fein, D. (Eds.) *The exceptional brain: Neuropsychology of talent and special abilities*. New York, NY, US: Guilford Press.

Rimland, B. (1978). Savant capabilities of autistic children and their cognitive implications.

Rinehart, N., Bradshaw, J., Moss, S., Brereton, A. and Tonge, B. (2000). Atypical interference of local detail on global processing in high-functioning autism and Asperger's disorder. *The Journal of Child Psychology and Psychiatry and Allied Disciplines, 41*(6), 769-778.

Robertson, P. (2004). Music and the Brain: A Musicologist's Viewpoint. *Neurology of the Arts: Painting, Music, Literature*, 307.

Robertson, E., Theoret, H. and Pascual-Leone, A. (2003). Studies in cognition: the problems solved and created by transcranial magnetic stimulation. *Journal of Cognitive Neuroscience*, 15(7), 948-960.

Rogers, T., McKimm, E., Dickson, P, Goldowitz, D., Blaha, C., and Mittleman, G. (2013). Is autism a disease of the cerebellum? An integration of clinical and pre-clinical research. *Frontiers in systems neuroscience, 7*, 15.

Roitman, J., Brannon, E. and Platt, M. (2007). Monotonic coding of numerosity in macaque lateral intraparietal area. *PLoS biology*, 5(8).

Rojas, J., Hermosilla, J., Montero, R. and Espí, P. (2009). Physical analysis of several organic signals for human echolocation: oral vacuum pulses. *Acta acustica united with acustica*, 95(2), 325-330.

Rommelse, N., van der Kruijs, M., Damhuis, J., Hoek, I., Smeets, S., Antshel, K., ... and Faraone, S. (2016). An evidenced-based perspective on the validity of attention-deficit/hyperactivity disorder in the context of high intelligence. *Neuroscience & Biobehavioral Reviews, 71*, 21-47.

Roth, I. (2020). Autism, Creativity and Aesthetics. *Qualitative Research in Psychology, 17*(4), 498-508.

Rush, B. (1789). Account of a wonderful talent for arithmetical calculation in an African slave, living in Virginia. *Am. Mus*, 5, 62-63.

Ruthsatz, J. and Stephens, K. (2016). *The Prodigy's Cousin: The Family Link Between Autism and Extraordinary Talent*. Current.

Ruthsatz, J., Petrill, S., Li, N., Wolock, S. and Bartlett, C. (2015). Molecular genetic evidence for shared etiology of autism and prodigy. *Human Heredity*, *79*(2), 53-59.

Sacks, O. (2012). *An anthropologist on Mars: Seven paradoxical tales*. Vintage.

Sacks, O. (2010). *Musicophilia: Tales of music and the brain*. Vintage Canada.

Sacks, O. (2009). *The man who mistook his wife for a hat*. London: Picador.

Sacks, O. (2007). *Musicophilia: Tales of Music and the Brain*. London: Picador.

Sacks, O. (2007b). A Bolt from the Blue. Where do sudden intense passions come from? The New Yorker, 23 July 2007. https://www.newyorker.com/magazine/2007/07/23/a-bolt-from-the-blue

Sacks, O. (2002). El hombre que confundió a su mujer con un sombrero. Editorial Anagrama: Barcelona.

Sacks, O., Schlaug, G., Jancke, L., Huang, Y. and Steinmetz, H. (1995). Musical ability. *Science-AAAS-Weekly Paper Edition*, *268*(5211), 621-622.

Sacks, O. (1985). *The Man Who Mistook His Wife for a Hat*. Gerald Duckworth & Co. London.

Safarova, B. (2013). George Widener: Secret Universe IV Paperback. Walther König, Köln; Bilingual edition.

Saffran, J. and Griepentrog, G. (2001). Absolute pitch in infant auditory learning: evidence for developmental reorganization. *Developmental psychology*, *37*(1), 74.

Sanderson, D. (2010). Autistic pianist's case heard in public after UK's last secret court opens. The Times. May 14, 2010. https://www.thetimes.co.uk/article/autistic-pianists-case-heard-in-public-after-uks-last-secret-court-opens-q72hrhdl92j

Schmidt, W. (1983). *Gifted Retardates: The Search for Clues to Mysterious Talent. The New York Times.* July 12, 1983. https://www.nytimes.com/1983/07/12/science/gifted-retardates-the-search-for-clues-to-mysterious-talent.html

Schumann, C. and Amaral, D. (2006). Stereological analysis of amygdala neuron number in autism. *Journal of Neuroscience*, *26*(29), 7674-7679.

Schulze, H. (2016). 10 Sonic Epistemology. *Sound as Popular Culture: A Research Companion*, 111.

Selfe, L. (2015). Nadia Chomyn obituary. The Guardian, 9 December 2015. https://www.theguardian.com/artanddesign/2015/dec/09/nadia-chomyn

Selfe, L. (2012). *Nadia revisited: A longitudinal study of an autistic savant.* Psychology Press.

Selfe, L. (1995). Nadia reconsidered. *The development of artistically gifted children*, 197-237.

Selfe, L. (1983). *Normal and anomalous representational drawing ability in children*. Academic Press, 1983.

Selfe, L. (1977). *Nadia: A case of extraordinary drawing ability in an autistic child*. Academic Press.

Semenza, C., & Benavides-Varela, S. (2018). Reassessing lateralization in calculation. *Philosophical Transactions of the Royal Society B: Biological Sciences, 373*(1740), 20170044.

Sergent, J. (1993). Music, the brain and Ravel. *Trends in neurosciences, 16*(5), 168-172.

Sforza, T. (2010). *The (Strangest) Song: One Father's Quest to Help His Daughter Find Her Voice*. Prometheus Books.

Sforza, T. (1998). Williams Syndrome. Chicago Tribune. September 18, 1998. https://www.chicagotribune.com/news/ct-xpm-1998-09-18-9809190188-story.html

Shin, S., Dixon, C., Okonkwo, D. and Richardson, R. (2014). Neurostimulation for traumatic brain injury: A review. *Journal of neurosurgery, 121*(5), 1219-1231.

Silberman, S. (2017). *Neurotribes: The legacy of autism and how to think smarter about people who think differently*. Atlantic Books.

Silberman, S. (2015). How Oliver Sacks helped introduce the world to autism. BuzzFeed. August 30, 2015. https://www.buzzfeed.com/ssilberman/how-oliver-sacks-introduced-the-world-to-autism

Silberman, S. (2015b). *Neurotribes: The legacy of autism and the future of neurodiversity*. Penguin.

Simola, A. (2015). *The Roving Mind: A Modern Approach to Cognitive Enhancement*. ST Press.

Singer, W. (2009). The brain, a complex self-organizing system. *European Review, 17*(2), 321-329.

Skudra, N. (2019). Journey Of The Heart: A Film About Blind, Autistic Musical Savant Tony DeBlois. The art of autism. https://the-art-of-autism.com/

journey-of-the-heart-a-film-about-blind-autistic-musical-savant-tony-dublois/

Slonimsky, N. (2002). *Perfect pitch: an autobiography*. Omnibus Press& Schirmer Trade Books.

Small, S., Hlustik, P., Noll, D., Genovese, C. and Solodkin, A. (2002). Cerebellar hemispheric activation ipsilateral to the paretic hand correlates with functional recovery after stroke. *Brain, 125*(7), 1544-1557.

Smith, D., Anderson, J., Zammit, S., Meyer, T., Pell, J. and Mackay, D. (2015). Childhood IQ and risk of bipolar disorder in adulthood: prospective birth cohort study. *BJPsych open, 1*(1), 74-80.

Smith, N., Tsimpli, I., Morgan, G. and Woll, B. (2010). *The signs of a savant: Language against the odds*. Cambridge University Press.

Smith, R. (2005). Untamed Art From the Fringes Is a Gust of Bracing Air. The Ney York Times. January 28, 2005. https://www.nytimes.com/2005/01/28/arts/design/untamed-art-from-the-fringes-is-a-gust-of-bracing-air.html

Smith, D. (2004). *Introduction to special education: Teaching in an age of opportunity* (pp. 85-86). Pearson/A and B.

Smith, N. and Tsimpli, I. (1995). *The mind of a savant: Language learning and modularity*. Blackwell Publishing.

Smith, N., Tsimpli, I. and Ouhalla, J. (1993). Learning the impossible: The acquisition of possible and impossible languages by a polyglot savant. *Lingua, 91*(4), 279-347.

Smolka, J. and Fox, D. (2002). The Inner Savant. Discover Magazine. February 1, 2002. https://www.discovermagazine.com/mind/the-inner-savant

Snyder, A. (2009). Explaining and inducing savant skills: privileged access to lower level, less-processed information. *Philosophical Transactions of the Royal Society B: Biological Sciences*, 364(1522), 1399-1405.

Snyder, A. (2007). Comment on Priming Skills of Autistic Twins and Yamaguchi (2006) Letter to the Editor: "Questionable Aspects of Oliver Sacks' (1985) Report", Journal of Autism and Developmental Disorders. *Journal of Autism and Developmental Disorders, 37*(7), 1398-1399.

Snyder, A., Bahramali, H., Hawker, T. and Mitchell, D. (2006). Savant-like numerosity skills revealed in normal people by magnetic pulses. *Perception*, 35(6), 837-845.

Snyder, A., Mulcahy, E., Taylor, J., Mitchell, D., Sachdev, P. and Gandevia, S. (2003). Savant-like skills exposed in normal people by suppressing the left fronto-temporal lobe. *Journal of integrative neuroscience*, 2(02), 149-158.

Snyder, A. (2001). Paradox of the savant mind. *Nature, 413*(6853), 251-252.

Snyder, A. and Mitchell, D. (1999). Is integer arithmetic fundamental to mental processing?: the mind's secret arithmetic. *Proceedings of the Royal Society of London. Series B: Biological Sciences, 266*(1419), 587-592.

Solomon, O. (2013). Autism and Affordances of Achievement. *The social life of achievement*, 2, 120.

Spencer, K. (2011). My stroke turned me into an artist. Express. August 23, 2011. https://www.express.co.uk/life-style/health/266585/My-stroke-turned-me-into-an-artist

Spitz, H. (1995). Calendar calculating idiots savants and the smart unconscious. *New Ideas in Psychology, 13*(2), 167-182.

Stambaugh, L. (1996). Special Learners with Special Abilities: Developing the special musical abilities of children and adults with Williams syndrome can be a rewarding experience that requires specialized teaching strategies. *Music Educators Journal, 83*(3), 19-23.

Stephenson, K. (2009). Kim Peek, Murray man who inspired 'Rain Man', dies. The Salt Lake Tribune. December 21, 2009. https://archive.sltrib.com/story.php?ref=/ci_14043625

Sternberg, R. J. (1985). *Beyond IQ: A triarchic theory of human intelligence.* CUP Archive.

Steven, M. and Pascual-Leone, A. (2006). Transcranial magnetic stimulation and the human brain: an ethical evaluation. In *21st Century neuroethics: defining the issues in research, practice and policy* (pp. 201-211). Oxford University Press, Oxford, UK.

Stewart, L., Walsh, V. and Rothwell, J. (2001). Motor and phosphene thresholds: a transcranial magnetic stimulation correlation study. *Neuropsychologia*, 39(4), 415-419.

Straus, J. (2014). Idiots Savants, Retarded Savants, Talented Aments, Mono-Savants, Autistic Savants, Just Plain Savants, People with Savant Syndrome, and Autistic People Who Are Good at Things: A View from Disability Studies.

Strickland, A. (2016). Portarit of a 6-year-old artist with autism and her therapy cat. CNN. March 11, 2016. https://edition.cnn.com/2016/03/11/health/turning-points-iris-grace-autism/index.html

Strong, M. (2020). Taiwan artist mixes art and technology at Café Astoria. Taiwan News. Jun 18, 2020. https://www.taiwannews.com.tw/en/news/3950227

Tammet, D. (2017). *Every Word Is a Bird We Teach to Sing.* Little, Brown Spark.

Tammet, D. (2017b). Languages Revealing Worlds and Selves. *The Times Literary Supplement.* TLS. https://www.the-tls.co.uk/articles/daniel-tammet-synaesthesia-languages/

Tammet, D. (2016). *Mishenka.* ARENES. French Edition.

Tammet, D. (2016b). Autism: a spectrum of speculation. *Brain, 139*(3), 999-1000.

Tammet, D. (2014). *Je suis né un jour bleu.* Les arènes.

Tammet, D. (2013). *Thinking in Numbers: On Life, Love, Meaning, and Math.* Little, Brown Spark.

Tammet, D. (2012). Olympics: Are the Fastest and Strongest Reaching Their Mathematical Limits. The Guardian. August 21, 2012. https://www.theguardian.com/sport/2012/aug/12/olympic-records-time-numbers-mathematics

Tammet, D. (2012b). What I'm thinking about... Tolstoy and maths. The Guardian. August 23, 2012. https://www.theguardian.com/books/booksblog/2012/aug/23/tolstoy-maths-daniel-tammet

Tammet, D. (2009). *Embracing the Wide Sky: A Tour Across the Horizons of the Mind.* Simon and Schuster.

Tammet, D. (2007). *Born on a blue day: Inside the extraordinary mind of an autistic savant.* Simon and Schuster.

Tammet, D. (2006). *Born on a blue day.* Hodder & Staughton.

Tantam, D. (1988). Asperger's syndrome. *Journal of child psychology and psychiatry,* 29(3), 245-255.

Thaler, L., Reich, G. M., Zhang, X., Wang, D., Smith, G., Tao, Z., ... and Antoniou, M. (2017). Mouth-clicks used by blind expert human echolocators–signal description and model based signal synthesis. *PLoS computational biology, 13*(8), e1005670.

Thomson, H. (2013). Mindscapes: Stroke turned ex-con into rhyming painter.

New Scientist. Health. May 10, 2013. https://www.newscientist.com/article/dn23523-mindscapes-stroke-turned-ex-con-into-rhyming-painter/

Tick, B., Bolton, P., Happé, F., Rutter, M. and Rijsdijk, F. (2016). Heritability of autism spectrum disorders: a meta-analysis of twin studies. *Journal of Child Psychology and Psychiatry, 57*(5), 585-595.

Tommaney, S. (2015). A Lawyer's Head injury unveils artistic talents. Houston Press. February 23, 2015. http://www.houstonpress.com/arts/a-lawyers-head-injury-unveils-hidden-artistic-talents-6375112

Torres, F., Villalon, E., Poblete, P., Moraga-Amaro, R., Linsambarth, S., Riquelme, R., ... and Stehberg, J. (2015). Retrospective Evaluation of Deep Transcranial Magnetic Stimulation as Add-On Treatment for Parkinson's Disease. *Frontiers in neurology, 6*, 210.

Townsend, J. and Westerfield, M. (2010). Autism and Asperger's syndrome: A cognitive neuroscience perspective. In *Handbook of medical neuropsychology* (pp. 165-191). Springer, New York, NY.

Tredgold, A. (1929). Idiot savants. Retrieved from Survival after. http://www.survivalafterdeath.info/articles/abnormal/tredgold.htm

Treffert, D. and Rebedew, D. (2015). The savant syndrome registry: a preliminary report. *WMJ, 114*(4), 158-162.

Treffert, D. (2015). Leslie Lemke: An Inspirational Performance. https://www.wisconsinmedicalsociety.org/professional/savant-syndrome/profiles-and-videos/profiles/leslie-lemke-an-inspirational-performance/

Treffert, D. (2014). Savant syndrome: Realities, myths and misconceptions. *Journal of Autism and Developmental Disorders, 44*(3), 564-571.

Treffert, D. (2014b). *Whatever Happened to Leslie Lemke?* Scientific American. June 17, 2014. https://blogs.scientificamerican.com/guest-blog/whatever-happened-to-leslielemke/#:~:text=I%20am%20asked%20so%20often,whatever%20happened%20to%20Leslie%20Lemke%3F&text=Leslie%20is%20alive%20and%20well,after%20May%20died%20in%201993.

Treffert, D. (2014c). Accidental genius. *Scientific American, 311*(2), 52-57.

Treffert, D. (2010). *Islands of genius: The bountiful mind of the autistic, acquired, and sudden savant.* Jessica Kingsley Publishers.

Treffert, D. (2010b). Kim Peek 1951-2009. *Wisconsin Medical Journal, 109*(2), 61.

Treffert, D. (2009). The savant syndrome: an extraordinary condition.

A synopsis: past, present, future. *Philosophical Transactions of the Royal Society B: Biological Sciences*, 364(1522), 1351-1357.

Treffert, D. (2007). Thristan "Tum-Tum" Mendoza. Agnesian. SSM Health. https://www.agnesian.com/page/thristan-tum-tum-mendoza

Treffert, D. (2006). "Richard Wawro – An Amazing Artist". https://www.wisconsinmedical society.org/professional/savant-syndrome/profiles-and videos/profiles/richard-wawro-anamazing-artist/

Treffert, D. and Christensen, D. (2005). Inside the mind of a savant. *Scientific American*, 293(6), 108-113.

Treffert, D. and Wallace, G. (2004). Islands of genius. *Scientific American Mind*, 14(1), 14-23.

Treffert, D. and Wallace, G. (2002). Islands of genius. *Scientific American*, 286(6), 76-85.

Treffert, D. (2000). Extraordinary people: Understanding savant syndrome. iUniverse. com.[rBC].

Treffert, D. (1999). The savant syndrome and autistic disorder. *CNS spectrums*, 4(12), 57-60.

Treffert, D. (1989). An unlikely virtuoso: Leslie Lemke and the story of savant syndrome. *The sciences*, 29(1), 28-35.

Tucker, R. (1999). A Global Perspective on Bilingualism and Bilingual Education. CSAL Online Resources: Digests. August, 1999. file:///C:/Users/Osvaldo%20 Cairo%20B/Downloads/AGlobalPerspectiveonBilingualism%20(1).pdf

Varga, K. (2018). From silence to sensation: Prodigy Matt Savage, born with autism, now a music veteran. Democratic & Chronicle. June 17, 2018. https://www.democratandchronicle.com/story/lifestyle/2018/06/17/matt-savage-autistic-savant-and-child-prodigy-plays-jazz-fest-xrijf-rochester-jazz/690534002/

Vargha-Khadem, F., Carr, L., Isaacs, E., Brett, E., Adams, C. and Mishkin, M. (1997). Onset of speech after left hemispherectomy in a nine-year-old boy. *Brain: a journal of neurology*, 120(1), 159-182.

Viscidi, E., Triche, E., Pescosolido, M., McLean, R., Joseph, R., Spence, S., and Morrow, E. (2013). Clinical characteristics of children with autism spectrum disorder and co-occurring epilepsy. *PloS one*, 8(7).

Vitelli, R. (2013). Creativity and the Healey Brain. Psychology Today. April 29, 2013.

https://www.psychologytoday.com/us/blog/media-spotlight/201304/creativity-and-the-healing-brain

Voineskos, D., Levinson, A., Sun, Y., Barr, M., Farzan, F., Rajji, T., ... and Daskalakis, Z. (2016). The relationship between cortical inhibition and electroconvulsive therapy in the treatment of major depressive disorder. *Scientific reports, 6,* 37461.

Volkmar, F. and Rutter, M. (1995). Childhood disintegrative disorder: results of the DSM-IV autism field trial. *Journal of the American Academy of Child & Adolescent Psychiatry, 34*(8), 1092-1095.

Vos, T., Allen, C., Arora, M., Barber, R. M., Bhutta, Z. A., Brown, A., ... and Coggeshall, M. (2016). Global, regional, and national incidence, prevalence, and years lived with disability for 310 diseases and injuries, 1990–2015: a systematic analysis for the Global Burden of Disease Study 2015. *The Lancet, 388*(10053), 1545-1602.

Walker, D., Thompson, A., Zwaigenbaum, L., Goldberg, J., Bryson, S., Mahoney, W., ... and Szatmari, P. (2004). Specifying PDD-NOS: a comparison of PDD-NOS, Asperger syndrome, and autism. *Journal of the American Academy of Child & Adolescent Psychiatry, 43*(2), 172-180.

Wallace, G, Happé, F. and Giedd, J. (2009). A case study of a multiply talented savant with an autism spectrum disorder: neuropsychological functioning and brain morphometry. *Philosophical Transactions of the Royal Society B: Biological Sciences, 364*(1522), 1425-1432.

Wallace, G. (2008). Neuropsychological studies of savant skills: Can they inform the neuroscience of giftedness? *Roeper Review, 30*(4), 229-246.

Wallis, C. and Goehner, A. (2006). A tale of two schools. *Time, 20,* 48-51.

Wang, B. (2018). Highly Superior Autobiographical Memory. https://www.nextbigfuture. com/2018/05/highly-superior-autobiographical-memory.html

Wang, L., Li, J., Shuang, M., Lu, T., Wang, Z., Zhang, T., ... and Wu, Z. (2018). Association study and mutation sequencing of genes on chromosome 15q11-q13 identified GABRG3 as a susceptibility gene for autism in Chinese Han population. *Translational psychiatry, 8*(1), 1-12.

Wansell, G. (2008). Revealed: How autistic genius Stephen Wiltshire drew his amazing picture of London's skyline. Daily Mail. April 8, 2008.

https://www.dailymail.co.uk/news/article-557942/Revealed-How-autistic-genius-Stephen-Wiltshire-drew-amazing-picture-Londons-skyline.html

Ward, J., Huckstep, B. and Tsakanikos, E. (2006). Sound-colour synaesthesia: To what extent does it use cross-modal mechanisms common to us all?. *Cortex, 42*(2), 264-280.

Warner, J. (2009). Franco Magnani and JG Ballard. Identity Theory. May 10, 2009. http://www.identitytheory.com/franco-magnani-and-jg-ballard/

Wassermann, E. (2002). Variation in the response to transcranial magnetic brain stimulation in the general population. *Clinical Neurophysiology*, 113(7), 1165-1171.

Wassermann, E. Wedegaertner, F., Ziemann, U., George, M. and Chen, R. (1998). Crossed reduction of human motor cortex excitability by 1-Hz transcranial magnetic stimulation. *Neuroscience Letters, 250*(3), 141-144.

Watt, N., Strauss, E. and Rodrigues, A. (2010). Daniel Tammet: Mathematical Genius Visualizes Numbers, Solves Problems in Blink of an Eye. ABC News. http://abcnews.go.com/2020/autistic-savant-daniel-tammet-solves-problems-blink-eye/story?id=10759598

Webb, S., Sparks, B., Friedman, S., Shaw, D., Giedd, J., Dawson, G. and Dager, S. (2009). Cerebellar vermal volumes and behavioral correlates in children with autism spectrum disorder. *Psychiatry Research: Neuroimaging, 172*(1), 61-67.

Weber, B. (2009). *Kim Peek, Inspiration for 'Rain Man,' Dies at 58.* December 26, 2009. The New York Times. https://www.nytimes.com/2009/12/27/us/27peek.html

Wexler, A. (2020). Autism and outsiderism: The art of George Widener. *International Journal of Education Through Art, 16*(1), 83-99.

White, R. (2005). Autism First-Hand: An Expert Interview with Temple Grandin. *Medscape Psychiatry, 10(1).* https://www.medscape.org/viewarticle/498153

White, B., Saunders, F., Scadden, L., Bach-Y-Rita, P. and Collins, C. C. (1970). Seeing with the skin. *Perception & Psychophysics, 7*(1), 23-27.

Wieser, H. (2003). Music and the brain. *Annals of the New York Academy of Sciences*, 999(1), 76-94.

Wilkinson, D. (2014). A Half Deaf Guy Had a Head Injury and Now He's Amazing at Piano. March 6, 2014. https://www.vice.com/da/article/rnvpgx/youneedtohearthis-a-half-deaf-guy-had-a-head-injury-and-now-hes-amazing-at-piano-derek-amato

Wilson, P. (2009). A savvy savant finds his voice. The Australian. http://www.theaustralian.com.au/archive/news/a-savvy-savant-finds-his-voice/news-story/a44b6937e96177cba2e67f7f51b3f6ec

Wiltshire, S. (1993). *Stephen Wiltshire's American Dream*. Michael Joseph Ltd; 1st edition (April 29, 1993).

Wiltshire, S. (1992). *Floating Cities: Venice, Amsterdam, Leningrad, and Moscow*. Summit Books; First Edition edition (January 1, 1992)

Wiltshire, S. (1988). *Cities*. Orion Publishing Co; 1st Edition edition (1988).

Wiltshire, S. (1987). *Drawings*. J. M. Dent & Sons (Canada).

Wing, L. (1981). Asperger's syndrome: a clinical account. *Psychological medicine, 11(1),* 115-129.

Winner, E. (2000). Giftedness: Current theory and research. *Current directions in psychological science, 9*(5), 153-156.

Winslow, F. (1860). *On obscure diseases of the brain, and disorders of the mind*. Blanchard & Lea.

Wolfe, C. (2013). Learning from Temple Grandin, or, animal studies, disability studies, and who comes after the subject. *Re-Imagining Nature: Environmental Humanities and Ecosemiotics*, 91-107.

Wolff, S. and Chick, J. (1980). Schizoid personality in childhood: A controlled follow-up study. *Psychological Medicine, 10*(1), 85-100.

Wood, A. (2016). *Temple Grandin: Voice for the Voiceless*. Skyhorse.

Woodruff, G., & Premack, D. (1981). Primative mathematical concepts in the chimpanzee: proportionality and numerosity. *Nature*, 293(5833), 568-570.

Wraw, C., Deary, I., Der, G. and Gale, C. (2016). Intelligence in youth and mental health at age 50. *Intelligence, 58*, 69-79.

Xu, J., Kemeny, S., Park, G., Frattali, C. and Braun, A. (2005). Language in context: emergent features of word, sentence, and narrative comprehension. *Neuroimage*, 25(3), 1002-1015.

Yamaguchi, M. (2009). Savant syndrome and prime numbers. *Polish Psychological Bulletin, 40*(2), 69.

Yamaguchi, M. (2007). Response to Snyder's "Comments on Priming Skills of Autistic Twins and Yamaguchi (2006) Letter to the Editor: 'Questionable Aspects of Oliver Sacks' (1985) Report,'" Journal of Autism and Developmental Disorders. *Journal of Autism and Developmental Disorders*, 37(7), 1401-1401.

Yeates, E. (2008). Disabled boy a musical genius. KSL. https://www.ksl.com/article/2664997/disabled-boy-a-musical-genius

Yirmiya, N., Shaked, M. and Erel, O. (2001). Comparison of siblings of individuals with autism and siblings of individuals with other diagnoses. *The research basis for autism intervention*, 59-73.

Made in the USA
Las Vegas, NV
04 November 2026

57428961R00186